Public Health Nutrition

Public Health Nutrition

Essentials for Practitioners

Edited by Jessica Jones-Smith

Johns Hopkins University Press
Baltimore

© 2020 Johns Hopkins University Press
All rights reserved. Published 2020
Printed in the United States of America on acid-free paper
9 8 7 6 5 4 3 2 1

Johns Hopkins University Press
2715 North Charles Street
Baltimore, Maryland 21218-4363
www.press.jhu.edu

Library of Congress Cataloging-in-Publication Data

Names: Jones-Smith, Jessica, 1977- editor.
Title: Public health nutrition : essentials for practitioners / edited by
    Jessica Jones-Smith.
Description: Baltimore : Johns Hopkins University Press, 2020. |
    Includes bibliographical references and index.
Identifiers: LCCN 2019047555 | ISBN 9781421438504 (paperback ;
    alk. paper) | ISBN 9781421438511 (ebook)
Subjects: MESH: Nutritional Physiological Phenomena | Public Health
    Practice | Nutrition Policy | Health Promotion | Nutrition Disorders—
    prevention & control
Classification: LCC RA601 | NLM QU 145 | DDC 362.17/6—dc23
LC record available at https://lccn.loc.gov/2019047555

A catalog record for this book is available from the British Library.

*Special discounts are available for bulk purchases of this book. For more
information, please contact Special Sales at specialsales@press.jhu.edu.*

Johns Hopkins University Press uses environmentally friendly book
materials, including recycled text paper that is composed of at least
30 percent post-consumer waste, whenever possible.

Contents

Contributors

Jeanne M. Barcelona, PhD
Assistant Professor
College of Education, Division of Kinesiology, Health,
    and Sport Studies
Wayne State University
Detroit, MI, USA

Alexandra L. Bellows, MS
Visiting Scientist
Harvard T. H. Chan School of Public Health
Harvard University
Boston, MA, USA

Sara N. Bleich, PhD
Professor
Harvard T. H. Chan School of Public Health
Harvard University
Boston, MA, USA

Melissa Chapnick, RD, MS, MPH
Research Manager, E3 Nutrition Lab
Brown School
Washington University in St. Louis
St. Louis, MO, USA

Damien de Walque, PhD
Senior Economist
Development Research Group
The World Bank

Rachael D. Dombrowski, PhD, MPH
Assistant Professor
College of Education, Division of Kinesiology, Health,
    and Sport Studies
Wayne State University
Detroit, MI, USA

Jessica Fanzo, PhD
Bloomberg Distinguished Associate Professor
Johns Hopkins University
Berman Institute of Bioethics, Nitze School of Advanced
    International Studies (SAIS) and Bloomberg School
    of Public Health
Washington, DC, USA

Johannah M. Frelier, MPH
Research Assistant
Harvard T. H. Chan School of Public Health
Harvard University
Boston, MA, USA

Valerie M. Friesen, MSc
Technical Specialist
Knowledge Leadership
Global Alliance for Improved Nutrition (GAIN)
Geneva, Switzerland

Paul Gertler, PhD
Li Ka Shing Professor
Haas School of Business
University of California
Berkeley, CA, USA

Lia C. Haskin Fernald, PhD
Professor
School of Public Health
University of California, Berkeley
Berkeley, CA, USA

Melissa Hidrobo, PhD
Senior Research Fellow
International Food Policy Research Institute (IFPRI)
Dakar, Senegal

Lora L. Iannotti, MA, PhD
Associate Dean for Public Health
Associate Professor
Director, E3 Nutrition Lab
Brown School
Washington University in St. Louis
St. Louis, MO, USA

Scott B. Ickes, PhD
Associate Professor
Department of Applied Health Sciences
Wheaton College
Wheaton, IL, USA

Lindsay M. Jaacks, PhD
Assistant Professor
Harvard T. H. Chan School of Public Health
Harvard University
Boston, MA, USA

Jessica Jones-Smith, PhD, MPH, RD
Associate Professor
School of Public Health
University of Washington
Seattle, WA, USA

A. Gita Krishnaswamy, MPH, MEd
Senior Lecturer
School of Public Health
University of Washington
Seattle, WA, USA

Noel Kulik, PhD, CHES
Associate Professor
College of Education, Division of Kinesiology, Health,
    and Sport Studies
Wayne State University
Detroit, MI, USA

Mduduzi N. N. Mbuya, PhD
Senior Technical Specialist
Knowledge Leadership
Global Alliance for Improved Nutrition (GAIN)
Washington, DC, USA

Kimberly B. Morland, PhD, MPH
Director, Public Health Research Institute of Southern
   California
Adjunct Associate Professor, Icahn School of Medicine
   at Mount Sinai
Los Angeles, CA, USA

Lynnette M. Neufeld, PhD, MSc
Director
Knowledge Leadership
Global Alliance for Improved Nutrition (GAIN)
Geneva, Switzerland

Vanessa M. Oddo, PhD, MPH
Assistant Professor
College of Applied Health Sciences
University of Illinois at Chicago
Chicago, IL, USA

Cynthia L. Ogden, PhD, MRP
Branch Chief and Epidemiologist
NHANES Program
CDC/NCHS
Hyattsville, MD, USA

Julie A. Reeder, PhD, MPH, MS, CHES
Senior Research Analyst
Oregon WIC Program
Portland, OR, USA

Colin D. Rehm, PhD, MPH
Assistant Professor
Department of Epidemiology & Population Health
Albert Einstein College of Medicine
Bronx, NY, USA

Scott A. Richardson, MBA
Doctoral Student
Harvard T. H. Chan School of Public Health
Harvard University
Boston, MA, USA

Sarah Ross-Viles, MPH
Clinical Instructor
School of Public Health
University of Washington
Seattle, WA, USA

Marie Ruel, PhD
Director, Poverty, Health and Nutrition Division
International Food Policy Research Institute (IFPRI)
Washington, DC, USA

Julie C. Ruel-Bergeron, PhD, MPH
Nutrition Specialist
The Global Financing Facility
Health, Nutrition and Population
The World Bank
Washington, DC, USA

Garrison J. Spencer, MDP
Public Health Analyst
Center for Global Noncommunicable Diseases
RTI International
Seattle, WA, USA

Marie L. Spiker, PhD, MSPH, RDN
Healthy and Sustainable Food Systems Fellow
Academy of Nutrition and Dietetics Foundation
Chicago, IL, USA

Andrew L. Thorne-Lyman, ScD, MHS
Associate Scientist
Johns Hopkins Bloomberg School of Public Health
Baltimore, MD, USA

Alison Tumilowicz, PhD, MPH, RD
Program Officer
Nutrition, Global Development Program
Bill & Melinda Gates Foundation
Seattle, WA, USA

Kelsey A. Vercammen, MSc
Doctoral Student
Harvard T. H. Chan School of Public Health
Harvard University
Boston, MA, USA

Marissa L. Zwald, PhD, MPH
Epidemiologist
Centers for Disease Control and Prevention
Atlanta, GA, USA

Public Health Nutrition

1

Introduction

Jessica Jones-Smith

Public health nutrition encompasses policies, programs, practices, interventions, and research that are aimed at understanding or improving nutrition, nutritional status, or nutrition-related disease of populations. Public health nutrition is a growing discipline but one with well-established roots. Practitioners of public health nutrition work in a plethora of different positions, including local, state, and federal health departments and agencies; community-based organizations; nongovernmental organizations; ministries of health; think tanks; universities; and health systems.

Public health nutrition practitioners are on the front lines of designing and implementing policies and programs aimed at improving the health of populations, and oftentimes with a focus on improving the health of the most nutritionally vulnerable among us. Research in this field is often aimed at elucidating relationships between dietary factors and disease, examining root causes of poor health and health inequities, and testing the effectiveness of interventions to improve health.

For students thinking about a career in public health nutrition, there are many different directions one can pursue, including a large number of nutrition-related diseases to study—ranging from diseases of deficiency and undernutrition to diseases associated with overconsumption of calories or specific foods. Additionally, the potential risk factors studied by public health nutritionists include dietary intake, eating behavior, food environments, food systems, socioeconomic environments, food marketing, and many others. Specific responsibilities of a public health nutrition practitioner might include assessing the nutrition-related health of a local community, planning environmental or systems-level changes aimed at improving the nutrition-related health of a community, evaluating a program designed and implemented by a government organization, designing programs to improve dietary intake or physical activity, running a community-based organization, advising on which nutrition programing to implement or scale up, providing technical nutrition expertise on a research team, or researching causes of and solutions for nutrition-related diseases and health inequities.

This book is designed to be a graduate-level introduction to public health nutrition. It covers fundamental topics in public health nutrition, but it assumes basic nutrition knowledge. It also can provide a much-needed resource for already-established practitioners of public health nutrition. The emphasis of this book is on providing essentials that will allow new graduate students of public health or public health nutrition to build their familiarity and comfort with a toolbox of skills most commonly used in public health nutrition research and practice. In particular, the primer on community health and needs assessment in chapter 4 can be used as a foundation for practitioners or researchers. The discussion of nutrition surveillance systems and methods will be of interest to practitioners and researchers seeking to better understand available data sources. In addition to focusing on tools of the public health nutrition practitioner or researcher, the book covers key content areas commonly encountered or studied in public health nutrition.

The book was designed to be used as a textbook in a semester- or quarter-long course. Chapters are authored by eminent experts in their field. We aimed to be selective in its topics, covering core, foundational topics and methods in the field, rather than providing an exhaustive scope of current research.

The book is divided into four parts. Part One covers key tools of public health nutrition, with chapters on nutrition surveillance, dietary assessment methods, community health assessment, program planning, and program evaluation. Part Two examines key nutrition-related diseases in high-income and low- and middle-income countries, including chapters on leading causes of disease and death, as well as chapters that take a deeper look at obesity, stunting, and the nutrition transition (or dramatic changes in dietary intake and physical activity patterns coinciding with economic development). Part Three discusses frameworks for thinking about the causes of nutrition-related diseases from a population health perspective. In particular, we discuss environmental and underlying contributors to nutrition-related disease. We also discuss systems thinking. Part Four outlines key nutrition-related policies and programs in high-income countries and low- and middle-income countries. We take a closer look at two particular programs or program types: in the United States, we explore WIC: The Special Supplemental Nutrition Program for Women, Infants, and Children, while in low- and middle-income countries, we examine cash transfer programs.

If using this book in a classroom, instructors can easily switch the ordering of the chapters presented. For instance, some instructors might want to begin the class with some foundational material about which diseases are most prevalent in high-income and low-and middle-income countries. They could start the course with the material presented in Part Two, then move into Part Three to present the frameworks and underlying causes of disease, followed by the tools of presented in Part One, and wrap up by presenting policies and programs in Part Four. In addition, each chapter is intended to stand alone, so instructors can pick and choose which chapters make the most sense to cover in their class. The chapters are rigorous and provide a foundation of knowledge. In my own classroom, this has provided a solid base off of which I can incorporate more active learning strategies in the classroom. Finally, each chapter contains learning objectives and reflection questions to facilitate learning.

PART ONE

Key Tools of Public Health Nutrition

2

Population Surveillance and Monitoring

Marissa L. Zwald and Cynthia L. Ogden

LEARNING OBJECTIVES

- To define public health surveillance and monitoring
- To describe the types and attributes of a public health surveillance system
- To define nutrition surveillance and monitoring in the United States
- To describe a major nutrition surveillance system in the United States and how its data have been used to address public health nutrition issues
- To identify additional selected national nutrition surveillance systems in high-income and low- and middle-income countries

Collecting and interpreting nutrition and health-related information from individuals and populations is crucial to promoting public health. These surveillance and monitoring data allow researchers, practitioners, advocates, and policy makers to develop, implement, and evaluate programs and policies that aim to improve nutritional status and health outcomes.[1-4] The range of nutrition surveillance and monitoring activities at the national level varies extensively across high-income and low- and middle-income countries, and in this chapter we aim to describe the efforts to collect, analyze, and utilize data on the nutritional status of populations in various countries. First, we provide a brief overview of important concepts related to public health surveillance. Second, we build upon this foundational information by describing core concepts of general nutrition surveillance and monitoring in the United States. A substantial portion of this chapter is devoted to presenting a national nutrition surveillance system in the United States, the National Health and Nutrition Examination Survey (NHANES). Through this case example, we describe the survey methods and share several vignettes about how nutritional surveillance data from this particular system have been used to monitor trends, inform programs and policies, and set research priorities. Following this in-depth analysis of NHANES, we provide several summaries of nutrition surveillance activities in various high-income and low- and middle-income countries. Specifically, we discuss selected examples of national nutrition surveillance systems and their applications to advance public health nutrition in Canada, Japan, Korea, and Australia. We then describe the nuances of conducting nutrition surveillance and monitoring activities in low- and middle-income countries and present two examples of nutrition surveillance systems, including the Mexican National Health and Nutrition Survey and the Demographic and Health Survey.

Background on Public Health Surveillance

In 1988, the National Academy of Medicine, formerly the Institute of Medicine, released a groundbreaking report that outlined the core functions needed to support the future of public health. This report identified **assessment** as one of the three core functions of public health (figure 2.1) and recommended that "every public health agency regularly and systematically collect, assemble, analyze, and communicate information on the health of the community, including statistics on health status, community health needs, and epidemiologic and other studies of health problems."[5] Public health surveillance, often considered the foundation of public health practice, is a vital part of the core function of assessment, and without it the other public

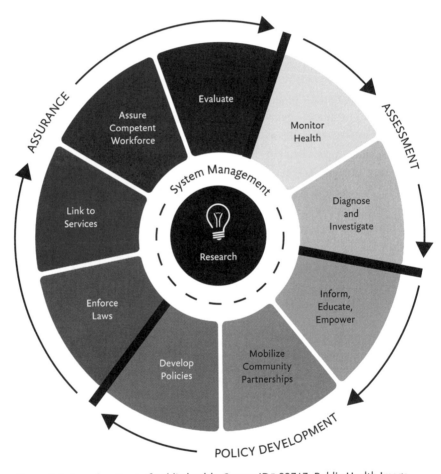

Figure 2.1. Core functions of public health. *Source:* ID#:22747. Public Health Image Library, Centers for Disease Control and Prevention. https://phil.cdc.gov/Details.aspx ?pid=22747.

health core functions of policy development and assurance could not be performed.[6]

Public health surveillance is typically defined as the ongoing and systematic collection, management, analysis, and interpretation of data, which is followed by the dissemination of these data to promote public health action.[7] Data collected from surveillance systems can cover a wide range of health events of interest, including diseases, conditions, injuries, or disabilities. Surveillance data can be collected on both infectious and noncommunicable diseases, such as cancer, diabetes, or heart disease; it can capture information on risk factors, protective behaviors, and other exposures, such as dietary intake (including breastfeeding), smoking, or sexual behavior;[8] and it can also track practices and programs that support various health behaviors, such school environmental supports that facilitate healthy eating.[9] Surveillance systems can also be developed and implemented at different levels, from local, state, regional, or global levels, and across single or multiple geographic locations. Typically, the level and location(s) in which information is collected for a surveillance system depends on the users of the surveillance data and its relevance and timeliness in addressing the health event of interest.[1,8,10]

Sources for public health surveillance data generally are considered either primary or secondary. **Primary data** sources represent data where an investigator conducts the data collection activities. Selected examples of primary data collection methods, where an investigator obtains data directly from an individual, include interviews, surveys, questionnaires, focus groups, or environmental assessments. **Secondary data** are already compiled, gathered, organized, and published by others.[10-12] Some examples of secondary data sources include reportable disease systems, electronic health records (e.g., hospital discharge data), vital records (e.g., birth and death certificates), or registries (e.g., national cancer registry).[8]

Public health surveillance data can be used for different purposes (table 2.1).[6,10,13] Surveillance data can be used to estimate the magnitude and scope of a public health problem, including the demographic and geographic distribution of certain health events. Data can be used to detect changes in individual health practices, monitor changes in infectious and environmental agents, evaluate prevention and control measures, describe the natural history of a health event of interest, generate hypotheses, and foster additional research.

An effective and efficient public health surveillance system is simple, timely, representative, flexible, and sensitive; has strong predictive value; and is acceptable to stakeholders and the public (table 2.2). Because surveillance systems can vary in purpose, scope, data collection methods, and objectives, certain attributes might be more important in one system and less important in another. For example, a surveillance system that prioritizes high

Table 2.1. Example Uses of Public Health Surveillance Data

- Guide immediate action for important public health issues
- Measure the burden of disease, including the identification of high-risk populations and new or emerging public health concerns
- Guide the planning, implementation, and evaluation of programs and policies to prevent and control disease
- Evaluate a public health policy or intervention
- Detect changes in health practices and the effects of these changes
- Prioritize the allocation of public health resources
- Describe the clinical course of a disease
- Provide a basis for epidemiologic research

Source: https://www.cdc.gov/mmwr/preview/mmwrhtml/rr5013a1.htm.

Table 2.2. Attributes of a Public Health Surveillance System

Attribute	Definition
Simplicity	Structure and ease of operation of surveillance system. System should be as simple as possible.
Timeliness	The speed or delay between steps, such as data collection and reporting, in a surveillance system.
Representativeness	Surveillance system accurately describes the occurrence of a health-related event over time and its distribution in the population by place and person.
Flexibility	Surveillance system can adapt to changing information needs or operating conditions with little additional cost in time, personnel, or allocated funds. System can also accommodate changes in case definitions and variations in reporting sources.
Sensitivity	Surveillance system can accurately classify cases according to a health event of interest and can also detect changes in the prevalence of a health event over time.
Predictive value positive	The proportion of persons identified as having cases who actually do have the condition under surveillance.
Acceptability	Willingness of individuals and institutions to participate in the surveillance system.
Data quality	Completeness and validity of the data recorded in the surveillance system.
Stability	Reliability and availability of the surveillance system.

Source: https://www.cdc.gov/mmwr/preview/mmwrhtml/rr5013a1.htm.

sensitivity by accurately identifying a health event of interest might undermine other attributes, such as simplicity or timeliness.[13]

Nutrition Surveillance in the United States

Surveillance and monitoring of nutritional status, an important determinant of health status, is essential to understanding complex nutrition and health-related issues, such as undernutrition, hunger, suboptimal growth, micronutrient deficiencies, over-nutrition and its associations with chronic diseases and obesity, and increasingly, the interplay of several of these problems.[1,3,14] Descriptions of key concepts related to surveillance and monitoring of some of the aforementioned nutrition and health-related issues are discussed below.

Nutrition surveillance has been defined as "to watch over nutrition, in order to make decisions that lead to improvement in nutrition in populations."[1,15] More specifically, nutrition surveillance has been described as the continuous assessment of dietary intake and nutritional status of a population or a selected population subgroup for the purposes of detecting changes and initiating public health action. **Nutrition monitoring**, while often used interchangeably with nutrition surveillance, also represents the assessment of diet and nutrition of a population or population subgroup for the purposes of detecting changes but does not necessarily result in public health action.[1,2,16,17]

Nutrition assessment is the collection and interpretation of data that examines dietary behaviors and intake and nutrition-related health status of individuals or groups of individuals.[2-4,18] Common nutritional assessment methods are **anthropometry, dietary intake assessment**, and **biomarker** data.[16,18] Anthropometric measures include measures of physical dimensions and body composition, such as height, weight, skinfold assessments, and waist circumference, which help assess body composition and growth. Dietary intake assessments collect data on food and nutrient intake of individuals. Commonly utilized methods for collecting individual dietary intake data include *food records, 24-hour dietary recalls*, and *food frequency questionnaires* (FFQs), which are typically used for nutrition surveillance. Food records or diaries measure dietary intake over a single time period and can include measuring or weighing consumed items. The 24-hour dietary recall includes asking participants to report on the kinds and amounts of all food and drinks consumed during the previous 24 hours. FFQs are typically self-administered questionnaires in which participants are presented with a list of food items and asked to report the usual frequency of their consumption over a lengthier period of time.[19,20] Lastly, biomarkers are defined by a work group led by the World Health Organization (WHO) as "any substance, structure, or process that can be measured in the body or its products and influence or predict the incidence of outcome or disease."[21] Nutritional biomarkers can provide information on nutritional exposures, susceptibility of diseases and conditions, and objective health outcomes. They include laboratory tests measured in biological specimens, such as urine or blood, and are often considered more objective than self-reported dietary intake.[3,16] Chapter 3 describes these tools and their use in more detail.

In the United States, nutrition surveillance and monitoring have helped to keep a pulse on the dietary, nutritional, and related health status of Americans, and provide information intersecting the full spectrum of food and health, including food production, supply, availability, and consumption. Nutrition surveillance and monitoring have also supported our understanding of factors that influence dietary intake and nutritional status, including upstream economic and societal determinants like housing or income level and individual factors like knowledge, attitudes, and practices around food and nutrition.[3,4] Additionally, data from nutrition surveillance systems have helped inform nutrition objectives, such as those included in Healthy People 2020; track progress toward these objectives; set nutrition research priorities; and guide federal public health policies, such as dietary guidance for Americans, food safety, and food fortification.[3,4,16]

As nutrition topics of concern evolved in the United States, from challenges associated with undernutrition toward the increased prevalence of obesity, surveillance and monitoring activities have had to be adapted to collect relevant and timely information for stakeholders.[14] Today, these activities span many surveillance systems, population-based surveys, and other monitoring activities across multiple national, state, and local organizations working in a variety of sectors, such as health, agriculture, education, economics, and labor.[4] At the national level and within the health sector, selected examples of nutrition surveillance systems that have shaped nutrition policy in the United States are listed in table 2.3.

While these varied national surveillance systems have provided important information on the nutritional status and health of people in the United States, in the next section, we provide an in-depth description of a case example of a US surveillance system, the National Health and Nutrition Examination Survey (NHANES).[22]

Case Example from the United States
Overview of NHANES

NHANES represents a program of studies designed to assess the health, nutritional status, and health behaviors of adults and children in the United States (https://www.cdc.gov/nchs/nhanes/). The NHANES program began in the early 1960s as the National Health Examination Survey, which collected limited information on nutritional status, including anthropometry and a few nutrition biomarkers. A nutrition component with dietary assessment was incorporated into the program in 1970, and it became known as the National

Table 2.3. Examples of Nutrition Surveillance Systems in the United States

Surveillance system	Sponsoring agency	Purpose	Selected examples of nutritional data collected	Website
Behavioral Risk Factor Surveillance System (BRFSS)	National Center for Chronic Disease Prevention and Health Promotion, Centers for Disease Control and Prevention	BRFSS assesses the prevalence of personal health practices that are related to the leading causes of death.	■ Frequency of fruit and vegetable consumption ■ Sugar-sweetened beverage consumption (select states) ■ Food security status	https://www.cdc.gov/brfss.html
National Immunization Survey (NIS)	National Center for Immunization and Respiratory Diseases, Centers for Disease Control and Prevention	NIS monitors vaccination coverage among children and teens, and also assesses breastfeeding behaviors.	■ Ever breastfed ■ Breastfeeding duration ■ Age child was first fed something other than breastmilk	https://www.cdc.gov/vaccines/imz-managers/nis/about.html https://www.cdc.gov/breastfeeding/data/nis_data/index.htm
National Health Interview Survey (NHIS)	National Center for Health Statistics, Centers for Disease Control and Prevention	NHIS is a basic health and demographic survey that addresses major current health issues through the collection and analysis of data on the civilian, non-institutionalized population of the United States.	■ Selected dietary information from Dietary Screener Questionnaire (for adults only and only in certain years) ■ Food assistance program participation	https://www.cdc.gov/nchs/nhis.htm

(continued)

Table 2.3 (continued)

Surveillance system	Sponsoring agency	Purpose	Selected examples of nutritional data collected	Website
National Health and Nutrition Examination Survey (NHANES)	National Center for Health Statistics, Centers for Disease Control and Prevention	NHANES is a program of studies designed to assess the health and nutritional status of adults and children in the United States. The survey is unique in that it combines interviews and physical examinations.	■ Anthropometry ■ Iron deficiency ■ Total food and nutrient intake ■ Food security ■ Frequency and types of meals away from home	https://www.cdc.gov/nchs/nhanes.htm
Pregnancy Risk Assessment Monitoring System (PRAMS)	National Center for Chronic Disease Prevention and Health Promotion, Centers for Disease Control and Prevention, and state health departments	PRAMS collects state-specific, population-based data on maternal attitudes and experience before, during, and shortly after pregnancy, including infant feeding practices.	■ Breastfeeding	https://www.cdc.gov/prams/index.htm
Youth Risk Behavior Surveillance System (YRBSS)	Division of Adolescent and School Health of the National Center for HIV/ AIDS, Viral Hepatitis, STD, and TB Prevention; Centers for Disease Control and Prevention	YRBSS monitors priority risk behaviors among adolescents through national, state, and local surveys.	■ Frequency of consumption of selected foods (e.g., fruits, vegetables, soda, milk) ■ Frequency of eating breakfast	https://www.cdc.gov/healthyyouth/data/yrbs.htm

Source: Directory of Federal and State Nutrition Monitoring and Related Research Activities, https://www.cdc.gov/nchs/data/misc/direc-99.pdf.

Health and Nutrition Examination Survey. In 1999, the survey became a continuous program that regularly adapts its health and nutrition surveillance to meet emerging public health concerns, and research needs and recommendations. Nutrition-related data from the continuous NHANES are currently used to describe prevalence estimates for undernutrition, obesity, and micronutrient deficiencies (e.g., folate, vitamin D, and iron); to describe dietary intake of Americans; and to monitor trends in certain diet-related behaviors and diseases.[16,23,24]

NHANES is unique in that it is a nationally representative survey that combines personal interviews with standardized physical examinations and laboratory tests. The examination component consists of medical, dental, and physiological measurements, in addition to laboratory tests administered by highly trained medical personnel.[22] The survey has a complex, multistage probability sampling design. It examines approximately 5,000 persons each year selected from 15 different locations that are chosen from a sampling frame of all counties in the United States, and data are released every two years. The 15 different survey locations selected each year are mostly single counties, or in some cases groups of contiguous counties, with probability proportional to a measure of size. Over the years, some groups have been oversampled to produce reliable estimates for various population subgroups. For example, in recent survey years, persons who identified as Asian American, Hispanic, non-Hispanic black, low-income white, and/or older adults were oversampled.[22]

Nutritional status is comprehensively examined through the combined assessment of dietary intake, anthropometric measurements, and laboratory tests. All participants complete a detailed in-person household interview where information is obtained on dietary behaviors and nutrition-related topics, such as supplement use, weight history, and weight control practices among adult participants, and breastfeeding and other childhood feeding practices for participants aged ≤6 years.[22] Following the interview, all participants are invited to complete a health examination, performed in a mobile examination center (MEC) where laboratory studies, anthropometric measurements, and additional interviews, including a dietary recall (Day 1), are conducted (figure 2.2). Following the health examination, participants are asked to complete a second dietary recall over the telephone.[22]

NHANES is the only nationally representative survey in the United States that collects dietary recall information on both adults and children.[16] The in-person 24-hour dietary recall is conducted by trained dietary interviewers who administer in either English or Spanish. Survey participants aged 12 years and older complete the dietary interview on their own; a proxy respondent (usually a parent) reports for participants aged 5 years and younger and for other persons who cannot self-report. Proxy-assisted interviews are conducted with children between the ages of 6 and 11 years. Since 2002, all

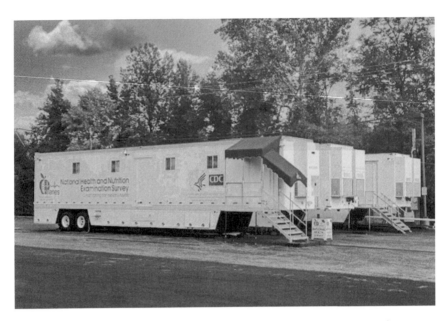

Figure 2.2. National Health and Nutrition Examination Survey. *Source:* National Center for Health Statistics. Centers for Disease Control and Prevention. https://www.cdc.gov /nchs/nhanes/participant-eligibility.htm.

participants are asked to complete two 24-hour dietary recall interviews to account for day-to-day variation in foods consumed. Table 2.4 describes types of data that are collected in NHANES dietary questionnaires, including information obtained during the two 24-hour recalls.

Interviewers administer the 24-hour recall using the United States Department of Agriculture's (USDA) Automated Multiple-Pass Method (AMPM). The AMPM is a computer-assisted multiple-pass format interview system with standardized probes to help estimate current dietary intake and to reduce misreporting. The five-step multiple-pass process aims to improve complete and accurate data collection, while also reducing participant burden by prompting the participant to recall food and beverages consumed during the 24-hour period with probes using three-dimensional food models and a food model booklet (for Day 2 recall over the telephone) to approximate portion size.[16,25] Figure 2.3 shows how the data are collected using the five standardized steps.

NHANES also collects food and nutrition data through an FFQ, as well as a diet behavior and nutrition questionnaire. In previous NHANES cycles an expanded version of an FFQ was used, but NHANES currently utilizes a targeted FFQ to collect data on specific foods and beverages, such as dairy, fish, and seafood consumption. Similar to the 24-hour recalls, survey participants aged 12 years and older complete the FFQ on their own and a proxy respondent reports for individuals 5 years and younger and for other persons who cannot self-report. Proxy-assisted interviews are conducted with children between 6 and 11 years of age.[16] The diet behavior and nutrition

Table 2.4. Types of Nutrition Data Collected from NHANES Dietary Questionnaires

Types of data collected	Description of data obtained
Data collected on food and beverages consumed on a recall day	■ Detailed description (type, form, brand name) ■ Additions to the food ■ Amount consumed ■ What foods were eaten in combination ■ Time eating occasion began ■ Name of eating occasion ■ Food source (where obtained) ■ Whether food was eaten at home ■ Amounts of food energy and more than 60 nutrients/food components provided by the amount of food (calculated)
Data collected specific to the recall day	■ Day of the week (recall day) ■ Amount and type of water consumed, including total plain water, tap water, and plain carbonated water ■ Recall day's consumption amount compared to typical diet ■ Daily total intakes of food energy and more than 60 nutrients/food components (calculated)
Data collected specific to a participant's overall diet	■ Source of tap water ■ Added salt: Frequency and type of salt added at the table and when preparing food ■ Whether on a special diet and type of diet ■ Frequency of fish and shellfish consumption (past 30 days)

Source: https://www.cdc.gov/nchs/tutorials/dietary/surveyorientation/dietarydataoverview/info2.htm.

Note: NHANES = National Health and Nutrition Examination Survey.

questionnaire is administered during the household interview and collects information on various dietary behavior and nutrition-related topics, such as infant feeding practices, community or government meal program participation, school meal program participation, eating away from the home, and use of nutritional information on restaurant menus.[16,22]

Objective assessments of nutritional status in NHANES include anthropometric and biochemical measurements. Anthropometric data collected in the mobile examination center include weight, recumbent length for children less than 4 years of age, and standing height for participants aged 2 years and older. Various body circumferences and skinfold thickness measurements are also assessed based on the age of participants.[26] In some NHANES cycles, body composition has been measured using bioelectric impedance and dual energy X-ray absorptiometry (DXA) on nonpregnant participants within a selected age group.[22] Biomarkers collected in NHANES include but

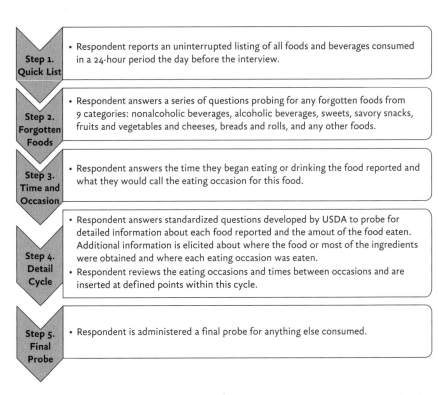

Step 1.
Quick List
- Respondent reports an uninterrupted listing of all foods and beverages consumed in a 24-hour period the day before the interview.

Step 2.
Forgotten Foods
- Respondent answers a series of questions probing for any forgotten foods from 9 categories: nonalcoholic beverages, alcoholic beverages, sweets, savory snacks, fruits and vegetables and cheeses, breads and rolls, and any other foods.

Step 3.
Time and Occasion
- Respondent answers the time they began eating or drinking the food reported and what they would call the eating occasion for this food.

Step 4.
Detail Cycle
- Respondent answers standardized questions developed by USDA to probe for detailed information about each food reported and the amout of the food eaten. Additional information is elicited about where the food or most of the ingredients were obtained and where each eating occasion was eaten.
- Respondent reviews the eating occasions and times between occasions and are inserted at defined points within this cycle.

Step 5.
Final Probe
- Respondent is administered a final probe for anything else consumed.

Figure 2.3. Continuous NHANES web tutorial. *Source:* Centers for Disease Control and Prevention, November 2010. https://www.cdc.gov/nchs/tutorials/dietary/surveyorientation /dietarydataoverview/info2.htm.

are not limited to blood, urine, and certain tissue samples. All samples are processed in the mobile examination center and subsequently shipped to partnering laboratories across the United States for analysis. Selected nutrition biomarkers assessed in NHANES that can help researchers better understand nutritional status include indicators like vitamin D, iodine, and folate.[22]

Examples of nutrition data, including dietary intake, anthropometry and biomarkers, collected from NHANES are presented in table 2.5.

Applications of NHANES to Inform Public Health Nutrition

Nutrition surveillance data from NHANES have been used in various ways to improve public health practice, including monitoring folate levels after food fortification, obesity prevalence in children and adults, and ***trans* fat** levels before and after national policies were implemented. In addition, NHANES data have also been used to develop dietary guidance, including the revision of food nutrition labels and the development of the Dietary Guidelines for Americans; assess patterns and trends in food and nutrition consumption; prioritize nutrition research; and monitor progress toward

Table 2.5. Examples of Nutritional Data Collected from NHANES by Data Collection Stage

NHANES data collection stage	Selected examples of nutrition collected
Household Interview	■ Demographic characteristics ■ Nutrition knowledge and behaviors ■ Infant feeding practices ■ Eating away from home ■ Weight history and weight control practices
Health Examination (including Clinical Assessments and Laboratory)	■ Eating away from home ■ Weight history and weight control practices ■ Anthropometric measurements ■ Body composition ■ Biological specimen collection and laboratory testing (nutrient status, such as vitamin D and folate) ■ 24-hour dietary recall
Post-Exam Components and Interviews	■ Nutrition knowledge and behaviors ■ 24-hour dietary recall

Source: Adapted from Ahluwalia N., J. Dwyer, A. Terry, A. Moshfegh, and C. Johnson. 2016. "Update on NHANES Dietary Data: Focus on Collection, Release, Analytical Considerations, and Uses to Inform Public Policy." *Advances in Nutrition* 7 (1): 121-134.

Note: NHANES = National Health and Nutrition Examination Survey.

health and nutrition goals and objectives, including those outlined in *Healthy People 2020*.[16,23,24]

Food fortification is a major example that highlights the use of NHANES as a nutrition surveillance system.[24] Prior research demonstrated that low intake of folate in women was associated with an increased risk of neural tube defects.[27-31] In 1992, based on this research, the United States Public Health Service recommended that food in the United States be fortified with folic acid to target women of childbearing age.[32] In 1998, this resulted in mandatory fortification of some enriched grain products with folic acid.[27-30,33] Using dietary intake data collected from NHANES, researchers were able to establish the amount of folic acid that needed to be added to the food supply to provide beneficial effects without causing harmful effects from potentially excessive intake. Using biomarker data of folate concentrations from NHANES (as measured by serum and RBC folate concentrations), researchers have reported that folate concentration levels among the US population significantly increased after fortication was implemented.[34] NHANES continues to assess folic acid intake and folate concentration levels. This information is used by researchers, policy makers, and public health professionals to support the monitoring of these fortification programs.[16,24,35,36]

Objectively measured height and weight data from NHANES have been used to calculate **body mass index (BMI)**, the most widely used measure of **obesity**. These data collected over many decades have allowed researchers to monitor trends in obesity among adults and children in the United States; assess patterns of obesity prevalence in specific population subgroups; examine associations between obesity and other diseases, health conditions, and risk of death; and identify individual, environmental, and socioeconomic factors that may contribute to obesity.[3,16] A recent analysis using NHANES data from 2007-2008 through 2015-2016 demonstrated obesity and severe obesity prevalence in adults linearly increased during this time period, although there was no significant change among youth.[37] Public health officials and policy makers regularly use information like this from NHANES to monitor obesity levels and to develop and implement prevention and control strategies to address obesity in the United States.[38] (Learn more about obesity in chapter 8.)

Because the consumption of *trans* fat is associated with an increased risk of coronary heart disease,[39] the Food and Drug Administration (FDA) required in 2003 that *trans* fat be declared on the Nutrition Facts label of processed foods. In 2015, the FDA took additional measures to remove *trans* fat from the food supply by announcing that any *trans* fat intentionally added to foods was subject to approval by the FDA.[40-44] Given the development and implementation of national policies around *trans* fat and the food supply, NHANES biomarker data have been used to examine changes in plasma *trans* fat concentrations among adults in the United States before and after these policies were enacted. Analysis of NHANES data from the 1999-2000 through the 2009-2010 survey cycles demonstrated that plasma *trans* fat concentrations in the NHANES adult population decreased 54% between the survey cycles, suggesting a potential impact of the FDA regulations around *trans* fat.[45]

These represent only a few selected applications of how NHANES surveillance data, which uniquely combines the collection of dietary intake, dietary knowledge and behaviors, anthropometry, and nutrition biomarker data, have been used to support public health nutrition and how national nutrition surveillance can help meet domestic public health practice needs.[6]

Nutrition Surveillance in International Settings: Selected Examples from High-Income Countries

Similar to the United States, a number of other high-income countries have made national efforts to strengthen and coordinate their diet and nutrition surveillance activities.[46,47] In the 1990s, there was an increase in nutrition surveys being implemented, as local governments and international organizations, including the World Health Organization (WHO) and the European Commission, called for the development of and improvements to nutrition surveillance systems.[48,49] As a result, most countries in Europe have a health and nutrition interview survey and several high-income countries have a health examination survey.[2,46,47] The nutrition and dietary information collected from these surveys and the methods used vary, which can limit comparability of nutrition and health information across countries.[50] A brief overview of the sponsoring agencies, methods used, and applications of selected surveillance systems, including the Canada Health Measures Survey, Japan National Health and Nutrition Survey, Korea National Health and Nutrition Examination Survey, and Australian Health Survey, are described below.

Canada Health Measures Survey (CHMS)

Canada's central statistical office, Statistics Canada, launched the CHMS in 2007 to collect information on the health of Canadians. Similar to the data collection methods utilized in NHANES, the CHMS conducts household interviews, in addition to physical examinations and biochemical assessments conducted at a mobile clinic (figure 2.4).[51] The CHMS uses a complex, multistage, cluster sampling design to achieve a nationally representative cross-sectional sample of the Canadian population aged 3 to 79 years. Anthropometric measures and nutrition biomarkers are collected during the physical examination and laboratory tests. Selected examples of nutrition biomarkers collected include vitamin B_{12}, vitamin D, iodine, sodium, and potassium.[51,52] The CHMS household interview incorporates an FFQ, which asks participants to recall their usual intake of specific food groups, including meat, milk, dairy, grains, salt, dietary fat, and fruits and vegetables. Nutrition data from CHMS have been used in a variety of ways by researchers,

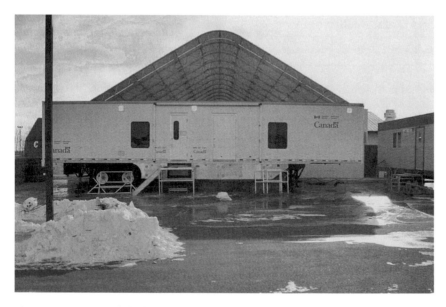

Figure 2.4. CHMS mobile clinic. *Source:* Statistics Canada, https://www.statcan.gc.ca /eng/start.

policy makers, and practitioners, including determining policy priorities, making financial and budgetary decisions, updating guidelines and regulations, and making international comparisons. Specifically, Statistics Canada highlights that the most recent nutrition biomarker data have been used to update national guidelines related to folic acid intake in women of childbearing age, based on results of vitamin B_{12} and folate levels, as well as inform the national update of recommended vitamin D intake guidelines.[53]

Japan National Health and Nutrition Survey (NHNS)

Organized and implemented by the Japanese Ministry of Health, the NHNS is a cross-sectional household interview and examination survey conducted annually.[54,55] It began after World War II as the National Nutrition Survey to investigate the nutritional status of the Japanese civilian population experiencing food shortages and to secure emergency food aid from countries abroad. After the end of the country's occupation in 1952, the survey continued as priority health issues changed. As the nutritional status of the Japanese population improved and the number of older adults rapidly increased, the focus of the survey shifted toward understanding the management and prevention of chronic diseases.[54] The survey currently aims to collect data on health, nutrition, physical activity, individual health behaviors, anthropometric measures, and biochemical and clinical profiles.[54,55] Similar to NHANES, data from the Japan NHNS are used to set national targets related to nutrition and dietary behaviors and monitor progress toward these

Table 2.6. Health Japan Indicators and Targets Related to Nutrition and Dietary Behaviors

Indicator 1. Increase percentage of individuals maintaining ideal body weight
a. Reduce the percentage of obese individuals and underweight individuals

Indicator 2. Increase the percentage of individuals who consume appropriate quality and quantity of food
a. Increase the percentage of individuals who eat a balanced diet with staple food, main dish, and side dish more than twice a day
b. Decrease the mean salt intake
c. Increase the consumption of vegetables and fruit

Indicator 3. Increase in dining with family regularly
a. Decrease the percentage of children who eat alone

Indicator 4. Increase in number of corporations in food industry that supply food product low in salt and fat

Indicator 5. Increase the in percentage of specific food service facilities that plan, cook, and evaluate and improve nutritional content of menu based on the needs of clients

Source: http://www.mhlw.go.jp/seisakunitsuite/bunya/kenkou_iryou/kenkou/kenkou nippon21/en/kenkounippon21/mokuhyou.html.

goals and objectives, or the "National Health Promotion Movement in the 21st Century" (Health Japan 21).[56] Example national targets from Health Japan 21 related to nutrition and dietary behaviors for 2011 to 2020 are presented in table 2.6, which highlight the varying nutrition priorities of another high-income country.

Korea National Health and Nutrition Examination Survey (KNHANES)

Since 1998, the Korea Centers for Disease Control and Prevention has conducted the KNHANES, a national surveillance system that assesses the health and nutritional status of Koreans. KNHANES is a nationally representative cross-sectional survey employed every year that includes a health interview, examination, and laboratory assessment, which are all conducted by trained medical personnel in a mobile examination center.[57] A nutrition survey is also implemented by trained dieticians in the home of participants after the health interview and examination, and incorporates a dietary behavior questionnaire, an FFQ, and a food intake questionnaire that utilizes a 24-hour recall method. Like NHANES, KNHANES nutritional data has been used by public health officials and researchers to develop and track national health and nutrition objectives, including the Dietary Reference Intakes for Koreans, and to produce growth charts for infants and children.[57] KNHANES data have also been used to research the associations between nutritional factors and noncommunicable diseases and to monitor the prevalence and trends in nutritional status among Korean adults and children.[52,57]

Australian Health Survey

Conducted by the Australian Bureau of Statistics, the Australian Health Survey incorporated the Australia National Nutrition and Physical Activity Survey (NNPAS) in 2011-2013 to collect detailed information on dietary intake and food consumption from over 12,000 Australian adults and children (aged 2 years and over), in addition to detailed physical activity data using reported and device-based methods.[58] Information for the nutrition component was collected using a 24-hour dietary recall on all foods and beverages consumed on the day prior to the interview and where possible, at least eight days after the first interview, respondents were contacted to participate in a second 24-hour dietary recall via telephone interview. In addition to the dietary intake assessments conducted during these years, the Australian Health Survey conducts a household interview and a voluntary biomedical component called the National Health Measures Survey, where participants are asked to provide blood and urine samples, which are assessed for biomarkers of nutritional status and chronic diseases. Unlike NHANES, which collects reported and objective nutritional data from participants every year, the NNPAS collects nutritional data from participants intermittently, where the last data collection occurred from 2011 to 2013. Food and nutrition data collected from this latest survey helped public health officials and researchers determine food and nutrient intakes in the population, enabled monitoring and reporting of the adequacy of food and nutrient intakes against national dietary guidelines, facilitated comparison of food and nutrient intakes to those reported in previous national surveys conducted in 1995 and 2007, and informed the development and evaluation of Australian food regulatory standards.[52,58]

Nutrition Surveillance in International Settings: Selected Examples from Low- and Middle-Income Countries

Earlier in this chapter, we described nutrition surveillance as the continuous assessment of dietary intake and nutritional status of a population or selected population subgroups for the purposes of detecting changes and initiating public health action.[1,2,16,17] This definition remains relevant for low- and middle-income countries, but the challenges in conducting nutrition surveillance in low- and middle-income countries can be numerous and differ from those of high-income ones for a number of reasons.[2] First, in most low- and middle-income countries, the prevalence of health problems related to dietary intake and nutritional status, particularly those associated with undernutrition, are higher than in high-income countries. The prevalence also varies substantially within and between regions and countries. Second, continuous national monitoring of dietary intake and nutritional status is not well established in many countries and resources are limited. Third, during the past decade, there has been a rise in the prevalence of obesity and overweight as well as their related comorbidities, which can heighten the need for nutrition surveillance systems to provide useful information to stakeholders.[2,12,59] Changes in disease burdens in low- and middle-income countries are described in more detail in chapters 9 and 10. Finally, logistical considerations are often different in low- and middle-income countries, and can include additional barriers such as: the lack of preexisting maps; populations living in remote, hard-to-reach locations; and unreliable electricity or Internet access for survey equipment.

The public health nutrition issues of international significance in low- and middle-income countries range from micronutrient deficiencies, the double burden of under- and over-nutrition, and challenges associated with food and economic crises.[2,46] These health problems, along with the surveillance challenges described above, heighten the need for nutrition surveillance systems that are able to provide useful information to stakeholders.[2,59,60] Two nutrition surveillance systems highlight these surveillance challenges and contrasting nutritional health priorities: the Mexican National Nutrition Survey and the Demographic and Health Survey.

Mexican National Nutrition Survey

To monitor the nutritional status and dietary intake of the Mexican population, the Mexican National Nutrition Survey was first administered in a nationally representative sample in 1988. Implemented by the National Institute of Public Health in Mexico and its Ministry of Health, the survey aimed to serve as a baseline for health measures and laid the foundation for current nutrition and health surveys administered in Mexico today.[61,62] Adaptations to the survey were implemented in 1999, 2006, and most recently in 2012.[61,63] Survey findings from 1988 facilitated the assessment of nutrition trends, and along with data collected in 1999, Mexican researchers identified pressing nutrition issues in Mexico at the time, including stunting, anemia, micronutrient deficiencies, and a rise in obesity and overweight in adults and children.[63] The survey administered in 2006 was modified to collect representative data at the state level and for all age groups to facilitate tailored public health initiatives for specific geographic areas and population subgroups.[63] The most recent survey, administered in 2012 and renamed the National Health and Nutrition Survey (ENSANUT-2012), represented a combination of previous health and nutrition surveys implemented in the country. It collected data on nutritional habits, physical activity behaviors, and overall health of children, adolescents, adults, and older adults through household and individual questionnaires collected from over 50,000 Mexican households. This version also incorporated blood samples and anthropometric measurements from selected participants.[61-63]

Since the inception of the Mexican National Health and Nutrition Survey, the country has experienced significant demographic, economic, environmental, and cultural changes that have influenced Mexicans' health and well-being.[63,64] Parallel to these shifts, nutrition surveillance data from the Mexican National Health and Nutrition Survey has revealed where Mexico has made progress in addressing existing public health nutrition issues, and helped to identify new nutrition priorities for the country. For example, since the late 1990s, the prevalence of undernutrition and anemia have decreased, but remain concerning for specific population subgroups, including children, women of reproductive age, and older adults. The prevalence of stunting has remained high, particularly among lower income and indigenous infants and children.[63] Lastly, data from all cycles of the survey have demonstrated that chronic diseases and obesity rates have increased and often coexist with health problems associated with malnutrition, particularly among adults and children living in poverty.[64]

Demographic and Health Survey

Nutrition surveillance across countries, including low- and middle-income countries, is possible too. Since 1984, the United States Agency for International

Development (USAID) has organized a program called the Demographic and Health Surveys (DHS), which aims to collect and disseminate nationally representative data on health in and across low- and middle-income countries.[2,65] Currently, the DHS program is comprised of nationally representative household surveys that collect information on a wide range of population, health, and nutrition issues using survey questionnaires, biomarker testing, and geographic information systems.[2,65,66]

The DHS program collects data on nutrition indicators for both women and children within the domains of infant and young child feeding practices, nutritional status, and micronutrient deficiencies. For infant and child feeding practices, the DHS surveys assess the breastfeeding status of infants, with special attention to exclusive breastfeeding. Guided by WHO guidelines, the DHS program also assesses complementary feeding of children aged 6 to 23 months, which includes continued breastfeeding, or feeding of milk or milk products to non-breastfed children; feeding children solids the minimum number of times; and feeding children solid foods from the minimum number of food groups. The DHS program collects anthropometric data on height, weight, mid-upper arm circumference (MUAC), and waist and hip circumferences which allows for the analysis of stunting, wasting, underweight, and overweight for women and children. For micronutrient deficiencies, the DHS program uses biomarker measurements, including hemoglobin to assess anemia, and serum retinol to assess vitamin A deficiency.[66,67]

Through the collection and dissemination of these data to individual countries and across multiple countries, data from the DHS program have been used to: assess trends in nutrition nationally and globally; identify health needs in specific population subgroups and geographic locations; develop nutrition, health, and demographic indicators; monitor progress towards national and global targets, such as the Millennium Development goals and Sustainable Development goals; and inform program, policy, and funding decisions by governments, donors, and international organizations.[2,60]

Conclusion

Surveillance represents the foundation for key decision makers and stakeholders to make informed public health decisions by providing timely and useful evidence.[10] Through ongoing and systematic nutrition surveillance activities and the availability of reliable, relevant, and current data at the national level, public health professionals can help address the public health nutrition needs of today and the future.[2,3,16] As mentioned throughout the chapter, in both high-income and low- and middle-income countries, national surveillance data can be used in a variety of ways, including to monitor and assess trends in nutritional status; to identify factors associated with complex nutrition and health-related issues; to inform the development, implementation, and evaluation of nutrition policies and programs; to track progress toward meeting national nutrition goals and objectives; and to make comparisons on nutrition and health outcomes across countries.[2]

In this chapter, we described how national-level nutrition data collected in the United States from NHANES, a major longstanding nutrition surveillance system, have been used by researchers, policy makers, and practitioners for all of these aforementioned purposes. More specifically, NHANES data have been used to examine folate levels after food fortification, monitor obesity prevalence in youth and adults, and assess *trans* fat levels before and after the implementation of national regulations. Additionally, we highlighted a few selected examples of nutrition surveillance systems in other high-income and low- and middle-income countries, including Canada, Japan, Korea, Australia, Mexico, and a cross-country nutrition surveillance system. National data from these nutrition surveillance systems have also been used to inform public health and nutrition in many of the ways described above. While data from these national nutrition surveillance systems have provided information on nutritional status both domestically and globally, the environments in which we conduct nutrition surveillance are likely to change, and public health nutrition issues and priorities will likely evolve. As such, the nutrition surveillance systems that capture data on these changing health issues will be required to adapt.[6]

Review Questions

1. How does surveillance align with the three core functions of public health of assessment, assurance, and policy development?
2. What are the main attributes of a public health surveillance system?
3. What are commonly used surveillance methods for collecting information on individual dietary intake in the United States?
4. How has nutrition surveillance data from the United States National Health and Nutrition Examination Survey been used to address public health nutrition challenges?
   a. Canada Health Measures Survey?
   b. Japanese Health and Nutrition Survey?
   c. Korea National Health and Nutrition Examination Survey
   d. Australian Health Survey?
   e. Mexico National Health and Nutrition Survey?
   f. USAID Demographic and Health Survey?
5. What do you view as limitations and emerging issues of the United States National Health and Nutrition Examination Survey that may influence public health nutrition?
   a. Canada Health Measures Survey?
   b. Japanese Health and Nutrition Survey?
   c. Korea National Health and Nutrition Examination Survey

    d. Australian Health Survey?

    e. Mexico National Health and Nutrition Survey?

    f. USAID Demographic and Health Survey?

6. What are some challenges to public health nutrition surveillance in low- and middle-income countries, relevant to both the health problems of low- and middle-income countries and the surveillance capacity of low- and middle-income countries?

References

1. Mason, J. B., and J. T. Mitchell. 1983. "Nutritional Surveillance." *Bulletin of the World Health Organization* 61 (5): 745-55. https://doi.org/D64.

2. Tuffrey, Veronica, and Andrew Hall. 2016. "Methods of Nutrition Surveillance in Low-Income Countries." *Emerging Themes in Epidemiology* 13 (1): 1-21. https://doi.org/10.1186/s12982-016-0045-z.

3. Briefel, Ronette R., and Margaret A. McDowell. 2012. "Nutrition Monitoring in the United States." In *Present Knowledge in Nutrition*, edited by J. J. Erdman, I. MacDonald, and S. Zeisel, 10th ed., 1082-1109. Oxford, UK: Wiley-Blackwell.

4. Interagency Board for Nutrition Monitoring and Related Research. 2000. "Nutrition Monitoring in the United States: The Directory of Federal and State Nutrition Monitoring and Related Research Activities." Hyattsville, Maryland: National Center for Health Statistics. https://www.cdc.gov/nchs/data/misc/direc-99.pdf.

5. Institute of Medicine. 1988. "The Future of Public Health." Washington, DC: National Academies Press. https://doi.org/10.17226/1091.

6. Thacker, Stephen B., Judith R. Qualters, and Lisa M. Lee. 2012. "Public Health Surveillance in the United States: Evolution and Challenges." *Morbidity and Mortality Weekly Report* 61: 3-9.

7. Porta, M. 2008. *Dictionary of Epidemiology.* 5th ed. New York: Oxford University Press.

8. Nsubuga, Peter, Mark E. White, Steven B. Thacker, Mark A. Anderson, Stephen B. Blount, Claire V. Broome, Tom M. Chiller, et al. 2006. "Public Health Surveillance: A Tool for Targeting and Monitoring Interventions." In *Disease Control Priorities in Developing Countries*, edited by D. T. Jamison, J. G. Breman, and A. R. Measham, et al., 3rd ed. New York: Oxford University Press.

9. Hoelscher, Deanna M., Nalini Ranjit, and A. Pérez. 2017. "Surveillance Systems to Track and Evaluate Obesity Prevention Efforts." *Annual Review of Public Health* 38: 187-214.

10. Thacker, S. B., and G. S. Birkhead. 2008. "Surveillance." In *Field Epidemiology*, edited by Michael B. Gregg, 38-64. Atlanta, GA: Centers for Disease Control and Prevention: Oxford Scholarship.

11. Centers for Disease Control and Prevention. 2012. "CDC's Vision for Public Health Surveillance in the 21st Century." *Morbidity and Mortality Weekly Report* 61: 1-40.

12. Lee, Lisa M., Steven M. Teutch, Stephen B. Thacker, and Michael E. St. Louis. 2010. *Principles and Practice of Public Health Surveillance.* 3rd ed. Oxford, UK: Oxford University Press.

13. Guidelines Working Group. 2001. "Updated Guidelines for Evaluating Public Health Surveillance Systems: Recommendations from the Guidelines Working Group." *Morbidity and Mortality Weekly Report* 50 (RR13): 1-35.

14. Briefel, Ronette R., and Clifford L. Johnson. 2004. "Secular Trends in Dietary Intake in the United States." *Annual Review of Nutrition* 24 (1): 401-31. https://doi.org/10.1146/annurev.nutr.23.011702.073349.

15. United Nations Administrative Committee on Coordination/Subcommittee on Nutrition. 1982. "Report of the International Workshop on Nutritional Surveillance." Cali, Colombia, July 14-17, 1981. Rome: ACC/SCN.

16. Ahluwalia, Namanjeet, Johanna Dwyer, Ana Terry, Alanna Moshfegh, and Clifford Johnson. 2016. "Update on NHANES Dietary Data: Focus on Collection, Release, Analytical Considerations, and Uses to Inform Public Policy." *Advances in Nutrition* 7 (1): 121-34. https://doi.org/10.3945/an.115.009258.

17. Ahluwalia, Namanjeet, Kirsten Herrick, Ryne Paulose-Ram, and Clifford Johnson. 2014. "Data Needs for B-24 and Beyond: NHANES Data Relevant for Nutrition Surveillance of Infants and Young Children." *American Journal of Clinical Nutrition* 99 (3): 747S-754S. https://doi.org/10.3945/ajcn.113.069062.

18. Elmadfa, I., and A. L. Meyer. 2014. "Developing Suitable Methods of Nutritional Status Assessment: A Continuous Challenge." *Advances in Nutrition: An International Review Journal* 5 (5): 590S-598S. https://doi.org/10.3945/an.113 .005330.

19. Gibson, R. 2005. *Principles of Nutritional Assessment.* Oxford, UK: Oxford University Press.

20. Willett, W. 1999. *Nutritional Epidemiology.* 2nd ed. New York: Oxford University Press.

21. WHO International Programme on Chemical Safety Biomarkers in Risk Assessment. 2001. "WHO International Programme on Chemical Safety Biomarkers in Risk Assessment."

22. Zipf, G., M. Chiappa, K. Porter, Y. Ostchega, B. Lewis, and J. Dostal. 2013. "National Health and Nutrition Examination Survey: Plan and Operations, 1999-2010." *Vital and Health Statistics* 56.

23. Woteki, C. E. 2003. "Integrated NHANES: Uses in National Policy." *Journal of Nutrition* 133: 585-89.

24. CDC National Center for Health Statistics. n.d. "National Health and Nutrition Examination Survey: An Overview."

25. Moshfegh, A. J., D. G. Rhodes, D. J. Baer, T. Murayi, J. C. Clemens, W. V. Rumpler, D. R. Paul, et al. 2008. "The US Department of Agriculture Automated Multiple-Pass Method Reduces Bias in the Collection of Energy Intakes." *American Journal of Clinical Nutrition* 88 (2): 324-32.

26. Fryar, Cheryl D., Qiuping Gu, and Cynthia L Ogden. 2012. *Anthropometric Reference Data for Children and Adults: United States, 2007-2010. Vital and Health Statistics. Series 11: Data from the National Health Survey.* https://doi.org/10.1186/1471 -2431-8-10.

27. Laurence, K. M., N. James, M. Miller, et. al. 1981. "Double Blind Randomized Controlled Trial of Folate Treatment before Conception to Prevent Recurrence of Neural-Tube Defects." *British Medical Journal* 282 (6275): 1509-11.

28. MRC Vitamin Study Research Group. 1991. "Prevention of Neural Tube Defects: Results of the Medical Research Council Vitamin Study." *The Lancet* 338: 131-37.

29. Smithells, R. W., N. C. Nevin, M. J. Seller, et al. 1983. "Further Experience of Vitamin Supplementation for the Prevention of Neural Tube Defect Recurrences." *The Lancet* 1 (8832): 1027-31.

30. Mulinare, J., J. F. Cordero, J. D. Erickson, and R. J. Berry. 1988. "Periconceptional Use of Multivitamins and the Occurrence of Neural Tube Defects." *Journal of the American Medical Association* 260: 3141-45.

31. Milunsky, A., H. Jick, S. Jick, et al. 1989. "Multivitamin/Folic Acid Supplementation in Early Pregnancy Reduces the Prevalence of Neural Tube Defects." *Journal of the American Medical Directors Association* 262: 2847-52.

32. Centers for Disease Control and Prevention. 1992. "Recommendations for the Use of Folic Acid to Reduce the Number of Cases of Spina Bifida and Other Neural Tube Defects." *Morbidity and Mortality Weekly Report* 41: RR-14.

33. Merserue, P., K. Kilker, H. Carter, E. Fassett, J. Williams, and A. Flores. 2004. "Spina Bifida and Anencephaly before and after Folic Acid Mandate: United States 1995-1996 and 1999-2000." *Morbidity and Mortality Weekly Report* 53 (17): 236-365.

34. Pfeiffer, Christine M., Rosemary L. Schleicher, Clifford L. Johnson, and Paul M. Coates. 2012. "Assessing Vitamin Status in Large Population Surveys by Measuring Biomarkers and Dietary Intake—Two Case Studies: Folate and Vitamin D." *Food and Nutrition Research* 56: 1-10. https://doi.org/10.3402/fnr.v56i0.5944.

35. Flannery, B., J. Clippard, R. K. Zimmerman, M. P. Nowalk, M. L. Jackson, L. A. Jackson, A. S. Monto, et al. 2015. "Updated Estimates of Neural Tube Defects Prevented by Mandatory Folic Acid Fortification—United States, 1995-2001." *Morbidity and Mortality Weekly Report* 64 (1): 10-15. https://doi.org/mm6401a4 [pii].

36. Dwyer, Johanna T., Catherine Woteki, Regan Bailey, Patricia Britten, Alicia Carriquiry, P. Courtney Gaine, Dennis Miller, Alanna Moshfegh, Mary M. Murphy, and Marianne Smith Edge. 2014. "Fortification: New Findings and Implications." *Nutrition Reviews* 72 (2): 127-41. https://doi.org/10.1111/nure.12086.

37. Hales, C. M., C. D. Fryar, M. D. Carroll, D. S. Freedman, and C. L. Ogden. 2018. "Trends in Obesity and Severe Obesity Prevalence in US Youth and Adults by Sex and Age, 2007-2008 to 2015-2016." *Journal of the American Medical Association* 319 (16): 1723-25. https://doi.org/10.1001/jama.2018.3060.

38. Kumanyika, Shiriki K., Eva Obarzanek, Nicolas Stettler, Ronny Bell, Alison E. Field, Stephen P. Fortmann, Barry A. Franklin, et al. 2008. "Population-Based Prevention of Obesity: The Need for Comprehensive Promotion of Healthful Eating, Physical Activity, and Energy Balance: A Scientific Statement from AHA Council on Epidemiology and Prevention, Interdisciplinary Committee for Prevention. *Circulation* 118 (4): 428-64. https://doi.org/10.1161/CIRCULATIONAHA.108.189702.

39. Yang, Quanhe, Zefeng Zhang, Fleetwood Loustalot, Hubert Vesper, Samuel P. Caudill, Matthew Ritchey, Cathleen Gillespie, Robert Merritt, Yuling Hong, and Barbara A. Bowman. 2018. "Plasma Trans-Fatty Acid Concentrations Continue to Be Associated with Serum Lipid and Lipoprotein Concentrations

among US Adults after Reductions in Trans-Fatty Acid Intake 1-4." *Journal of Nutritional Epidemiology* 147: 896-907. https://doi.org/10.3945/jn.116.245597.

40. Department of Health and Human Services. 2013. "Tentative Determination Regarding Partially Hydrogenated Oils; Request for Comments and for Scientific Data and Information." *Federal Registry* 78: 67169-75.

41. "CFR 570.38—Determination of Food Additive Status." n.d. *Code of Federal Regulations*.

42. "CFR 570.30—Eligibility for Classification as Generally Recognized as Safe (GRAS)." n.d. *Code of Federal Regulations*.

43. McCarthy, Michael. 2015. "US Gives Food Manufacturers Three Years to Ban Trans Fats." *British Medical Journal* 350 (7): h3315. https://doi.org/10.1136/bmj.h3315.

44. McCarthy, Mike. 2013. "US Moves to Ban Trans Fats." *British Medical Journal* 347: f6749. https://doi.org/10.1136/bmj.f6749.

45. Vesper, H. W., S. P. Caudill, H. C. Kuiper, Q. Yang, N. Ahluwalia, D. A. Lacher, and J. L. Pirkle. 2015. "Plasma Trans-Fatty Acid Concentrations in Fasting Adults Declined from NHANES 1999-2000 to 2009-2010." *American Journal of Clinical Nutrition* 344 (6188): 1173-78. https://doi.org/10.1126/science.1249098.Sleep.

46. Friedman, Gregg. 2014. *Review of National Nutrition Surveillance Systems. The Science of Improving Lives*. Washington, DC: FHI 360/FANTA.

47. World Health Organization. 2014. "Food and Nutrition Surveillance Systems: A Manual for Policymakers and Programme Managers." Geneva, Switzerland.

48. United Nations Administrative Committee on Coordination/Subcommittee on Nutrition. 1987. "First Report on the World Nutrition Situation." In *ACC/SCN*. Rome.

49. United Nations Administrative Committee on Coordination Subcommittee on Nutrition. 1989. "Update on the Nutrition Situation—Recent Trends in Nutrition in 33 Countries." Geneva, Switzerland: Author.

50. Sahyoun, N. R. 2013. "Nutrition Surveillance in Developed Countries." In *Encyclopedia of Human Nutrition*, edited by B. Cabellero, 3rd ed., 363-71. Elsevier Ltd. https://doi.org/10.1016/B978-0-12-375083-9.00205-1.

51. StatCAN. 2018. "Canada Health Measure Survey."

52. Keyzer, Willem de, Tatiana Bracke, Sarah A. McNaughton, Winsome Parnell, Alanna J. Moshfegh, Rosangela A. Pereira, Haeng Shin Lee, Pieter van't Veer, Stefaan de Henauw, and Inge Huybrechts. 2015. "Cross-Continental Comparison of National Food Consumption Survey Methods—A Narrative Review." *Nutrients* 7 (5): 3587-3620. https://doi.org/10.3390/nu7053587.

53. Statistics Canada. 2013. "The Canadian Health Measures Survey 2007/2008 to 2012/2013 Evaluation Report."

54. Ikeda, Nayu, Hidemi Takimoto, Shino Imai, Motohiko Miyachi, and Nobuo Nishi. 2015. "Data Resource Profile: The Japan National Health and Nutrition Survey (NHNS)." *International Journal of Epidemiology* 44 (6): 1842-49. https://doi.org/10.1093/ije/dyv152.

55. "Japan National Health and Nutrition Survey." n.d. Japan Ministry of Health, Labour, and Welfare.

56. "Health Japan 21 (Second Term)." n.d. Japan Ministry of Health, Labour, and Welfare.

57. Kweon, Sanghui, Yuna Kim, Myoung Jin Jang, Yoonjung Kim, Kirang Kim, Sunhye Choi, Chaemin Chun, Young Ho Khang, and Kyungwon Oh. 2014. "Data Resource Profile: The Korea National Health and Nutrition Examination Survey (KNHANES)." *International Journal of Epidemiology* 43 (1): 69-77. https://doi.org/10.1093/ije/dyt228.

58. "Australian National Nutrition and Physical Activity Survey." 2016. Australia Bureau of Statistics.

59. Neufeld, L. M., and L. Tolentino. 2013. "Nutrition Surveillance in Developing Countries." In *Encyclopedia of Human Nutrition*, edited by B. Caballero, 3rd ed., 371-81. Elsevier Ltd.

60. St. Louis, M. 2012. "Global Health Surveillance." *Morbidity and Mortality Weekly Report* 61: 15-19.

61. Rodríguez-Ramírez, Sonia, Verónica Mundo-Rosas, Alejandra Jiménez-Aguilar, and Teresa Shamah-Levy. 2009. "Methodology for the Analysis of Dietary Data from the Mexican National Health and Nutrition Survey 2006." *Salud Pública de México* 51 (1): 523-29. https://doi.org/10.1590/S0036-36342009001000007.

62. Resano-Pérez, E., I. Méndez-Ramírez, T. Shamah-Levy, J. A. Rivera, and J. Sepúlveda-Amor. 2003. "Methods of the National Nutrition Survey 1999." *Salud Publica de Mexico* 45 (4): S558-64.

63. Rivera, Juan A., Laura M. Irizarry, and Teresa González de Cossío. 2009. "Overview of the Nutritional Status of the Mexican Population in the Last Two Decades." *Salud Publica de Mexico* 51 (4): 645-56. https://doi.org/10.1590/S0036-36342009001000020.

64. Aceves-Martins, Magaly, Elisabet Llauradó, Lucia Tarro, Rosa Solà, and Montse Giralt. 2016. "Obesity-Promoting Factors in Mexican Children and Adolescents: Challenges and Opportunities." *Global Health Action* 9 (1): 1-13. https://doi.org/10.3402/gha.v9.29625.

65. United States Agency for International Development (USAID). n.d. "Demographic and Health Survey Overview."

66. Croft, Trevor N., Aileen M. J. Marshall, Courtney K. Allen, et al. 2018. *Guide to DHS Statistics*. Rockville, MD: ICF International.

67. US Agency for International Development (USAID). 2012. "Biomarker Field Manual: Demographic and Health Surveys Methodology." Calverton, MD: ICF International.

3

Nutrition Epidemiology and Assessment of Dietary Intake

Jessica Jones-Smith and Vanessa M. Oddo

LEARNING OBJECTIVES

- Develop a basic understanding of the complexity of collecting and analyzing dietary intake data
- Better understand the challenges of establishing diet–disease relationships
- Describe common dietary assessment tools, including their appropriate use, advantages, and disadvantages

Case Study: Sodium and Blood Pressure

An estimated 103 million US adults have high blood pressure, which is a leading risk factor for cardiovascular diseases.[1] A number of studies on the effect of salt intake on blood pressure have been carried out over the past several decades. One of the first was conducted in 1948 by Watkin and colleagues, who reported blood pressure lowering effects of a low-salt diet.[2] A large number of observational and experimental studies have since confirmed that salt intake is an important factor in elevating blood pressure. The first double-blind controlled study of moderate salt restriction was performed in the early 1980s by MacGregor and colleagues. But it was the well-conducted landmark study, Dietary Approaches to Stop Hypertension (DASH) sodium trial, that provided the best evidence about the effect of salt intake on blood pressure.[3] DASH was a 12-week, multicentered clinical trial that studied three levels of sodium intake (150, 100, and 50 mmol/day) on approximately 400 individuals with and without hypertension. Participants were randomly assigned to eat either a control diet, typical of intake in the United States, or the DASH diet, which is rich in fruits, vegetables, and low-fat dairy products. Within both diets, participants ate foods with high, intermediate, and low levels of sodium for 30 days each. Reducing sodium intake from the high to the intermediate level reduced systolic blood pressure by 2.1 mm during the control diet and by 1.3 mm Hg during the DASH diet. Reducing sodium intake from the intermediate to the low level caused additional reductions of 4.6 mm Hg during the control diet and 1.7 mm Hg during the DASH diet, respectively. In other words, lower-sodium diets, irrespective of other macro- or micronutrient intake, reduced blood pressure and the effects of lower sodium were observed in participants irrespective of race/ethnicity or gender.

Nutrition epidemiology is the science of identifying relationships between dietary intake and disease outcomes. Early discoveries of the role of diet in disease risk were primarily focused on diseases that result from a deficiency of nutrients. For example, the discovery that the deficiency of vitamin C caused scurvy or that the deficiency of vitamin B$_3$ caused pellagra are some of the first documented relationships between dietary factors and disease outcomes. Ensuing research over the next 50 years identified the essential nutrients, or nutrients that are necessary to sustain life.

Today, rather than focusing on essential nutrients, all of which have been identified to the best of our knowledge, most nutrition epidemiologic research focuses on relationships between differing levels of consumption of dietary factors (i.e., nutrients, nutrient-like substances, foods, food groups, or dietary patterns) and risk for disease. Many times, the goal is to identify whether higher or lower intake of a certain dietary factor results in increased or decreased risk for a specific disease outcome. This is true in both higher- and lower-income countries; however, often the diseases of primary interest and their suspected nutritional risk factors vary by setting. For instance, in high-income countries, nutrition epidemiologists are often pursuing questions about which dietary patterns increase risk for heart disease or other leading noncommunicable diseases. Whereas in low- and middle-income countries (LMIC), researchers are often pursuing whether micronutrient supplementation or supplemental foods during infancy and early childhood can decrease risk of stunting, or other diseases related to chronic undernutrition and/or communicable diseases. (See chapter 9 for more about nutrition-related disease burdens in LMIC. See chapter 10 for a discussion of the nutrition transition.)

In this chapter, we discuss the elements of nutrition epidemiology that are most relevant to public health nutrition practitioners. Specifically, we focus on the measurement of dietary intake with an eye toward its importance in assessing diet-disease relationships. This is a cornerstone topic of nutrition epidemiology and one of importance to multiple aspects of public health nutrition. We begin with a discussion of some of the difficulties involved in measuring diet and identifying causal diet-disease relationships. We then provide an overview of the most commonly used dietary assessment methods, including a discussion of strengths and weaknesses of each, as well as recommendations about when to use each of the assessment methods. We briefly cover the use of biomarker data.

Difficulties in Accurately Measuring Dietary Intake

If you are a consumer of the news, it may feel like nutrition advice is constantly changing—something that is a "superfood" today may lose its magical powers by next year. While this occurs in other fields as well, the field of nutrition epidemiology is often singled out for having ever-changing recommendations. Certainly, some of this apparent "flip-flopping" is attributable to oversimplification and the search for catchy headlines by nonscientists; however, undoubtedly, a contributing factor is that diet is an incredibly complex exposure and is difficult to measure, analyze, and relate to health outcomes. In this section, we briefly describe some factors that contribute to the difficulty of accurately measuring diet.

Difficulty in Recalling Dietary Intake

Take a moment to consider what you have eaten in the last 24 hours, the last 48 hours, or last week. Can you recall all of the foods you ate and beverages you drank? Could you estimate the portion size of every food that you ate? Do you know what was in the foods you consumed at a restaurant or what method of cooking was used prepare the food? Was yesterday a typical day? Can you estimate the number of times you consumed green leafy vegetables on average in the past 30 days? Over the past year? Understandably, it is difficult to recall with accuracy everything we eat in a day and our average intake over a month or a year. This difficulty can be even more pronounced when parents are asked to recall a school-aged child's intake or in populations with memory declines.

To overcome this difficulty with recall, you might suggest that recording your intake in real time—either using an app or paper and pencil would increase the accuracy (especially if you were to also measure your foods for portion size). However, recording our intake typically makes us become more aware of our eating and can induce behavior change in and of itself (thereby limiting our ability to capture your typical diet—or what you would eat were you not recording your intake). Additionally, social desirability, or the tendency to report more socially acceptable/encouraged foods and omit foods that are viewed as unhealthy or "bad" foods, may influence our behavior (i.e., we may choose to eat, but not record, items that we perceive to be less healthy for fear of being judged by the researcher). Relatedly, even when using recall (rather than food diary methods), in the context of an intervention, we can choose to not report the foods targeted in the intervention. For example, participants in a weight loss trial in which the intervention consists of a low-carbohydrate diet may decide to omit a bout of nonadherence to the diet due to social desirability bias.

Translating What We Eat to Nutrients, Phytochemicals, Food Groups, and Other Components

Beyond the obstacles to obtaining accurate dietary recall, additional complexity in measuring dietary consumption stems from the fact that for many applications, we need to translate the foods reported in dietary recalls to nutrients and other food constituents. Each food or beverage reported needs to be matched to an entry in a nutrient database, which contains the estimated nutrient composition for that food. For foods reported in a dietary recall, the first issue is matching to an appropriate food in the nutrient database. Consider that the average supermarket sells approximately 40,000 to 50,000 products and that between 2010 and 2016 an average of 20,000 new foods (mostly snacks and baked goods) and beverages were introduced in the United States each year.[4] This represents a 120% increase from 1998, when approximately 12,000 new foods and beverages were introduced to the US market annually. A popular, research-level nutrient database, the Nutrition Data System for Research (NDSR), contained 18,000 different foods, including 8,000 brand-name foods in 2019. By necessity, researchers must attempt to make the best match possible, but this means the nutrient content assigned to that food and to an entire day's worth of food is an estimate rather than an exact measure. Moreover, researchers should consider whether the database contains the appropriate foods for subpopulations within the United States or for analyzing dietary data from other countries, for whom many regularly consumed foods may not be represented in the database.

It is also important to consider where the nutrient information in a nutrient database comes from. It can come from either a chemical analysis of the food or through an estimate based on a recipe of ingredients that make up that food and their chemical composition. For fruits and vegetables, multiple samples of the food are typically assessed, since growing conditions can influence nutrient composition. An average of the values from the different samples at different times of year and from different parts of the country is then used, which can be different then from the average in any one location.

Additionally, the number of nutrients, phytochemicals, and other food constituents reported in a nutrient database for each food varies. Although all foods will have macronutrient content and vitamins/minerals included on the nutrition label, not all foods are analyzed for various phytochemicals or specific fatty acid composition. This limits our ability to assess relationships among food components that are not included in the nutrient databases for all foods.

One final concern worthy of mention is that there are additional estimations and assumptions involved for assigning nutrient compositions to foods collected from a food frequency questionnaire (FFQ). Some of the questions on popular FFQs will ask participants to report intake of a whole category of food. For example, "how often did you drink soda or soft drinks?" To translate entries like this into nutrient composition, an average or a weighted average of the nutrient composition of sodas and soft drinks is used.

Complexity in Measuring Usual Intake

As we have seen, accurately measuring and assessing the nutrient content of just one day of dietary intake is hard in and of itself, but for most applications in public health nutrition, we are not interested in just one day of intake but rather usual or habitual intake. This is because for most diseases, we hypothesize that it is **usual dietary intake** that influences disease risk rather than intake on a single day. For example, your heart disease risk is not influenced by your dietary intake last week, but it may be influenced by your dietary intake in the last year, 10 years, 20 years, or longer. Ideally, we would periodically assess dietary intake using multiple days of dietary recall during different times of the year, repeated over multiple years. This would allow us to capture usual dietary intake over a long period of time and also account for normal day-to-day variability in diet; for example, many people may not eat meat on a given day. Some of those people do not consume meat ever, and other people consume meat with varying frequency. We cannot distinguish between these differences in habitual consumption if we only have one or two days of data. However, since collecting multiple days of dietary recall is extremely costly and burdensome for participants, we typically rely on an FFQ to ask people to recall their typical intake of a list of 60 to 150 foods or food groupings or are limited to collecting one to three days of dietary recalls. These data collection tools are described in detail below.

Establishing Diet-Disease Relationships

We have now established that dietary intake is difficult to measure and, as a result, suffers from measurement error (i.e., it is measured imperfectly). There are few additional factors that should be considered as we evaluate the relationship between dietary intake and disease.

First, nutrients and foods can be highly correlated, making it difficult to determine what the causal agent is in any diet-disease relationship. For instance, energy intake is highly correlated with fat intake, as is fruit and vegetable intake. Energy intake, is, in turn, associated with variations in body size, activity levels, and metabolism across individuals. Furthermore, isolating particular nutrients or phytochemicals that appear to increase or decrease risk of diseases and administering them as supplements has generally not yielded benefits to noncommunicable disease (i.e., vitamin C, vitamin E, omega-3 fatty acids, beta-carotene).[5-9] These findings over many years have led to greater recognition that the whole food "package" may be important for achieving health impacts because nutrients in foods come packaged with other substances that may be required for achieving health benefits. Beyond foods, the whole dietary pattern, rather than single foods or food groups, is likely a more reasonable exposure and, recently, there has been a shift in the field of nutrition epidemiology toward studying the effects of whole dietary patterns rather than attempting to isolate the impacts of specific nutrients, phytochemicals, or foods.[10]

A second factor that contributes to difficulty in establishing the role of dietary factors in disease development is the disease that the latency period, or time between being exposed to something that causes disease and the development of disease, is thought to be long (e.g., coronary artery disease) or unknown (e.g., breast cancer). Therefore, following individuals for long periods of time and repeatedly collecting dietary information is oftentimes necessary. Furthermore, even when dietary data have been collected for long periods of time on cohorts of individuals, it is unclear how to best analyze repeated dietary assessments measured over long periods of time when the relevant latency period remains unknown and when dietary habits can change over such long periods.

Third, as discussed in chapter 7, randomizing populations to a particular dietary pattern or food exposure and following them until they develop disease is typically not feasible due to long latency periods, the inability to stay on a prescribed diet for an extended period, and the cost of such trials. Randomized trials can be used to study intermediary biomarkers associated with disease endpoints (instead of the disease endpoint itself), but evidence from these intermediary markers is less compelling since the disease endpoint is not directly observed. This implies that, instead, researchers must rely on observational research and therefore, pay special attention to controlling for confounding (the possibility that an observed relationship is actually due to a different exposure) and reverse causality (the possibility that the "outcome" causes the "exposure" rather than the other way around), two key factors that can result in spurious associations between diet and disease. Dietary intake is correlated with many other characteristics and risk factors, such as exercise, smoking, drinking, and socioeconomic status. Therefore, residual confounding and unmeasured confounding are often a threat to validity of findings from observational cohort studies. In addition, often individuals change their diet in response to being newly diagnosed with a disease. For this reason, reverse causality is a potential threat to unbiased associations, particularly in cross-sectional studies.

We explain these limitations so that public health nutrition practitioners can become more critical consumers of the nutrition epidemiology literature. These limitations do not invalidate findings from nutrition epidemiological studies. However, we review these potential limitations and complexities to emphasize the importance of utilizing validated dietary assessment measures, using the most appropriate dietary assessment measure for the re-

search question, employing rigorous study designs, addressing the same research question with multiple methods (in multiple populations), employing
rigorous sensitivity analyses, and utilizing meta-analytic techniques to summarize multiple studies on the same topic. Public health nutrition practitioners can evaluate how robust the literature on a particular association between dietary factors and disease is by carefully considering these factors.

Key Dietary Assessment Tools

In this section, we discuss three of the most commonly used tools to assess diet: the 24-hour recall, the FFQ, and dietary screeners. Each dietary
assessment tool varies in terms of its appropriate use, and each has strengths
and weaknesses.

24-Hour Recall

The **24-hour recall** is a detailed report of all food and beverages consumed
in the preceding 24 hours. It includes information about method of food preparation and portion size. It is open-ended and is meant to capture all foods
and beverages eaten.

The most common method for administering a 24-hour recall is via
trained interviewer (in-person or telephone), often done with the assistance
of interactive computer software, like the USDA Automated Multiple Pass
Method (AMPM). The AMPM is a multiple-pass approach employing five
steps designed to enhance accurate food recall and reduce respondent burden:
(1) quick list of foods, (2) interviewer probes for forgotten foods, (3) interviewer collects the time and occasion of foods eaten, (4) the interviewer
goes through the detailed cycle to review the 24-hour day and collect specific information including food details and portion size, and (5) there is a
final probe. This multiple-pass method is considered the gold standard for
24-hour recalls and is used in *What We Eat in America*, the dietary interview
component of the National Health and Nutrition Examination Survey
(NHANES). The 24-hour recall typically takes about 20 to 60 minutes to complete.[11] In an effort to decrease the cost of interviewer-assisted data collection,
researchers at the National Cancer Institute have developed an online version
of the 24-hour recall, called the ASA24, which can be self-administered, although it requires an Internet connection.

When to Use It

The 24-hour recall captures mean usual dietary intake for populations.
The 24-hour recall is the most appropriate dietary assessment method to estimate the mean dietary intakes of a population. For instance, one day of
24-hour recall data from the NHANES survey can be used to estimate the
mean intake of foods, food groups, and macronutrients, such as energy or
protein intake. If information about dietary supplements is also incorporated,

this can be used to estimate total nutrient intakes for the overall population in the United States. In addition, the 24-hour recall is also the preferred dietary assessment measure for evaluating whether an intervention changed dietary intake. One day of 24-hour recall can be used to assess whether an intervention changed population mean intakes;[11] however, two days of 24-hour recalls can allow for more precise estimates on smaller samples since they can be used to assess and adjust for day-to-day variation within the same individual.

Two days of 24-hour recalls with statistical adjustment to derive the distribution of mean usual intake are needed to estimate the proportion of consumption above or below a certain threshold (i.e., meeting Dietary Reference Intakes).[11] When collecting two days of 24-hour recalls, including a weekday and weekend day is preferred. To estimate longer-term intake, we need additional recalls (e.g., three or four recalls in each of the four seasons of the year). Because of this, FFQs are usually used for longer-term intake.

Advantages and Disadvantages

An advantage of a traditional, interviewer-administered 24-hour recall is that it does not require literacy and it is appropriate for more culturally diverse populations (you can accommodate any food or food combination in the recall, as opposed to food frequency questionnaires that ask about a set list of foods). The respondent burden is relatively low. In addition, the 24-hour recall provides analytical flexibility since you can analyze the data for total diet as well as by meal, in addition to being able to analyze data for nutrients, individual foods, food groups, or dietary patterns. Portion size is collected, and the time of day and type of eating occasion can also be collected.

Disadvantages of the 24-hour recall include the tendency toward underreporting of total energy intake due to forgotten or intentionally omitted foods. In addition, 24-hour recalls rely on specific memory rather than general memory (but by using highly trained interviewers and providing a list of commonly forgotten foods, you can reduce the chance that foods will be forgotten). The recall captures short-term, current intake, unless it is repeated throughout different times of the year. For this reason, seasonal differences in intake will not be captured. This can be particularly important in LMIC, where dietary intake may vary greatly depending on the season. The cost of administering 24-hour recalls can be substantial since it involves calling participants (usually repeatedly until they are reached), and then a trained professional administering the recall for at least 20 to 60 minutes per person for each 24-hour recall. The ASA24 is a lower-cost alternative that is a self-administered 24-hour recall. Currently, the US ASA24 is only available in English and Spanish, and only the ASA24 for adults is being maintained and updated.

Food Frequency Questionnaire

The FFQ is a structured questionnaire that contains a list of usually 60 to 150 commonly consumed foods. Determining which foods are included on the FFQ is an important aspect of developing the questionnaire. Typically, the choice of foods is informed by considering foods that are consumed regularly by at least some of the population, contain nutrients of interest, and vary in consumption from person to person.[12] FFQs ask participants to report frequencies of foods consumed during a specified period, most commonly the preceding month, six months, or year. Semi-quantitative FFQs ask participants to report usual portion size of the foods consumed, either in the question or in the response options. Other FFQs ask only about frequency and do not specifically ask about portion size. FFQs are typically self-administered; however, they can be interviewer administered. Typically, the self-administered FFQs can take 30 to 60 minutes to complete. Since FFQs are not open-ended but rather ask about only certain foods, the food list should be adapted to reflect the intake of the population of interest, otherwise key foods could be missed entirely.

When to Use It

The FFQ is designed to assess longer-term usual dietary intake. When paired with a nutrient database, the FFQ can also be used to rank the intake of nutrients and other food constituents, in addition to foods and food groups. The FFQ is most appropriate for ranking dietary intake of individuals (i.e., low, medium, high intake), rather than estimating the absolute levels of intake. The FFQ is appropriate for examining associations between diet and disease because it assesses usual, longer-term dietary intake (which is typically the most relevant dietary exposure in relationship to chronic disease) and because, in examining associations between diet and disease, it is meaningful to examine people with lower versus higher intake of a food or nutrient (i.e., ranking of individual intakes). Because FFQs can suffer from systematic error (as opposed to random error), due to the reliance on complex cognitive tasks and food lists (rather than being open-ended), the FFQ is not the preferred method for estimating population group means.[13]

Advantages and Disadvantages

FFQs are substantially less expensive than 24-hour recalls and they can assess long-term dietary intake. They are fairly quick to complete, so they represent a relatively low burden to participants. They also depend on generic rather than specific memory, which is believed to be easier for participants.[12] However, it is also argued that participants have to perform cognitively complex averaging and make an assessment about typical intake for a large number of foods.[13] Response options are limited and reliant on the foods listed, which means that different FFQs should be developed when the food list is not reflective of the consumption of a population. Developing an appropriate FFQ for a new study population is a nontrivial task and requires validation.

Screeners

Dietary screeners are short dietary assessment instruments that often focus on one aspect or a few aspects of the diet (e.g., fruit and vegetable intake, beverage intake, dietary fat intake). Most dietary screeners ask about the frequency of eating specific foods, but they do not always collect information on portion size. One of the most commonly used screeners is the Dietary Screener Questionnaire (DSQ), developed by the National Cancer Institute (NCI). The DSQ is a 26-item screener that assess intakes of fruits and vegetables, dairy, added sugars, whole grains/fiber, red meat, and processed meat.[14] These 26 items were selected because of their relationship to one or more dietary factors of interest in the Dietary Guidelines for Americans (DGA). While the DSQ asks about a few aspects of the diet, the 15-item beverage questionnaire (BEVQ-15) focuses only on beverage consumption. Respondents are asked to indicate "how often" and "how much" of a beverage they consumed in the past month for 15 commonly consumed beverages in the United States. Estimates of intake from these short dietary assessment instruments are generally not as accurate as those from more detailed methods, such as 24-hour dietary recalls or FFQs.

When to Use It

Oftentimes, researchers would prefer to assess the whole diet, but due to cost and participant burden they must opt for a screener. Screeners may be useful in situations that do not require assessment of the total diet. They can be appropriate to use when trying to characterize a population's mean or median intake or identifying individuals or populations with regard to higher versus lower intakes.[14] They are often used in intervention research targeted at particular foods. Additionally, screeners can be useful when comparing findings from a smaller study to a larger population, like those surveyed in the National Health Interview Survey (which uses only a few questions about dietary consumption), or when a researcher is aiming to add diet questions to a longer health survey, where there may be very limited room for questions.

Advantages and Disadvantages

Dietary screeners are much less expensive than both the 24-hour recall and FFQ methods. They also have a very low respondent burden and may be easier for lower-literacy populations. Therefore, screeners may be the dietary assessment method used when a larger sample size is needed and other methods are cost-prohibitive, or when conducting a telephone or intercept survey where minimizing participant burden is critical for participation. However, screeners are considered a more crude dietary assessment tool, compared to 24-hour recalls or FFQs, as they are not appropriate to use for an assessment of the total diet.

Additional Considerations for Dietary Assessment in LMIC

The 24-hour recall, FFQs, and dietary screeners can be used in LMIC, if appropriately adapted to the country (or world region). But when doing so, additional considerations and complexity arises. Most importantly, the nutrition-related disease burden differs in the United States versus LMIC, so dietary assessment methods must be adapted accordingly. In LMIC, it is common for dietary assessment methods to focus on micronutrient intake, compared to the United States, where macronutrient intake is typically of interest (i.e., carbohydrates, fats, protein, total calories). For example, FFQs and dietary screeners in LMIC often focus on vitamin A or iron-rich foods, in addition to including questions about commonly consumed staples (e.g., rice, beans). Seasonality is likely to be more important in LMIC, compared to higher-income countries where most foods are available year-round and famine or food deprivation due to droughts or floods is not common. Therefore, depending on the question of interest, data collection may need to coincide with the season (e.g., harvest or rainy season). In addition, household-level food sharing (i.e., family-style meals) is more common, posing challenges to assessing individuals' intake. Finally, in some contexts there is no reliable food database with nutrient composition, making the translation of dietary data into nutrients and other food constituents difficult.

Dietary Assessment in Special Populations

Dietary assessment can be additionally complex among infants, children, adolescents, and elderly populations, therefore it is important to consider the limitations of these dietary data. Dietary assessment among breastfed infants is extremely difficult and rare. In the rare cases researchers do attempt to assess intake among infants, they typically do so using the weighing method. The weighing method simply consists of weighing the baby before and after each feed. The researcher should obtain 12-hour weighed intakes, with some collection of nighttime feeds. This method allows one to obtain the volume/weight of breast milk consumed, but no information is available on total energy or nutrient intakes.

The interview-administered 24-hour recall is the most accurate method to assess children's dietary intake.[15] When assessing children's diets, parents are relied upon as proxy reporters for capturing their intake because young children (i.e., those 11 years of age and younger) generally have limited ability to estimate portion sizes, incomplete concepts of time, and potentially limited knowledge of food names and preparation methods.[16,17] For example, the NHANES uses proxy reporting for children under age 5 and assisted reporting for children aged 6-11 years. In general, parents are able to report what their young children eat and drink fairly accurately; however, the accuracy of portion size estimates is lower.[18] If using an FFQ or screener with young children it is often necessary to adapt the food list and portion sizes. There is limited development of new methods that are suitable for assessment of dietary intake among children; however, using image-based assessment for children aged 3-10 years shows promise.[19]

Adolescents can typically report their own diet, but like younger-aged children, if using an FFQ, the food list and portion sizes may require adaptation and there is some evidence that adolescents are prone to underreporting.[20] Typically, adolescents are more adept with technology and public health nutrition practitioners could consider using a more diverse range of newer methods of dietary assessment that are available for examining the patterning (i.e., frequency, spacing, regularity) and nutrient content. For example, several studies have shown that apps and camera functions via mobile phones or computers fitted with webcams are promising methods for data collection, which may be particularly well-suited for this population.[21]

Finally, the appropriateness of dietary assessment methods also warrants additional consideration among elderly populations. For example, special diet recommendations may bias reporting, and neither 24-hour recalls nor FFQs are appropriate if an individual is memory impaired. If these methods are used, being administered by an interviewer is preferred. Among elderly populations, considering common micronutrient deficiencies (e.g., vitamin B_{12}) and capturing supplement use are also important.

Diet Quality

We often use composite measures to summarize the quality of diet. This is in part due to an increasing interest in the whole dietary patterns rather than attempting to isolate the impacts of specific nutrients or foods. In the United States, most commonly these include the Healthy Eating Index (HEI) and the Mean Adequacy Ratio. The HEI is a measure of diet quality that assesses how well individuals' diet aligns with the DGA, which advises the US population on diet composition, aimed at maintaining health and preventing diseases. The 2015 DGA emphasized that a healthy dietary pattern includes a variety of vegetables (e.g., dark green, red, orange), whole fruits, whole grains, fat-free or low-fat dairy, a variety of protein foods (e.g., lean meats and poultry, eggs), and vegetable oils (e.g., olive, soybean, sunflower), and one should limit added sugar, *trans* fat, saturated fat, and sodium. Because the DGA informs the HEI score, the score has changed over time as the DGA has evolved; for example, in 2015, the "empty calories" component was replaced with saturated fat and added sugar, since this was a focus of the DGA in 2015. However, the core aspects of a healthful diet (e.g., green vegetables, dairy, grains) have remained consistent. The HEI is a 12-component score that assesses adequacy (nine items) and moderation (three items). A key feature of the HEI is that the scoring separates dietary quality from quantity using a density approach. In other words, the components are calculated as a food group amount per 1,000 calories in the total mix of foods. This allows researchers to apply the HEI in a variety of research settings.

The Mean Adequacy Ratio is also a common measure of dietary quality, which examines the adequacy of the diet for each individual, for two to 15 nutrients, with respect to the Recommended Dietary Allowance (i.e., nutrient reference values for the population). Similar to the HEI, one strength of this indicator is that it allows public health nutrition researchers to consider and communicate a population's overall nutritional adequacy, rather than focusing on specific nutrients that alone may not indicate a healthy diet.

In addition to measuring healthful diet quality, we also measure unhealthful diet quality by estimating an indicator of energy density. Energy density is the amount of energy (or calories) per gram of food. Lower energy density foods (e.g., soups, salads) have a higher water content and thus provide fewer calories per gram of food—this means that one can eat larger portions of these foods, with a relatively low calorie content. High-energy density foods tend to include foods that are high in fat and have a low water content (e.g., potato chips, butter, and cheese).

Diet quality is also of interest in lower-income country settings, particularly among children aged 6 to 23 months and women of child-bearing age. In LMIC, dietary diversity scores are used to assess diet quality, with one point for each food or food group among children aged 6 to 23 months: grains, roots, and tubers; meat; eggs; vitamin A–rich fruits and vegetables; dairy products, legumes, and nuts; and other fruits and vegetables.[22] Among women, similar food groups are used to assess diet diversity, but the 10-item score also includes the addition of dark-green leafy vegetables and other fruits and vegetables as separate groups.[23]

Technological Advancements and Potential Future Trends in Dietary Assessment

Newer technologies using electronic and mobile methods, such as handheld personal digital assistants and mobiles phones, have the potential to overcome some of the limitations associated with traditional dietary assessment methods. To date, applying technology to dietary assessment has primarily focused on introducing improvements relating to data entry and mode of administration (e.g., mobile phones and tablets). These technologies can allow real-time data collection, improvements relating to coding and analyzing food intake, and accuracy of the data.[21] More recently, a number of devices have come to market that augment the data collection process and rely on image-based data collection (e.g., use of wearable devices and/or cameras).[24-29] For example, the SenseCam is a camera worn on a lanyard around the neck that automatically captures point-of-view images in response to movement, heat, and light (about every 30 minutes).[26,27] The eButton is a similar product, which automatically takes pictures of consumed foods for objective dietary assessment. From the acquired pictures, the food portion size can be calculated semi-automatically with the help of computer software.[28] Preliminary research has suggested that wearable cameras may reduce underreporting of energy intake in self-reported dietary assessment.[26-29]

Biomarkers for Diet Measurement

Biomarkers can sometimes be used to validate other forms of dietary assessment (e.g., FFQs) and as a surrogate for dietary intake. They are often categorized into short-term (reflecting intake over past hours/days), medium-term (reflecting intake over weeks/months), and long-term markers (reflecting intake over months/years) and can be collected via blood, hair, and adipose tissue. There is no perfect measure of dietary intake, including biomarkers. But biomarkers can offer some advantages: they are less subject to certain kinds of bias that is common in dietary assessment (e.g., recall bias, social desirability bias) and in some cases smaller sample sizes are required. Importantly, the measurement error that occurs in biomarkers should be uncorrelated with dietary questionnaires; thus, they are often used to validate other forms of dietary assessment.

Although biomarkers offer some advantages over recall-based assessment methods, biomarkers are also subject to misclassification and bias, unrelated to dietary intake, but due to the absorption and metabolism of nutrients, levels of binding proteins, and techniques used in the lab to analyze the data; however, lab-based error can be minimized, both by training lab technicians, by having a larger number of samples, and by using statistical techniques to adjust for error. The use of biomarkers is further limited by the fact that for many dietary factors there is not a marker of interest. For example, there are not biomarkers for total fat, total carbohydrate, sucrose/sugar, or fiber. Sensitivity of biomarkers to intake is also a problem. Sensitivity to intake is related to the degree of homeostatic control of the nutrient and the bioavailability, as well as genetic, environmental, and lifestyle factors. For plasma levels of cholesterol, retinol, and calcium, homeostatic regulation is strong, so their association with intake is very weak.

Although some biomarkers are considered weak, largely due to low sensitivity to intake, there are a few biomarkers that are consistently and more strongly associated with intake. These biomarkers are sometimes termed "recovery" biomarkers because the time between dietary intake and recovery (or excretion) is known.[30] These markers include doubly labeled water

(DLW) for the assessment of energy expenditure[31] which, assuming that the study subject is in energy balance, measures energy intake and 24-hour urinary nitrogen excretion, which measures protein intake. The DLW method is a technique used to measure average daily energy expenditure and involves the administration of water containing enriched quantities of deuterium, a stable isotope. Over time, the deuterium is eliminated from the body in the form of water and the oxygen is eliminated as both water and carbon dioxide. The difference in the elimination rates is used to calculate total energy expenditure. DLW is accurate, noninvasive, and can provide data over a period of weeks. However, it can be costly and requires more than one sample per individual.

Urinary nitrogen is a valid method of assessing total protein intake and is among the most robust diet biomarkers, although several limitations persist.[32,33] A comparison of a 28-day feeding study with multiple 24-hour urine nitrogen outputs produced a very high correlation (0.99). But when only collecting one day of data, the correlation is cut in half (0.50).[32] To obtain the most accurate measurements, individuals should be in nitrogen balance (i.e., nitrogen [or protein] in = nitrogen out) and multiple 24-hour urine samples are needed to appropriately assess protein status.

Conclusion

Nutrition epidemiology is central to the field of nutritional sciences and to the knowledge base of public health nutrition. Most research focuses on relationships between differing levels of consumption of dietary factors, often food groups or dietary patterns, and risk for disease. Typically, the goal is to identify whether higher or lower intake of a dietary factor results in increased or decreased risk for a specific disease. But as discussed throughout this chapter, there are a number of difficulties involved in measuring diet and identifying causal diet-disease relationships. Accurately measuring and assessing the nutrient content of just one day of dietary intake is hard in itself, but we are often interested in usual dietary intake that influences disease risk. The latency period is thought to be long or unknown; therefore, following individuals for years or even decades and repeatedly collecting dietary information is often necessary. In addition, researchers must rely on observational research and pay special attention to controlling for confounding and reverse causality.

We most often collect diet data using 24-hour recalls, FFQs, and screeners. The 24-hour recall is the most appropriate dietary assessment method to estimate the mean dietary intakes of a population. The FFQ is appropriate for examining associations between diet and disease because it assesses usual, longer-term dietary intake and for ranking the dietary intake of individuals (i.e., low, medium, high intake), rather than estimating the absolute levels of intake. Dietary screeners are short dietary assessment instruments that ask about the frequency of eating specific foods. They are often used when assessment of the whole diet is cost prohibitive or too burdensome to participants, and are useful in situations that do not require assessment of the total diet.

Despite some challenges in the investigation of diet–disease relationships, over the last century nutrition epidemiologists have documented many diet–disease relationships: sodium and blood pressure, folic acid and neural tube defects, vitamin A and night blindness, vitamin C and scurvy, vitamin D and rickets, iodine and goiter, beta carotene and lung cancer in smokers, and fat and sugar and heart disease, among others. The study of diet–disease relationships and the field of nutrition epidemiology informs nutrition policy, such as food fortification, the DGAs, food labeling policies, and nutrition standards for school meals.

Review Questions

1. Describe three difficulties in accurately measuring dietary intake.
2. Discuss two challenges public health nutritionists face when trying to establish diet-disease relationships.
3. List the three most common dietary assessment tools. For each tool, briefly describe their appropriate use, as well as one advantage and one disadvantage of using said tool.
4. Describe two additional considerations for dietary assessment in low- and middle-income countries.
5. Briefly explain the appropriateness and/or adaptations of common dietary assessment methods for children, adolescents, and elderly populations.
6. Describe the overall goal(s) of summarizing the quality of diet.
7. Name one advantage and one disadvantage of using biomarkers to assess diet.

References

1. Benjamin, E. J., S. S. Virani, C. W. Callaway, et al. 2018. "Heart Disease and Stroke Statistics—2018 Update: A Report From the American Heart Association." *Circulation* 137 (12). doi:10.1161/CIR.0000000000000558.

2. Watkin, D. M., H. F. Froeb, F. T. Hatch, and A. B. Gutman. 1950. "Effects of Diet in Essential Hypertension: II. Results with Unmodified Kempner Rice Diet in Fifty Hospitalized Patients." *American Journal of Medicine* 9 (4): 441-93. doi:10.1016/0002-9343(50)90200-2.

3. Sacks, F. M., L. P. Svetkey, W. M. Vollmer, et al. 2001. "Effects on Blood Pressure of Reduced Dietary Sodium and the Dietary Approaches to Stop Hypertension (DASH) Diet." *New England Journal of Medicine* 344 (1): 3-10. doi:10.1056/NEJM200101043440101.

4. USDA ERS. 2017. "New Products." https://www.ers.usda.gov/topics/food-markets-prices/processing-marketing/new-products/. Accessed March 14, 2019.

5. Huang H.-Y., B. Caballero, S. Chang, et al. 2006. "The Efficacy and Safety of Multivitamin and Mineral Supplement Use to Prevent Cancer and Chronic Disease in Adults: A Systematic Review for a National Institutes of Health State-of-the-

Science Conference." *Annals of Internal Medicine* 145 (5): 372-85. http://www.ncbi
.nlm.nih.gov/pubmed/16880453. Accessed March 14, 2019.

6. Fortmann, S.P., B. U. Burda, C. A, Senger, J. S. Lin, and E. P. Whitlock. 2013.
"Vitamin and Mineral Supplements in the Primary Prevention of Cardiovascular
Disease and Cancer: An Updated Systematic Evidence Review for the US Preventive Services Task Force." *Annals of Internal Medicine* 159 (12): 824-34. doi:10.7326
/0003-4819-159-12-201312170-00729.

7. Mozaffarian D. 2016. "Dietary and Policy Priorities for Cardiovascular
Disease, Diabetes, and Obesity." *Circulation* 133 (2): 187-225. doi:10.1161
/CIRCULATIONAHA.115.018585.

8. Rizos, E. C., E. E. Ntzani, E. Bika, M. S. Kostapanos, and M. S. Elisaf. 2012.
"Association Between Omega-3 Fatty Acid Supplementation and Risk of Major
Cardiovascular Disease Events." *JAMA* 308 (10): 1024. doi:10.1001/2012.jama.11374.

9. Wu, J. H. Y., and D. Mozaffarian. "ω-3 Fatty Acids, Atherosclerosis Progres-
sion and Cardiovascular Outcomes in Recent Trials: New Pieces in a Complex
Puzzle HHS Public Access." *Heart* 100 (7): 530-33. doi:10.1136
/heartjnl-2013-304421.

10. US Department of Health and Human Services, US Department of Agriculture. 2015. *2015-2020 Dietary Guidelines for Americans.* Washington, DC. https:
//health.gov/sites/default/files/2019-09/2015-2020_Dietary_Guidelines.pdf. Accessed
March 14, 2019.

11. National Institutes of Health, National Cancer Institute. "Dietary Assessment Primer, 24-hour Dietary Recall (24HR) At a Glance." https:/dietassess
mentprimer.cancer.gov/profiles/recall/. Accessed March 14, 2019.

12. Willett, W. C. 2012. "Food-Frequency Methods." In W. Willet, ed. *Nutritional Epidemiology*, 70-95. Oxford, UK: Oxford University Press. doi:10.1093/acprof
:oso/9780195122978.003.05.

13. National Institutes of Health, National Cancer Institute. "Dietary Assessment Primer, Evaluating the Measurement Error Structure of Self-Report Dietary
Assessment Instruments." https://dietassessmentprimer.cancer.gov/concepts/error
/error-affecting.html. Accessed March 14, 2019.

14. National Institutes of Health, National Cancer Institute. Short Dietary
Assessment Instruments. https://epi.grants.cancer.gov/diet/screeners/. Accessed
March 14, 2019.

15. Centers for Disease Control and Prevention. 2015. "NHANES: Measuring
Guidelines for Dietary Recall Interview." https://www.cdc.gov/nchs/nhanes
/measuring_guides_dri/measuringguides.htm. Accessed March 14, 2019.

16. Burrows, T. L., R. J. Martin, and C. E. Collins. 2010. "A Systematic Review
of the Validity of Dietary Assessment Methods in Children When Compared with
the Method of Doubly Labeled Water." *Journal of the American Dietetic Association*
110 (10): 1501-1510. doi:10.1016/J.JADA.2010.07.008.

17. National Collaborative on Childhood Obesity Research. 2016. "Key Considerations in Measuring Dietary Behavior Among Children—NCCOR Measures
Registry User Guides." https://www.nccor.org/tools-mruserguides/individual-diet
/key-considerations-in-measuring-dietary-behavior-among-children/. Accessed
March 14, 2019.

18. Wallace, A., S. I. Kirkpatrick, G. Darlington, and J. Haines. 2018. "Accuracy of Parental Reporting of Preschoolers' Dietary Intake Using an Online Self-Administered 24-h Recall." *Nutrients* 10 (8): 987. doi:10.3390/nu10080987.

19. Aflague, T., C. Boushey, R. Guerrero, et al. 2015. "Feasibility and Use of the Mobile Food Record for Capturing Eating Occasions among Children Ages 3-10 Years in Guam." *Nutrients* 7 (6): 4403-15. doi:10.3390/nu7064403.

20. Livingstone, M. B. E., P. J. Robson, and J. M. W. Wallace. 2004. "Issues in Dietary Intake Assessment of Children and Adolescents." *British Journal of Nutrition* 92 (S2): S213. doi:10.1079/BJN20041169.

21. Pendergast, F. J., R. M. Leech, and S. A. McNaughton. 2017. "Novel Online or Mobile Methods to Assess Eating Patterns." *Current Nutrition Reports* 6 (3): 212-27. doi:10.1007/s13668-017-0211-0.

22. World Health Organization. 2007. *Indicators for Assessing Infant and Young Child Feeding Practices: Part 1 Definitions.* Washington, DC. https://www.who.int/maternal_child_adolescent/documents/9789241596664/en/. Accessed March 6, 2020.

23. FAO, USAID, FANTA. 2016. "Minimum Dietary Diversity for Women: A Guide to Measurement." www.fao.org/publications/en. Accessed March 14, 2019.

24. Boushey, C. J., M. Spoden, F. M. Zhu, E. J. Delp, and D. A. Kerr. 2017. "New Mobile Methods for Dietary Assessment: Review of Image-Assisted and Image-Based Dietary Assessment Methods." *Proceedings of the Nutrition Society* 76 (3): 283-94. doi:10.1017/S0029665116002913.

25. Ptomey, L. T., E. A. Willis, J. J. Honas, et al. 2015. "Validity of Energy Intake Estimated by Digital Photography Plus Recall in Overweight and Obese Young Adults." *Journal of the Academy of Nutrition and Dietetics* 115 (9): 1392-99. doi:10.1016/J.JAND.2015.05.006.

26. Gemming, L., A. Doherty, P. Kelly, J. Utter, and C. N. Mhurchu. 2013. "Feasibility of a SenseCam-Assisted 24-h Recall to Reduce Under-reporting of Energy Intake." *European Journal of Clinical Nutrition* 67 (10): 1095. doi:10.1038/ejcn.2013.156.

27. Gemming, L., E. Rush, R. Maddison, et al. 2015. "Wearable Cameras Can Reduce Dietary Under-Reporting: Doubly Labelled Water Validation of a Camera-Assisted 24 h Recall." *British Journal of Nutrition* 113 (2): 284-291. doi:10.1017/S0007114514003602.

28. Jia, W., H.-C. Chen, Y. Yue, et al. 2014. "Accuracy of Food Portion Size Estimation from Digital Pictures Acquired by a Chest-Worn Camera." *Public Health Nutrition* 17(08): 1671-81. doi:10.1017/S1368980013003236.

29. Pettitt, C., J. Liu, R. M. Kwasnicki, G.-Z. Yang, T. Preston, and G. Frost. 2016. "A Pilot Study to Determine Whether Using a Lightweight, Wearable Micro-Camera Improves Dietary Assessment Accuracy and Offers Information on Macronutrients and Eating Rate." *British Journal of Nutrition* 115 (1): 160–67. doi:10.1017/S0007114515004262.

30. Kaaks, R., P. Ferrari, A. Ciampi, M. Plummer, and E. Riboli. 2002. "Uses and Limitations of Statistical Accounting for Random Error Correlations, in the Validation of Dietary Questionnaire Assessments." *Public Health Nutrition* 5 (6a): 969-76. doi:10.1079/PHN2002380.

31. Schoeller, D. A. 1988. "Measurement of Energy Expenditure in Free-Living Humans by Using Doubly Labeled Water." *Journal of Nutrition* 118 (11): 1278-1289. doi:10.1093/jn/118.11.1278.

32. Bingham, S. A. 2003. "Urine Nitrogen as a Biomarker for the Validation of Dietary Protein Intake." *Journal of Nutrition* 133 (3): 921S-24S. doi:10.1093/jn/133.3.921S.

33. Hedrick, V. E., A. M. Dietrich, P. A. Estabrooks, J. Savla, E. Serrano, and B. M. Davy. 2012. "Dietary Biomarkers: Advances, Limitations and Future Directions." *Nutrition Journal* 11: 109. doi:10.1186/1475-2891-11-109.

4

Community Health Assessment

A. Gita Krishnaswamy and Sarah Ross-Viles

LEARNING OBJECTIVES

- Practice ethical conduct during community health assessments
- Plan an assessment of a place, population, or health issue for health education and promotion purposes
- Defend the investment in conducting community health assessments prior to program planning
- Engage communities respectfully and effectively in designing, implementing, and interpreting health assessments
- Identify existing sources of secondary information on behavioral, environmental, and social determinants of health
- Select and adapt methods to collect and manage primary quantitative and qualitative data
- Determine needs and assets for health education and promotion based on assessment findings
- Interpret data and assessment findings to inform the development and evaluation of health promotion and health education programs

Case Study: How Can a Community Kitchen Promote Health and Social Cohesion in a Diverse Neighborhood?

Note: Names and other identifying information have been removed to protect the privacy of individuals and organizations involved.

Recently, a nonprofit public health–related organization launched a successful community kitchen serving an unincorporated area in an urban county. In partnership with a local hospital system, the community kitchen offers a shared cooking space where community members can take cooking lessons together, meal plan, cook meals, and take shared meals home to their families. The community kitchen primarily serves a neighborhood that has been home to many newly arrived immigrants as well as more established, low- to middle-income families. The goals of such an initiative are multifold: (1) to provide a welcoming environment for community members, particularly those unfamiliar with American cookware or the language to learn how to cook nutritious, familiar, or novel meals for their families; (2) to enable community members to produce large-scale, shareable meals to reduce the financial burdens of meal preparation; (3) to contribute one strategy to nutrition-related disease burden; and (4) to provide a fun, purposeful way for neighbors to interact and build community cohesion. Leaders of the nonprofit have heard positive anecdotal feedback from community kitchen users and the executive director of the neighborhood community development association. As such, they have started exploring the possibility of launching another community kitchen in a second location in the county.

The nonprofit's stated mission includes an emphasis on social justice and equity, referring both to how the organization conducts its internal operations and how it engages with the communities it serves through various programs and projects. The first community kitchen was largely made possible and driven by the local hospital, which had grant funding available and a staff advocate who was enthusiastic about providing cooking lessons to the local community. While the anecdotal feedback suggests the project is a success, the current project leadership wants to conduct a community health assessment to determine how to make another community kitchen successful—or perhaps to determine whether a community kitchen is even the best way to address some of the nutrition-related health issues in the new neighborhood of interest.

Short on staff capacity and time, they recruited a project intern from a local university to complete the community health assessment over the course of nine months. The student spent the first few months making several visits to the neighborhood, familiarizing herself with the layout of the neighborhood; exploring various area resources such as restaurants, parks, schools, and banks; and introducing herself to a handful of community stakeholders who agreed to provide key informant interviews—leadership of the nonprofit organization who requested the assessment, leadership, and staff of the neighborhood community development association, a group leader of an ethnic affinity group, and a school leader. During this time, she also conducted a literature review to explore what was currently known about the links between nutrition and chronic disease, risk and protective factors for nutrition-related diseases, and successful policy interventions to improve environmental conditions that influence nutrition-related disease. She also conducted research to determine whether particular ethnic groups in the United States are disproportionately affected by nutrition-related disease burden and what useful contextual information existed about the history, development, and health status of the unincorporated area she intended to serve.

The bulk of the student's time was spent on recruiting and interviewing community members through focus groups. In total, she conducted five focus groups in the top five languages spoken in the area, using translation and interpretation services arranged by the local neighborhood development association. Staff there also assisted the student in recruiting at least six participants to each focus group, primarily by posting translated flyers in and around the association's offices and on their social media pages. The student obtained the contact information for all people who expressed interest in participating and confirmed attendance through personal phone calls, done by herself or a local volunteer interpreter. Her focus group questions focused on whether community members were aware of the community kitchen and its goals; what successes or challenges they have had in providing nutritious meals to their families or themselves; what local changes would facilitate their choice or access to nutritious meals; whether the community kitchen created neighborly relationships; and how the nonprofit organization could engage community members more effectively.

After analyzing focus group transcripts with specific qualitative data analysis methods and software, the student organized her findings in to an elegantly designed report that she shared with the entire nonprofit staff. She prioritized recommendations based on her research and her own instincts, and she highlighted key differences in responses between each focus group, leading to some important understandings about the way one group's cultural practices mediated their interest and interaction with the community kitchen. The findings yielded generally positive sentiments about opening a second community kitchen, along with very useful policy, institutional, interpersonal, and environmental recommendations for the community kitchen project staff to use in promoting healthy nutrition access and choice. The student and nonprofit staff agreed that their own expertise nor the research alone would have led them to the same incisive recommendations that community members themselves proposed.

As a concluding step in the assessment process, the student created and published a video recording summarizing her findings. She had subtitles made in the four non-English languages used by participants, and the videos were circulated across various neighborhood organization websites and social media. The student also ensured that her final written report is available online for any community member who wishes to read about her findings and recommendations. While the student has concluded her work, the community kitchen project staff intend to incorporate her recommendations into the planning phases of the second kitchen.

This chapter introduces the role of assessment in planning for community health improvement. You will explore the role of assessment in identifying health disparities and patterns of health inequities; learn about participatory methods for community health assessment; consider ethical and efficient ways of assessing how determinants of health influence a specific community; review various methods to find and collect quantitative and qualitative data; and consider strategies for interpreting and disseminating assessment findings to describe the health resources, risks, and outcomes in a community.

Why We Use the Phrase *Community Health Assessment*

You may have noticed that we use the phrase *community health assessment* in this chapter, rather than *community needs assessment*. The Community Tool Box[1] simply describes a **need** as "the gap between what is and what should be," and Wright defines it as an "existing capacity to benefit."[2] Problems arise from unmet needs and are typically identified in the early stages of the assessment process. **Assets**, meanwhile, are individuals, organizations, material resources, and existing policies that support and positively influence the health of communities. Identifying community assets acknowledges that communities have strengths that can be leveraged to tackle problems. While public health practitioners often have good intentions in wanting to identify unmet needs and solve problems, this can unintentionally lead to a deficiency-based approach in which an assessment team focuses exclusively on problems, challenges, and frustrations stemming from unmet needs. Because assessment should focus on *both* needs and assets that influence community health, we avoid terms that place an undue emphasis on needs alone.

As described in more detail later in this chapter, we define a ***community*** as a group of people with common characteristics or interests, not necessarily restricted by geographical location, in which membership occurs mutually through self identification and group consensus; we define ***community health assessment*** as a systematic process for summarizing the needs and assets in a community, undertaken specifically for the purpose of taking action to improve health.

The Basics of Community Health Assessment

We measure what we value, and value what we measure.

- Why do public health practitioners conduct community health assessments?
- How are community health assessments different from individual health assessments?
- How do public health practitioners use assessment findings?
- What are the consequences of avoiding assessment work?

Writing for *The Lancet* in 2011, editor in chief Richard Horton reflected on the current and future state of public health in England. "Public health is the science of social justice," he wrote, "overcoming the forces that undermine the future security of families, communities, and peoples."[3] He urged public health leaders in England to recommit to evidence-based policy and advocacy and shift away from a focus on "management, administration, structure, bureaucracy."[3] To overcome the forces that undermine the health of communities—in other words, to eliminate inequities that unjustly distribute health risk factors—public health practitioners require specific knowledge of the root causes of poor and good health, an understanding of a community's current health status, unmet community needs associated with poor health outcomes, and, importantly, community members' perceptions of what steps should be taken to improve the health of their community.

Enter the *community health assessment (CHA), a systematic process for summarizing the needs and assets in a community, undertaken specifically for the purpose of taking action to improve health.* The second half of this definition is essential; assessments that merely describe a community's needs and resources are likely to collect dust on a shelf (or the proverbial digital equivalent). When assessments provide clear, community- and data-driven recommendations to legislators, program designers, and other decision makers, they facilitate informed action steps to positively influence health outcomes. Public health programs and interventions are less likely to be successful or viewed as credible if they are developed and implemented without an evidence base derived from both scientific literature and a participatory health assessment process.

The concept of health assessment is neither complex nor unfamiliar to most of us. Individual health assessments, for example, are quite common. During a routine visit to the doctor's office, a medical assistant usually starts by taking your weight, height, heart rate, temperature, and blood pressure. Your physician may also administer the PHQ-9, a health questionnaire that screens for the presence and severity of depression. These assessments help identify an individual patient's health status and possible needs, whereas a community health assessment identifies, among other things, unmet health needs that can benefit from changes to policy, systems, and environment rather than individual-level interventions.[2,4] These differences reflect the differences in the public health and medical models of health, with the latter being more concerned with individual-level assessment and intervention and the former concerned with improving the health of populations through more "upstream" change.[2,5]

Still, federal legislation has long required not-for-profit hospitals to conduct community health needs assessments to maintain tax-exempt status. The law specifically requires that not-for-profit hospitals "explicitly and publicly demonstrate community benefit by conducting a community health needs assessment (CHNA) and adopting an implementation strategy to meet the identified community health needs."[6] And, as of 2012, the Patient Protection and Affordable Care Act requires these hospitals to conduct a CHNA at least once every three years and to report progress in improving community health status on an annual basis. Hospital systems and other health-related organizations may also complete community health assessments when required as a condition for grant funding.

While such regulatory drivers of community health assessment exist, they need not be a perfunctory step toward meeting donor requirements or demonstrating regulatory compliance. As Chang emphasizes, "[a] community assessment process is not just a matter of surveying what people need, but it is a community organizing strategy. By rigorously and creatively assessing community needs, the process gives real 'voice' to individuals in the community . . . voices that can significantly influence [program design and health interventions]."[7] In this view, the process itself of conducting a community health assessment can provide a basis for strengthening relationships in a community; raise broader awareness of a community's needs, assets, challenges, and successes; and increase the sense of ownership and investment that individuals feel in their communities. Public health leaders who conduct regular community health assessments not only stay up to date on the health status of the communities they serve but also deepen their understanding of the social and cultural contexts within which they operate.[8]

Despite compelling reasons to conduct regular community health assessment, many organizations have not institutionalized assessment as a crucial part of the health planning process. The Community Tool Box[8] (an excellent, publicly accessible resource on community health assessment) identifies some common reasons that organizations avoid needs assessment surveys—one component of the overall health assessment process—and offers some strategies to counter resistance (table 4.1).

As the saying goes: we measure what we value, and we value what we measure. Investing in a participatory community health assessment process is one way to demonstrate that as a public health practitioner, you want your efforts to address the genuine needs and concerns prioritized by the community itself.

Understand and Partner with the Community You Will Serve

Community health assessments are done with *a community, not* on *a community.*

- What is the *community* in community health assessment?
- How do you get a lay of the land when working with new or unfamiliar communities?
- Who should be a part of a community health assessment team?
- What considerations should you make to successfully facilitate an assessment team?

It's probable that at some point in your life, as a member of a particular group or community, you were informed of a change and thought to yourself, "who thought *that* would be a good idea?" That sentiment often arises when community members have not been asked to provide input on changes, but you also run the risk of provoking that reaction if you haven't clearly defined "the community." The concept of community seemingly has as many definitions as "need," and the word is often mistakenly used interchangeably with other terms like population, neighborhood, and society. While there is no single accepted definition of community, we suggest that a

Table 4.1. Common Myths and Realities about the Community Health Assessment Process

Assessment myth	Reality
"I already know what the needs are in this community."	It's possible that you may be familiar with some needs of a community, but without having done a current, systematic, inclusive assessment, it would be unwise to think that you are aware of all needs in a community.
"We're busy, we just need to get started with the work."	It's true that we are often operating under tight deadlines. If that's the case, why risk spending time on work that a community doesn't actually care about? Best to find out their concerns and priorities first.
"We don't have time to survey people."	The beauty of a survey is that it is a tool designed to rapidly collect information from many people at once. Sometimes the work of developing the survey is what takes the most time, but collecting the information is rapid.
"We aren't qualified to do an assessment."	Many guides exist to assist people with performing health assessments, including this chapter. And, oftentimes, organizations can consult with assessment professionals and academics who offer guidance and other resources.
"People are already surveyed to death, they'll resent being asked to do yet another survey."	Most people do not resent being asked to give their input, and in fact, more often, organizations implement new projects with people feeling like their input was never solicited.

Source: Adapted from Community Tool Box, "Conducting Needs Assessment Surveys." https://ctb.ku.edu/en/table-of-contents/assessment/assessing-community-needs-and -resources/.

community consists of a group of people with common characteristics or interests, not necessarily restricted by geographical location, in which membership occurs mutually through self-identification and group consensus. This definition accounts for ethnic diasporas spread worldwide, online communities, and other types of communities not bound by location. By including criteria for membership, this definition also distinguishes community from related terms like population or neighborhood, in which individuals have de facto membership. In the opening case study for this chapter, both the protagonist and community kitchen managers are likely to be using community and neighborhood interchangeably. In this case, while it's possible that the two are synonymous—residents of unincorporated neighborhoods typically share a shared sense of identity due to shared challenges— our student would be well-served by taking steps to define the community and identify community affiliation of all assessment participants. Peck also suggests that communities make decisions together, which necessitates an interest in or ability to participate in decision-making.

Even if you are conducting an assessment with a community you know well—or perhaps especially when—getting a lay of the land ensures that you, and eventually your assessment team, understand basic facts about the community. These may include population size, racial and ethnic composition, languages spoken, population density, transportation infrastructure, and other factors that help you understand who is in the community, where they live, and how they live.[8] You should also review important social, political, or economic changes that have influenced this community[9] and have an awareness of influential organizations, cultural groups, and economic sectors in the community. You can derive some of this information from secondary data sources such as the United States Census or American Community Survey, but don't overlook the importance of reading local news and actually visiting the area—not as a tourist but with specific purpose as a public health practitioner. Later in this chapter, you will learn about common primary data collection techniques used to collect assessment data, many of which can be used at this early stage to help you engage with a community, deepen your understanding of the community, and ultimately refine your assessment approach.

Developing this basic understanding of a community also strengthens your credibility as you recruit your assessment team. Since community health assessments begin and end with the community (see table 4.2), this requires collaboration with and leadership from community stakeholders throughout the process. Community health assessment is intrinsically a team-based process when equity and inclusion are a priority.

You are more likely to garner interest if you demonstrate that you have done your homework on the community. Your assessment team could include, but doesn't have to be limited to:

- those most affected by the health issue you are interested in,
- civic leaders,
- neighborhood representatives,
- faith or cultural group leaders,
- community health workers,
- teacher or school district representatives, and
- community advocates.

When building your assessment team, carefully consider how you will recruit team members in an inclusive and equitable way, whether the overall composition of the team is representative of different demographics and community sectors, and whether you will have diverse perspectives on the team. You will also need to gauge the level of commitment each member can make and anticipate your own role in facilitating others' engagement with the process.

Table 4.2. How to Conduct a Community Health Assessment

I. Understand and partner with the community you will serve

Review ethical principles and cultural considerations to guide assessment work

Engage the community your assessment will serve

Assemble an assessment team that includes key community stakeholders

Learn about current health status, assets, problems, challenges, and successes

II. Plan and organize the assessment

Identify the purpose and scope of the assessment

Develop the overarching assessment question

Develop an assessment timeline and agree upon assessment methods

III. Develop data collection instruments and collect assessment data

Identify, review, and analyze secondary data related to the assessment question

Develop evidence-based primary data collection tools

Develop a strategy for primary data collection, participant recruitment, and analysis

Conduct primary data collection

IV. Analyze and interpret assessment data

Analyze primary data

Review all assessment findings to summarize needs and assets and prioritize recommendations

V. Plan for the future and disseminate assessment findings

Create an actionable plan with recommendations to address needs

Disseminate assessment findings and recommendations in an accessible format for the community

Decide an appropriate timeframe and suggested scope for future health assessment to monitor changes and progress within the community

---

Notes: You will find these steps organized differently in various texts, with some authors consolidating or omitting steps, and others describing steps not presented here. In addition, you will find relevant information for each "how-to" step above distributed throughout this chapter, not just in a single section. When conducting a community health assessment, use your best judgment in designing an assessment plan that is systematic, intentional, feasible, and ethical.

Often, serving on an assessment team will be additional and voluntary work for community members, thus the assessment process will need to feel "worth it." They are more likely to feel that they are contributing to a successful effort and actionable results if you start with a plan, develop logical timelines, communicate with team members and community stakeholders consistently and transparently, use secondary and primary data incisively, present findings in an engaging and accessible way, and most importantly, work respectfully with community members in a way that honors their history, community context, and agency.

Plan and Organize the Assessment

- How can an assessment team identify a specific issue or issues to assess?
- Why is it important to start by articulating an overarching assessment question?
- How can you apply a health model to help you clarify the scope of your assessment?

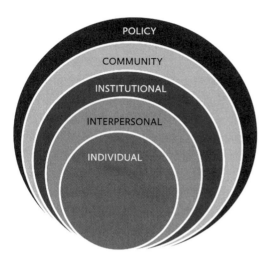

THE SOCIAL
ECOLOGICAL MODEL

The individual knowledge,
attitudes, and beliefs;
interpersonal relationships;
institutional environments;
community norms; and policies
that influence population health
outcomes over time

TIME

Figure 4.1. The social ecological model.

Before any data collection occurs, your assessment team must be clear on the purpose and scope of your assessment and agree on an overarching assessment question. Community health assessments vary widely in the breadth and depth of issues assessed—for example, a broad two-year assessment of Durham County's health status[10] is much broader and comprehensive in scope than the Health and Wellness Coalition of Wichita's assessment of food deserts in Wichita, Kansas.[11] In practice, community health assessments also vary by who actually determines which health issues or concern will be addressed—the public health practitioner or members of the community. This section assumes that specific health concerns have already been identified, due to the practitioner's professional interests, concerns originating from the community, or through participatory, collaborative methods in which community members and practitioners have worked together to identify concerns.

During the planning and organizing stages of assessment, applying a health model to your issues of interest can help clarify the purpose and scope of your assessment as well as identify potential health domains to assess. The social ecological model (figure 4.1), for example, is an explanatory model that illustrates how individual knowledge, attitudes, and beliefs; interpersonal relationships; institutional environments; community norms; and policies influence population health outcomes over time.

With your assessment team, you should discuss ways that factors of each of these levels positively and negatively influence your health issues of interest. Your background research on the community and a literature review would help inform this step. A root-cause analysis would also be a systematic way of identifying likely what factors, at multiple levels, are associated

---

Box 4.1. Why Is Jason in the Hospital? A Simple Root-Cause Analysis

---

"Why is Jason in the hospital?"
Because he has a bad infection in his leg.

But why does he have an infection?
Because he has a cut on his leg and it got infected.

But why does he have a cut on his leg?
Because he was playing in the junk yard next to his apartment building and there was some sharp, jagged steel there that he fell on.

But why was he playing in a junk yard?
Because his neighborhood is kind of run down. A lot of kids

play there and there is no one to supervise them.

But why does he live in that neighborhood?
Because his parents can't afford a nicer place to live.

But why can't his parents afford a nicer place to live?
Because his dad is unemployed and his mom is sick.

But why is his dad unemployed?

---

with your identified health concerns.[12] One simple technique for conducting a root-causes analysis is informally known as the "but why?" technique.[13] This "deceptively simple technique" starts by observing or identifying an individual health concern and then continually asking "but why?" until you have exhausted all possible explanations (box 4.1).[14]

While the focus of a community health assessment naturally considers needs, assets, and priorities at the community level, understanding downstream effects and upstream causes serves two purposes: (1) you can establish realistic parameters for the scope and limits of a community-level assessment and intervention; and (2) with a team that is fully aware of the full spectrum of factors associated with an observable health problem, you now have the opportunity to share that information with other stakeholders, community members, and decision makers who are prepared to act farther upstream or downstream.

At this point, you should feel prepared to articulate the *purpose* of your assessment, which explains the rationale for undertaking such an effort and assures that assessment outcomes will help direct resources toward addressing community needs. The *scope* of your assessment should clearly identify the community being assessed, descriptive inclusionary criteria, location, and the length of time under consideration. The purpose and scope should both be clear in your overarching assessment question, which is necessarily

Table 4.3. Poor and Better Assessment Questions

Poor assessment question	Better assessment questions
Why don't students at the University of Washington get enough sleep?	What modifiable academic and social factors influence sleep duration and quality of undergraduate students at the University of Washington during the regular academic year (September–June)?
What is causing an increase in graduate student debt in Washington State?	How have graduate student debt loads changed in the last 10 years for in-state resident students and nonresident students in Washington State?

broad yet specific enough to guide the subsequent development of data collection instruments and a data analysis plan. After all, you don't want to end up with information that, in the end, does not actually help answer your assessment question (table 4.3).

Develop Data Collection Instruments and Collect Assessment Data

To question or not to question . . . that is the question.

Secondary Data Collection and Analysis

- What role does secondary data collection and analysis serve during the assessment process?
- How do validity, reliability, and credibility influence your interpretation of secondary data?
- What are some inherent limitations of secondary data?
- How does a gap analysis of secondary data help inform primary data collection?

Community health assessments provide an excellent opportunity to gather and analyze information about specific communities, but before embarking on interviews or surveys, ask whether existing secondary data can shed at least partial light on your assessment question. Consider, after all, that one of the essential public health services is to monitor and surveil the distribution of risk factors and health outcomes in a population.[15] Early secondary data collection and analysis on your health issue of interest will allow you to be well-informed and efficient during primary data collection. Prior health assessments, heat maps, peer-reviewed research studies, vital statistics reports, and national and local health databases are all examples of traditional secondary data sources—that is, data that another entity has collected and/or analyzed, rather than data you yourself collected directly. Keep in mind that some secondary data are obtainable through data sharing agreements with organizations, even if not publicly available. In these cases, your assessment timeline must account for the time required to formulate and execute the terms of the data sharing agreement.

Secondary data collection and analysis typically provides a quick way of locating relevant information that uses fewer resources than primary data collection. After all, the time that community members spend as participating in primary data collection is a very valuable resource. Findings from secondary data analysis can clarify misconceptions about health issues or lead you to novel factors associated with your health issues of interest. This facilitates further refinement of your assessment question, if needed, and the design of primary data collection tools that focus on obtaining the information most needed from community members. Secondary data analysis also strengthens your credibility when presenting overall assessment findings, demonstrating that the assessment team has considered comparative national data, trends over time (within the same community if possible), and known indicators related to the assessment topic at hand. At times, if primary data collection is truly unfeasible, local or near-local secondary data sources become fundamental for determining priorities and next steps.

While it may seem odd to examine national-level data as part of a local community health assessment, these data are useful in understanding trends and providing comparative benchmarks for the local data you gather (see box 4.2 for sources of national secondary data). In addition, you may find localized data in the form of the following:[15]

- County Health Rankings
- Child Opportunity Index
- Metropolitan area quality of life indices
- State-level "report cards"
- State- and local-level community health indicators
- Community health profiles from local health departments
- School-based or school district-based "report cards"
- Law enforcement reports
- Hospital and health care system reports
- Other local-level health surveys

Yet, whether secondary data are your sole source of information or not, you should consider the validity and reliability of any data source. A simple way of thinking about validity is, "does your data measure what you intended to measure?" **Validity** is influenced by who is included or excluded during data collection (intentionally or not), the structure of questions used to obtain the data, the method of data collection, and biases in data collection design and analysis. **Reliability** means that findings are repeatable, and reliability is also influenced by the structure of questions and methods of data collection. Data must be reliable to be valid, but not all reliable data are also valid.

To further help you understand reliability and validity and how they influence our understanding of the health of populations, consider the examples of racial categories on the US Census and the failing of research studies

National Health and Nutrition Evaluation Survey
Behavior Risk Factor Surveillance System
Youth Risk Behavior Surveillance System
National Vital Statistics System
National Health Interview Survey
United States Census
American Community Survey
Cancer registries
Other national-level health survey

to appropriately include sexual and gender minorities. The US Census is a count of every resident in the United States, occurring every 10 years, the results of which help determine how federal funding will be directed to states and communities every year.[16] The US Census survey is constructed to *intentionally* produce invalid data based upon outdated, unscientific concepts of race.[17] The current Census uses racial categories (White, Black or African American, American Indian or Alaska Native, Asian, Native Hawaiian or Pacific Islander) that were delineated in the 18th century and used to justify actions like the Atlantic slave trade and "civilizing" American Indian children in boarding schools away from their families.[17] The rationale behind these five racial categories has been widely discredited as unscientific and racist, yet they persist in the Census and in public health research.

Ultimately, participants' responses to race-related questions and analyses by racial category will lead to results that cannot be properly interpreted. People of Middle Eastern ancestry, for example, are forced to select "White" on the Census as well as some health surveys.[18] Given that individuals of European and Middle Eastern ancestry experience social determinants of health quite differently in the United States, conclusions drawn from the "White" category may be skewed and also obscure important findings about those who identify as Middle Eastern. Along these lines, "Asian" encompasses an extremely diverse group of people who have some of the highest and lowest levels of income and educational attainment in the United States. The inability to disaggregate data on Asians by country or subregion prevents attention and resources from reaching Asian communities with the highest needs. Individuals who identify as biracial or multiracial are often overlooked or erased in data altogether if researchers re-assign these individuals to a single racial category based on what is presumed to be their "dominant" race.[19,20]

Similar problems exist when collecting data on sexual and gender minorities. When exclusive categories fail to account for the diversity of sexual orientations and gender identities, data collection methods may yield reliable (repeatable) yet inherently invalid results, as they do not sufficiently measure what is meant to measured.[21]

As you identify secondary data sources, develop a habit of asking yourself these questions:

- Who collected these data and for what purpose?
- From whom was data collected or not collected, and why?
- Who "owns" these data, and what stake did they have in the reported findings?
- What role did the public have in determining the data to be collected or interpretation and dissemination of results?
- What forms of bias could have influenced the collection, analysis, or interpretation of these data?

Even the most valid, reliable, and inclusionary sources of secondary data may have limitations in their usefulness for your assessment. First, depending on your specific assessment question, you may find closely related secondary data but not the specific measures you desire to answer your assessment question in an actionable way. Secondary data also may not be as recent as you'd like. With some geographical areas experiencing rapid demographic shifts, available data may not even be current after one year. If a community health assessment has been initiated to respond to recent or novel health concerns, prior assessment findings or health data may not be as representative of the community's current health status as you'd like.

A crucial step in secondary data analysis involves identifying remaining information gaps. Suppose that a county-level survey reveals that over 60% of adults do not meet the recommended daily physical activity guidelines. The survey report provides measures of the prevalence of known risk factors for decreased physical activity and also stratifies some results that indicate disparities in physical activity by ethnicity. This leads you to research other existing data that shed light on some measures of community safety, the number of public transportation stops in the area, and the number of public recreation areas, all of which lead you to some informed speculation on why so many adults in the county do not achieve the recommended daily physical activity guidelines (figure 4.2).

These data build your knowledge base but would not be sufficient to act on if trying to dedicate financial and human resources toward an intervention that increases physical activity levels. At this point, you would be missing answers to questions like:

- How important is physical activity to members of this community, and why?
- In addition to risk factors, what protective factors for health exist in this community, even if people are not meeting physical activity requirements?

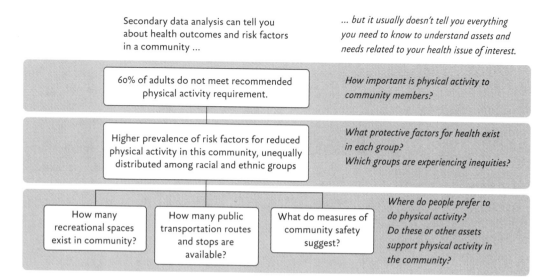

Figure 4.2. Secondary data gaps.

- Which risk factors do community members care most about, and are their others that haven't been identified?
- Although there are observable *disparities* in physical activity frequency, which subgroups are experiencing *inequities* leading to those disparities?

With secondary data analysis complete, including a gap analysis, you have a foundation to start the next step in community health assessment: planning for primary data collection.

Ethical Considerations for Primary Data Collection

- How can you conduct ethical, culturally competent, and equitable community health assessments?
- How can the practice of reflexivity enhance your assessment design and process?

Though community health assessments are typically not conducted with the same rigor as scientific research studies, the principles that guide ethical, culturally competent, equitable research apply just as well to assessment work. Before initiating any primary data collection efforts, which explore human experience and perception, know how you will protect the dignity, legal rights, and human rights of your participants.[22]

Articulating ethical primary data collection and analysis plans fosters trust within your assessment team and participants and ultimately contributes to public confidence in your methods and findings. If you have assembled a diverse, representative assessment team, they can provide a level of accountability and oversight for creating a primary data collection plan that avoids exploitative or disrespectful practices. Some additional resources at the end of this chapter provide excellent guidance on ethical principles for social research, forms of bias, public health critical race methodology, and the health educator's code of ethics. And, beyond what one can glean from a single textbook, public health practitioners should independently seek knowledge and training on new perspectives and methods to support socially just approaches to health equity.

One particularly challenging concern for public health practitioners is how to approach as an "outsider" to a community; or, the implications of "insiders"—a recognized member of the community being served—conducting work within their own communities. In a collection of short essays, Lewontin wrote that "science is a social institution about which there is a great deal of misunderstanding, even among those who are part of it. We think that science is an institution, a set of methods, a set of people, a great body of knowledge that we call scientific, is somehow apart from the forces that rule our everyday lives and that govern the structure of our society."[23] The concept of *reflexivity* helps public health practitioners and researchers to reconcile their relative position to those they aim to serve. **Reflexivity** is defined as "the process of a continual internal dialogue and critical self-evaluation of researcher's positionality as well as active acknowledgement and explicit recognition that this position may affect the research process and outcome."[24] Similar to Lewontin's sentiment, reflexivity supports the idea that researchers should not see their work as being independent from the economic, social, or political forces that shape society. Knowledge produced from efforts like primary data collection in community health assessment are undeniably influenced by the relative positioning of practitioner and participant. By habitually reflecting on the way factors like your age, gender, ethnicity, immigration status, and educational attainment influence the assessment process and participants' experience of that process, you will come to design more effective and ethical assessment questions, data collection methods, and plans for analysis and dissemination of findings.

Primary Data Collection and Analysis

- How does primary data differ from secondary data?
- What are some common ways of collecting primary data, and when are they best used?
- How do you develop evidence-based survey and focus groups questions?

Primary data—that is, original quantitative or qualitative data created directly by you—can be obtained using a number of different techniques, using a number of different channels. Consider the survey, which is probably the most common technique people think of for primary data collection. Surveys can be administered through face to face interviews, by phone or text message, or as online questionnaires, to name just a few channels. Each of these channels presents benefits and challenges that influence how you can interpret assessment findings, and each is vulnerable to forms of bias and threats to validity and reliability. Knowing the benefits and limits of the primary data collection techniques you select facilitate more accurate interpretation of the results and allow you to be transparent about limitations.

Five commonly used primary data collection techniques are:[25,26]

- Nominal group process (or nominal group technique)
- Direct and/or participant observation
- Key informant interviews
- Surveys
- Focus groups

Nominal Group Technique

The **nominal group technique (NGT)** is a "structured method for group brainstorming that encourages contributions from everyone."[27] The NGT is particularly useful at the start and end of a community health assessment process, as it is an effective way of gathering ideas, opinions, and suggestions from a large number of people. While the basic steps of the NGT remain the same, you can facilitate creatively to get feedback from a group as small as 10 people or an auditorium full of hundreds of community members. Because the NGT is not a full consensus-making process, individuals may contribute conflicting ideas and the group does not have to be derailed by differences in perspectives.

In the first part of the nominal group process, all participants individually brainstorm and contribute as many ideas as they have in response to specific prompts ("What things make you feel safe in your neighborhood?" or, "what things get in the way of you getting more physical activity?"). You might collect ideas written on index cards, submitted electronically, or have participants put sticky notes on a large piece of poster paper. All ideas are eventually displayed for all participants to see, and the facilitator can lead a discussion about those ideas, taking care not to allow for arguments or derogatory comments. Ideas can be modified if the original contributor agrees, but ideas can only be struck from the list through full consensus.

In the second part of the process, participants get a set number of votes which are used to prioritize issues for immediate attention. One of the simplest voting methods is to distribute a specific number of stickers to each participant, who can then place a sticker next to the issues they wish to prioritize. If done electronically, you can create a multiple choice question and restrict the maximum number of choices for participants. The ideas with the most number of votes are the ones that will be highlighted for immediate attention. When used at the beginning of an assessment process, it can help your assessment team understand the assets, needs, problems, and challenges the community perceives and cares about the most. At the end of the assessment process, it is a way of obtaining community input to prioritize action steps based on assessment findings.

Direct and Participant Observation

Direct and participant observation involve physically traveling to the area or community that your assessment will serve.[26] In direct observation, you develop or select a systematic way to observe specific activity or items within a community. You might conduct a "windshield survey," a systematic neighborhood observation conducted from a moving vehicle, or use a walkability audit tool while exploring a neighborhood; or, you might stay in a fixed location and count the specific number of times you witness a particular behavior. Direct observation does not involve interacting with community members intentionally or disclosing the purpose of your observation; you are a "fly on the wall." As with the nominal group technique, direct observation can be useful when trying to get a "lay of the land."

On the other hand, participant observation requires engaging directly with the activities, customs, and culture of the people you are observing. Participant observers identify their purpose for being there and may ask community members a variety of questions, just as you might when getting to know a new neighbor or friend. Participant observation can be an excellent way of establishing credibility and building trust with community members. However, it typically requires much more time than other primary data collection techniques, should be done as a reflexive practice, and yields qualitative results that are often difficult to generalize.

Key Informant Interviews

Key informants are typically people who, due to their professional training or life experience, have particularly in-depth knowledge about the health issue you are interested in. Key informant interviews can be the most prone to bias, as those selected as "key" may exclude community members who have valuable insight but are not identified as particularly influential or powerful. Key informants are also limited to a relatively small number of people, to make interviewing and analysis more manageable. Strategies exist, however, to create a pool of representative key informants.[25]

The results from key informant interviews are often useful in informing the development of subsequent primary data collection tools, such as surveys and focus groups. Key informant interviews can be done in person, by phone, or even by email, with each posing different benefits and challenges. For example, an emailed response allows the subject to respond freely within their own schedule but does not give you much opportunity to interact or clarify responses. On the other hand, a subject may feel more comfortable responding to difficult questions by phone if they don't have to interact with you face to face.

Surveys and Focus Groups

Surveys and focus groups are two of the most common techniques for gathering quantitative and qualitative information about community members' knowledge, attitude, beliefs, behaviors, and opinions related to your assessment question. Surveys are an effective way to rapidly gather quantitative data and concise qualitative data from a large number of individuals. Focus groups encourage community members to share nuanced insights about health needs and assets. Each technique could be the subject of their own textbook, and we have provided excellent resources on survey design and focus group facilitation at the end of this chapter.

Because you may have participated in surveys or focus groups yourself, you may be tempted to think that you have a good sense of how to design and administer a survey or focus group. However, novice survey and focus group administrators almost always underestimate the number and length of steps that must occur before they can even begin writing questions, let alone engage directly with participants. Surveys require rigorous planning and design that accounts for cost, sampling methods, literacy levels, linguistic considerations, administrator bias, recruitment strategies, field testing, and much more. Similarly, focus groups also require thoughtful planning that anticipates participant compensation, facilitator experience and confidence, recruitment strategies, group size and composition, equitable representation, translation and interpretation services, and facilities, amongst other elements.

With both methods, you will rarely work alone. Paper surveys typically require a trained team of individuals who have been trained to administer the survey and respond to challenges in identical ways. For instance, all survey administrators should be trained to allow any participant to abandon the survey without being pressured to continue or being asked why they prefer to end the survey. When differences occur in survey administration, the validity and reliability of your data can be compromised. Focus group administration requires a note taker, which allows a skilled facilitator to focus on the conversation and interaction between participants. With permission of the participants, focus groups should be recorded, and planning for recording, transcription, and analysis requires good foresight.

Constructing Good Questions

Most of the primary data collection methods above rely on the development of good questions—that is, questions that are easy for participants to understand and answer, without being subject to bias, and that yield valid and reliable data. Survey questions, in particular, should not require interpretation by the survey administrator. The questions included in your data

Table 4.4. Survey Constructs

Main constructs: What information do you want to gather about your assessment topic?	Evidence: What literature did you review that suggested this is a relevant construct?	Definitions: How would you specifically define the information you want to gather?	Measures: How can you measure each piece of information you want to gather?	Response type: Describe how the question will be formatted, or the format by which participants can respond	Potential problems: What issues might you anticipate with question delivery, reception, or analysis?	Analytical approach: How do you imagine using the responses about this construct? Will you summarize, compare, stratify, and correlate these data?
Do people eat enough fruits and vegetables?	*U.S. Dietary Guidelines for Adults, 2015–2020*	*Estimated average number of servings of fruits and vegetables per day*	*24-hour recall or screener for fruit and vegetable intake in previous 30 days*	*Multiple-choice options for frequency of intake*	*Difficulty understanding definition of "serving," difficulty recalling food consumption from previous month*	*Summarize for entire population and compare population subgroups*

Table 4.5. Focus Group Constructs

Main construct: What information do you want to gather about your assessment topic?	Evidence: What literature did you review that suggested this is a relevant construct?	Definitions: How would you specifically define the information you want to gather?	Prompts: What potential questions would you ask participants to respond to in order to gather the information you need about this construct?	Extensions: What potential follow-up or guiding questions would you ask participants to get more detail about a construct or encourage discussion among participants about this construct?	Potential problems: What issues might you anticipate with question delivery or reception?
Perceived access to healthy foods	Freedman, D. A., and B. A. Bell. 2009. "Access to Healthful Foods among an Urban Food Insecure Population." *Journal of Urban Health* 86 (6): 825–838. https://link .springer.com/article/10 .1007/s11524-009-9408-x.	Beliefs, practices, and confidence in obtaining fresh fruits and vegetables for self and family	Where do you get fresh fruits and vegetables? How easy is it to get fresh fruits and vegetables? How important is it to you to have fresh fruits and vegetables? How confident are you that you can get as many fresh fruits and vegetables as you'd like?	What is good about the places you get fresh fruits and vegetables from? Is there anything you don't like about these places? If you don't eat as many fruits and vegetables as you'd like, what prevents you from doing so?	Defining *fresh*; getting fresh foods for family could a be a sensitive topic for some participants; they may want suggestions or resources on healthy eating

Box 4.3. Bad Questions

You should avoid questions that are

- are oppressive, noninclusive, or offensive;
- have been previously identified as a low priority for the community;
- are leading or loaded;
- are too vague or open ended to provide useful information;
- collect information unrelated to your overall assessment question;
- collect demographic information that you will not actually use in your analysis;
- have unclear or imbalanced scales; or
- do not provide a "prefer not to answer" option or other way of knowing why a question wasn't answered.

Box 4.4. Unanswerable Questions

You should also steer clear of questions that cannot be answered, because they

- have response choices that overlap,
- ask two questions at the same time,
- do not have enough response options or an "other" option,
- require remembering an event too far in the past, and
- require a definition or result in different interpretations.

collection instruments shouldn't come from thin air; as with any intentionally designed tool, there should be an evidence base for the content and structure of your questions. Prior to writing survey or interview questions and developing data collection instruments, invest time in reviewing the literature on your health issue of interest, identifying already validated questions and measures, and using the literature to help structure and format your questions. Once you have designed a draft instrument, conducting a field test of survey questions, in which a small sample of participants take the survey and provide feedback about confusing or difficult words, concepts, or questions, is a good way to work out any lingering issues with your survey structure. In tables 4.4 and 4.5, we provide sample "construct tables" to use for questionnaire construction. Box 4.3 and box 4.4 give examples of bad questions and unanswerable questions.

Analyze and Interpret Assessment Data

- *How can your data analysis plan affect the design of your data collection instruments?*
- *What are commonly reported findings in assessment reports?*

While the exact statistical methods for data analysis are beyond the scope of this chapter, there are some basic considerations to make before even reaching the analysis and interpretation stages of your assessment work. Most importantly, you should understand the relationship between the data you want to collect, the structure and methods you will use to collect those data, and how you will analyze and present the data. Having an analytic plan in advance of designing survey instruments will help ensure that you collect data that is defined and operationalized the way you want. For example, if you want to report on the frequency with which people eat breakfast each week (number of breakfast meals consumed per week), you would not be well served by a survey question that only asks, "Do you eat breakfast every day?" Or, if you want to know what mode of transportation individuals use to get to the grocery store, you should consider how an open-ended, single-choice, or multiple-choice response will affect your methods for analyzing response options and displaying the findings. A word cloud, for example, requires a very different question structure than a pie chart.

Most often, you will use simple **descriptive statistics** to summarize your assessment data. These statistics include measures of central tendency (mean, median, mode), frequencies, trends over time, and relationships (correlation). You should know in advance whether you intend to make comparisons between measures from your community and similar state- or national-level measures, whether you want to stratify your own primary data and compare responses between different demographic groups, and whether any baseline measures exist against which you can compare your findings. In most cases, no specialized statistical software is necessary for analyzing assessment data. Should you find that you are interested in more sophisticated analyses than you can perform yourself, you may be able to secure low- or no-cost assistance from local universities or statistics associations.

Plan for the Future and Disseminate Assessment Findings
Determine Priorities, Share Information, Start Planning for the Next Assessment

Previously, this chapter emphasized the importance of developing a specific assessment question so that you do not collect data that you will not use. After collecting and interpreting the data, you will have a set of findings that answer the assessment question. Often, assessment reports will provide specific recommendations, to connect explicitly connect assessment data to its use in a project or program. As with the other steps of assessment, identifying and prioritizing findings involves the assessment team rather than an individual practitioner. It is extremely rare to do an assessment where community members have a single shared experience and share one, uniting view. Formal prioritization processes, like the nominal group technique described previously, and other formal decision-making tools can help your team select a final set of recommendations. The National Association of City and County Health Officials publishes a guide that lists different team prioritization processes and is a good reference for this step.[28]

The main goal in disseminating assessment findings is to provide important and actionable information to diverse audiences. In order to be useful, the findings need to be of value and make sense to that audience—another reason it matters to begin with an assessment question of value to the community you are serving. You will likely find that different modes of dissemination work for different audiences. The student in the case study at the start of this chapter used subtitled videos in multiple languages to share a summary of information collected from the community in addition to other key findings of the assessment. Other stakeholders, including your employer, may desire a technical written report with a clear index they can refer to when developing future related projects and programs.

Communities and community health issues change will never be completely captured in a one-time assessment, since the makeup of communities change over time, as do the distribution of health determinants. Your assessment work will have more value if you plan for the *next* assessment period as you wrap up your current assessment. Throughout the process and especially at the end, document lessons learned, stakeholders involved in the current assessment and others that could be involved in the future, unanticipated questions that came up during the process, and lingering questions that would be worth exploring in the next assessment. Given what you know about the community, how many years should you wait to update the assessment? Will it be necessary to collect entirely new data, or are some items unlikely to change? What baseline data from your current assessment requires follow up data collection? What new data would you recommend collecting? Along with answering these questions, save your data collection instruments and assessment plan.

Conclusion

In this chapter we introduced the role of assessment in planning for community health improvement. We explored the role of community health assessment in identifying health disparities and patterns of health inequities. We additionally considered ethical and efficient ways of assessing how determinants of health influence a specific community. Various methods that are commonly used to find and collect quantitative and qualitative data were explored, including participatory methods for community health assessment. The usefulness of the nominal group process, direct observation, key informant interviews, surveys, and focus groups were put into perspective. The characteristics of good versus bad survey and interview questions were identified. Relatedly, creating an analytic plan that matches the goals of the health assessment was considered; it is an important first step to have this plan in place so that data collected will be pertinent to the questions of interest. Finally, we considered strategies for interpreting and disseminating assessment findings to describe the health resources, risks, and outcomes in a community.

Review Questions

1. Review the opening case study on the community health assessment conducted prior to opening a new community kitchen. What *strengths* do you identify in the assessment methods used? If you had the opportunity to consult with the student or nonprofit organization that initiated the assessment, what *suggestions* would you give them for strengthening the assessment?

2. Reflect on the communities you are likely to work with as a public health practitioner or related position. If you are likely to be an outsider, what steps will you take to engage with other communities in a way that respects their knowledge, practices, and agency? If you are likely to be an insider, what steps will you take to ensure that your professional endeavors and community relationships are not compromised by personal knowledge or interactions?

3. This chapter states that assessment work begins and ends with the community. When leading assessment work, what specific strategies would you implement to ensure that you communicate about your progress consistently and transparently, in a way that is accessible to community members? What modifications would you make for community members who are not fluent in English, have lower literacy rates, are differently abled, or have other factors restricting their ability to receive or comprehend common forms of information dissemination?

4. What aspects of survey administration could compromise the validity and/or reliability of survey data, and what steps would you take during the survey design stage to minimize those issues in your survey formatting, question structure, or survey staff training?

5. Identify aspects of community health assessment work you anticipate being most challenging. If internal (lack of knowledge, skills, or confidence), identify some steps you would take to better situate you to lead assessment work. If external (capacity, logistics, interest), identify some specific strategies you would take to alleviate those factors.

Key Resources for Community Health Assessment

Community Tool Box: Assessing Community Needs and Resources[8] https://ctb.ku.edu /en/table-of-contents/assessment/assessing-community-needs-and-resources

Research Ethics https://warwick.ac.uk/fac/cross_fac/ias/activities/accolade /resources/ecu_research_ethics.pdf

Public health critical race methodology[29] https://www.sciencedirect.com/science /article/pii/S0277953610005800

Code of Ethics for the Health Education Profession[30] https://www.sophe.org/careers /ethics/

Survey design Designing and Conducting Survey Research: A Comprehensive Guide[31,32] https://coast.noaa.gov/data/digitalcoast/pdf/survey-design.pdf

Focus groups[33,34] https://ctb.ku.edu/en/table-of-contents/assessment/assessing -community-needs-and-resources/conduct-focus-groups/main https://coast.noaa.gov/data/digitalcoast/pdf/focus-groups.pdf

References

1. Heaven, Catie. 2018. "Developing a Plan for Assessment: Local Needs and Resources." Community Tool Box, Chapter 3, Section 1. Center for Community Health and Development, University of Kansas.

2. Wright, J., R. Williams, and J. R. Wilkinson. 1998. "Development and Importance of Health Needs Assessment." *BMJ* 316 (7140): 1310-13.

3. Horton, Richard. 2011. "Offline: Where Is Public Health Leadership in England?" *The Lancet* 378 (9796): 1060.

4. Centers for Disease Control and Prevention. 2013. "Community Needs Assessment: Participant Workbook." Atlanta, GA.

5. Glass, Thomas A., and Matthew J. McAtee. 2006. "Behavioral Science at the Crossroads in Public Health: Extending Horizons, Envisioning the Future." *Social Science and Medicine.* https://doi.org/10.1016/j.socscimed.2005.08.044.

6. "Community Benefit/ Community Health Needs Assessment." 2018. National Institutes of Health, U.S. National Library of Medicine.

7. Chang, H. N. L., et al. 1994. "Drawing Strength from Diversity: Effective Services for Children, Youth and Families." Los Angeles, CA: California Tomorrow.

8. Berkowitz, Bill, and Jenette Nagy. 2018. "Conducting Needs Assessment Surveys." Community Tool Box, Chapter 3, Section 7. Center for Community Health and Development, University of Kansas.

9. Goodman, Robert M., Marjorie A. Speers, Kenneth Mcleroy, Stephen Fawcett, Michelle Kegler, Edith Parker, Steven Rathgeb Smith, Terrie D. Sterling, and Nina Wallerstein. 1998. "Identifying and Defining the Dimensions of Community Capacity to Provide a Basis for Measurement." *Health Education & Behavior* 25 (3): 258-78. https://doi.org/10.1177/109019819802500303.

10. Durham County Department of Public Health. 2014. "2014 Durham County Community Health Assessment."

11. Health and Wellness Coalition of Wichita. 2013. "Wichita Food Deserts: Why We Should Care." Wichita, KS.

12. Berkowitz, Bill. 2018. "Analyzing Community Problems." Community Tool Box, Chapter 3, Section 5. Center for Community Health and Development, University of Kansas.

13. Lopez, Christine. 2018. "Analyzing Root Causes of Problems: The 'But Why?' Technique." Community Tool Box, Chapter 17, Section 4. Center for Community Health and Development, University of Kansas.

14. "What Makes Canadians Healthy or Unhealthy?" 2013. Government of Canada.

15. "Ten Essential Public Health Services." 2018. Community Tool Box, Chapter 2, Section 7. Center for Community Health and Development, University of Kansas.

16. US Census Bureau. 2019. "2020 Census: About the Census." Washington, DC.

17. Prewitt, Kenneth. 2013. "Fix the Census' Archaic Racial Categories." *New York Times*, August 2013.

18. US Census Bureau. 2017. "Race & Ethnicity." Washington, DC.

19. Pew Research Center. 2015. "Multiracial in America: Proud, Diverse and Growing in Numbers." Washington, D.C.: June, pp. 19–31.

20. Liebler, Carolyn A, and Andrew Halpern-Manners. 2008. "A Practical Approach to Using Multiple-Race Response Data: A Bridging Method for Public-Use Microdata." *Demography* 45 (1): 143–55.

21. Sell, Randall L. 2017. "Challenges and Solutions to Collecting Sexual Orientation and Gender Identity Data." *American Journal of Public Health* 107 (8): 1212–14.

22. ECU. 2017. Ethics in Primary Research (Focus Groups, Interviews and Surveys). Equality Challenge Unit, London. https://www.advance-he.ac.uk /knowledge-hub/ethics-primary-research-focus-groups-interviews-and-surveys.

23. Lewontin, Richard C. 1991. *Biology as Ideology: The Doctrine of DNA.* New York: HarperCollins.

24. Berger, Roni. 2015. "Now I See It, Now I Don't: Researcher's Position and Reflexivity in Qualitative Research." *Qualitative Research* 15 (2): 219–34. https://doi .org/10.1177/1468794112468475.

25. Carter, Keith A., and Lionel J. Beaulieu. 1992. "Conducting A Community Needs Assessment: Primary Data Collection Techniques." Gainesville: University of Florida, IFAS Extension.

26. Rabinowitz, Phil. 2018. "Qualitative Methods to Assess Community Issues." Community Tool Box, Chapter 3, Section 15. Center for Community Health and Development, University of Kansas.

27. "Nominal Group Technique (NGT)." 2018. American Society for Quality.

28. The National Connection for Local Public Health. n.d. "Guide to Prioritization Techniques." NACCHO: National Association of County & City Public Health.

29. Ford, Chandra L., and Collins O. Airhihenbuwa. 2010. "The Public Health Critical Race Methodology: Praxis for Antiracism Research." *Social Science & Medicine* 71 (8): 1390–98. https://doi.org/10.1016/j.socscimed.2010.07.030.

30. "Code of Ethics for the Health Education Profession." n.d. SOPHE: Society for Public Health Education.

31. Louis, Rea M., and Richard A. Parker. 2005. *Designing and Conducting Survey Research: A Comprehensive Guide.* 3rd ed. San Francisco, CA: Jossey-Bass.

32. Office for Coastal Management. 2015. "Social Science Tools for Coastal Programs: Introduction to Survey Design and Delivery." Silver Spring, MD: NOAA.

33. Berkowitz, Bill. 2018. "Conducting Focus Groups." Community Tool Box, Chapter 3, Section 6. Center for Community Health and Development, University of Kansas.

34. Office for Coastal Management. 2015. "Social Science Tools for Coastal Programs: Introduction to Conduction Focus Groups." Silver Spring, MD: NOAA.

5

Program Planning

Noel Kulik, Rachael D. Dombrowski, and Jeanne M. Barcelona

LEARNING OBJECTIVES

- Differentiate between **program planning** steps in the generalized model
- Create measurable goals and objectives for public health nutrition interventions
- Strategically plan public health nutrition interventions
- Develop logic models for public health nutrition interventions
- Understand and apply theories used in public health nutrition interventions

Case Study: Healthy Chicago Public Schools—Increase Access to Water

Research shows that consuming water in place of sugar-sweetened beverages and juice can help combat obesity, since substituting water for other beverages can result in lower caloric intake.[1,2] Encouraging and making water readily available in Chicago Public Schools (CPS) was a key strategy identified to improve healthy consumption of water and decrease other alternate beverages youth may consume throughout the school day.[3]

Water Consumption Pilot Intervention

The intervention took place within 10 elementary schools throughout the district and aimed to impact 4,000 students from kindergarten to eighth grade. The intervention was modeled after a similar approach within the New York Public School District. Schools were selected for inclusion in the intervention based on current student body mass index (BMI) levels and demographics as well as geographic location within the City of Chicago. Schools that were included in the intervention comprised a significant number of youth populations who were disproportionately affected by health disparities.

Development of the intervention included creating a logic model, which is presented later in this chapter. Additionally, this intervention was grounded in the social cognitive theory (SCT), also explained later in this chapter. Within this case it is important to note SCT was utilized to consider the dynamic interaction between student water consumption and the school environment. Specifically, the SCT illustrated the need to consider how students' personal factors including their attitude toward water consumption and knowledge of its importance as well as their behavioral capacities, such as skills and awareness to respond to thirst cues, could be fostered through the schools' environmental investment in resources to provide access to potable water and ultimately create a normative acceptance of water consumption. All schools throughout the district were provided with water dispensers during breakfast and lunch to comply with the Chicago Public Schools wellness policies[4,5] as well as US Department of Agriculture regulations for the National School Lunch Program.[6] Ten elementary schools were selected and then provided with more intensive nutrition education regarding water consumption, including its effects on the reduction of obesity and its impact on student health. Reusable water bottles were also provided for all youth (n = 4,000) to utilize within their classrooms. Some schools also established partnerships with community organizations (e.g., Purple Asparagus) to assist in the filling, cleaning, and maintenance of the water bottles. Schools were onboarded at the beginning of the school year (September–October) and were provided with nutrition education and the water bottles at the beginning of the third quarter (January–February). Assessments of the youth to determine impact of the project on water intake were completed at baseline (October) and at the end of the school year (May–June).

The evaluation of the project found no effect on water intake of the youth populations within the schools, although youth knowledge of the health effects of water did significantly improve. The lack of impact of the intervention may have been due to a number of factors, including the inability of three schools to fully complete the intervention, the burden the water bottles posed on teachers and staff when provided in classroom settings, and the lack of partnerships to assist schools in completing the intervention (as community organizations assisted only three schools). Given that a number of the schools selected had significant populations disproportionately affected by health disparities and poor academic outcomes, it was also difficult for schools to shift their prioritization to the water access project when improving curriculum and instruction was their more primary and urgent concern.

The results from this case study may further suggest that school-based interventions must consider multiple factors at the individual, interpersonal, and environmental level, especially during the planning process of school-based programs. Future interventions may want to consider the provision of social support within the school setting as well as embedding intervention activities into the curricular priorities. Additionally, the needs assessment process conducted with schools should assess their readiness and capacity for implementing complex interventions that include a focus on healthy eating behaviors, such as increasing water consumption among younger-aged populations. Although this intervention was not successful in changing water intake among youth, it did enable schools to improve their delivery of health and nutrition education and strengthen the overall Healthy CPS initiative, which still exists today.

Importance of Program Planning

Use of a planning process, or approach, is important to ensure effective nutrition intervention programming for priority populations. In a nutshell, planning is a rational and participatory approach to developing a set of activities that are designed and selected to address a particular health problem and implemented to reach a specific set of health goals. Good health promotion programs focused on nutrition are not created by chance but are the result of careful foresight and planning.

There are four key reasons why planning should be done intentionally and systematically before implementation, according to Hunnicutt in *The Power of Planning*.[7] First, planning allows you to think through the details of a program or intervention in advance. While this can seem like a daunting task, forgoing the planning process and moving straight into implementation might waste valuable resources, time, energy, and personnel if your program is not successful. The key is to plan in small doses—an entire intervention does not come together in a matter of hours, or even days. Often, key **stakeholders** (e.g., members of the priority population, administrators, funders, partners) or an advisory board can provide multiple perspectives and assistance in thinking through how the program can be successful. This type of input is usually solicited during the needs and assets assessment (see chapter 4) but can be helpful throughout the entire planning process. Second, planning makes a program transparent so that everyone understands how the program works and how success will be measured. This is helpful because stakeholders who have a vested interest in the program will be informed, and if something does happen to go wrong, the scapegoat for failure will not entirely fall on the planners themselves but on the myriad of other factors that go into effective programming. A plan is like a contract, so transparency ensures that all parties understand what needs to be done and who is going to do it. Third, planning is empowering. Once a plan is developed, stakeholders are on board, and the green light is given, the momentum to implement is powerful. Getting bogged down in a piecemeal plan that requires approval for each component as it is developed can affect employee (and participant) morale. Fourth, planning creates alignment. When the plan is approved from the "powers that be" (e.g., administrators, governing board, president, chief executive officer), organizational alignment is created and sends a message that people at all levels are committed to the program and understand how it fits within the organization's mission.

The preplanning process, while not explicit in many program planning approaches, can include such things as defining the community and the outcomes, determining what level or levels (individual, organizational, policy) the program will address, how partners will be selected and involved, how resources will be secured, and what deliverables will result. Often during the preplanning process, it is helpful to think about resistance to the program and how such challenges might be addressed or circumvented.

The Planning Process

Health promotion professionals use several models, which are visual representations and descriptions of the steps in the planning process. There are several factors to consider when selecting a planning model, such as how much time and resources are available; the preferences of stakeholders, funders, or the community; and how involved partners and the priority population will be. For the purposes of this book, we will use the generalized model[8] to describe the process, as it encompasses what is within most planning models in five steps:

1. Assessing needs
2. Setting goals and objectives
3. Developing an intervention
4. Implementing the intervention
5. Evaluating the results

Assessing needs is covered in chapter 4 of this book; however, it is important to point out that needs may change throughout the planning process, making it a cyclical rather than linear process that may warrant revisions to the program. For example, advances in knowledge, a change in policy, or new community-level data may become available that require program expansion or revision, depending on the needs of the community. Planners often loop back to earlier "steps" in the process to ensure that their program is on track.

Setting goals and **objectives** occurs after examining data, assessing needs, and understanding the scope of the problem. Goals and objectives serve as a solid foundation that guides the work of planners, and they highlight what is expected to be achieved during the program. Goals are often more global, broad, and general statements about what will be affected and what will change as a result of the program compared to objectives, which represent smaller steps on the way to achieving each goal. An example of a program goal might be "to prevent and reduce obesity among elementary school youth enrolled in the Building Healthy Communities program." Objectives are written on different levels and represent the building blocks leading toward the overall goal. One level of objectives, also called **outputs** in the **logic model**, can be focused on the use of intervention resources, attendance, participant satisfaction, or fidelity of the program (process). Another level of objectives, also called **outcomes** in the logic model include changes in knowledge, intention, motivation, attitude or behavior (impact), or health status, quality of life, or disease risk (outcome). Impact objectives can be comprised of changes in learning, behavior, or the environment and should be able to be realized during the course of the intervention. Impact and outcome objectives often fit into the logic model as short-, intermediate- and long-term outcomes. This is discussed further in the logic model section of this chapter.

Both program objectives and logic model outcomes use the **SMART format: S**pecific, **M**easurable, **A**ttainable, **R**ealistic, and **T**imed.[9] This means that the change desired should be explicitly stated and able to be measured using a questionnaire, observation, self-assessment tool, or other evaluation method. The expected changes from a health promotion program should also be attainable and realistic such that participants should be expected to change to a certain degree. Assuming that 100% of the priority population will change in the expected direction of your intervention is not realistic given that these programs exist in the real world, with complex and competing influences, and are often intended to reach a diverse audience. And finally, objectives should include a time period for the change to occur. In other words, objectives (and outcomes) should be explicit in what exactly will change, when it will change, the criterion for deciding whether the change is sufficient, and who will change. Table 5.1 shows the types of objectives, an example SMART output or objective for each type, and the associated outcomes.

After a thorough needs and assets assessment and the process of developing goals and objectives are completed, planners can begin to develop the intervention and convert goals and objectives into intended actions and **implementation** procedures. The key decision at this point is whether or not to use an existing, evidence-based program and tailor it to the needs of your priority population or create your own program altogether. When looking for an evidence-based, existing program (which are often called "interventions"), one can search for scholarly articles by priority population or type of intervention that provide a thorough review of the evidence to support the adoption of a specific intervention or program. There are also several global to local resources available online:

1. World Health Organization e-Library of Evidence for Nutrition Actions (eLENA)[10] (http://www.who.int/elena/en/; accessed May 28, 2018). This site is an online library of evidence-informed guidelines for an expanding list of nutrition interventions.
2. Healthy People 2020[11] (https://www.healthypeople.gov/2020/topics -objectives/topic/nutrition-and-weight-status/ebrs#ebr_header; accessed May 28, 2018). This site contains evidence-based nutrition education resources and rates each intervention on the strength of the evidence available.
3. Missouri Department of Health and Senior Services[12] (https://health.mo .gov/data/interventionmica/Nutrition/index_5.html; accessed May 28, 2018). This site provides an evidence-based nutrition education matrix sorted by strategy: provide education, group education,

Table 5.1. SMART Objectives

Type of objective	Example SMART outputs and objectives	Outcomes measured
Process (Output)	By the end of the 2018–2019 school year, the Building Healthy Communities Program will hold eight sessions in 20 schools, serving 8,500 youth.	Number of sessions held, student attendance
Impact (Short-Term and Intermediate)		
Learning	By the end of the 2018–2019 school year, 90% of youth in the Building Healthy Communities Program will have increased their knowledge of fruits and vegetables by 2 points on a 10-point scale.	Knowledge
Behavioral	By the end of the 2018–2019 school year, 75% of youth in the Building Healthy Communities Program will have increased their daily fruit and vegetable consumption by 1.5 servings.	Fruit and vegetable consumption
Environmental	By the end of the 2018–2019 school year, 95% of schools in the Building Healthy Communities Program will have implemented all components of the smarter lunchroom programming.	Number of environmental components implemented
Outcome (Long-Term)	By the end of the 2018–2019 school year, 50% of youth in the Building Healthy Communities Program will have maintained a healthy weight or reduced their body mass index (BMI) if overweight or obese.	Height and weight

Note: SMART = Specific; Measurable; Achievable; Realistic, Time-Bound.

individual education, campaigns and promotions, environments and policies, and more.

In creating your own intervention or program, the use of evidence-based strategies and approaches tailored to the priority population is key. Furthermore, successful intervention development hinges on a thorough understanding of the intervention literature, the population of interest, as well as an ability to establish key points of intervention within your proposed setting. As such, intervention development begins with identification of a health problem and the risk factors within the population of interest. Next, it becomes important to understand the parameters of the health problem within the contextual environment—meaning an in-depth consideration for the contributory factors across the structural and social environment where the intervention will take place. This is especially important when conducting community-level interventions as they are often occurring within complex systems of social norms, values, and cultural influence already present within local settings.[13] This was evident in the case study presented above within Chicago Public Schools, as a thorough understanding of the capacity and priorities of participating schools within the water consumption intervention was not completed prior to implementation. This likely had an effect on project outcomes (i.e., youth water consumption) as well as willingness of the schools to implement a complex intervention that was not grounded in curriculum or instructional standards. Guided by this foundational knowledge, an intervention can then begin to be developed. It is important to note that successful interventions are comprehensive and therefore may be comprised of multiple components. Therefore, you may discover that an evidenced-based program can be used for one of your intervention components while also finding out that you must develop other components. For example, a comprehensive school-based health intervention may use evidence-based physical and nutrition education programming, but one may discover that there is a lack of access to professional development for teachers or that established, culturally relevant family-based nutrition programs do not meet the needs of the target population. When existing programming cannot support a specific component of your intervention, it becomes necessary to develop your own, guided by the program planning process. Once all the components have been established and the intervention is fully developed, it is time for the interventionist to consider an implementation plan.

The next phase in the generalized model is implementation. This refers to putting an intervention into action, and the key to successful implementation is thorough planning, organization, and marketing. As an interventionist transitions from development to implementation, it is important to establish a detailed and concrete "plan of action." First, the interventionist must coordinate with individuals and organizations who will spearhead implementation. Often this will consist of formulating teams of people, either through direct hires or subcontracts with experts, who have the skills and motivation to move forward a specific intervention component. For example, a school district may wish to hire a registered dietitian to lead an intervention that aims to improve the delivery of nutrition education throughout the district. Additionally, they may wish to partner with local agencies to increase the use and monitoring of school gardens throughout a school district. After staffing and partner needs have been solidified, the interventionist should then use their logic model and program timelines to develop action plans across each intervention component. These can come in many forms, but most follow a quarterly cycle and state the specific action steps needed to complete the intervention, partners and staff responsible for implementation, and start and end dates of each action step. This "action planning" of the intervention is extremely important in ensuring the program is successful and all staff and partners understand what is expected of them. Finally, the interventionist will want to either develop an implementation management plan or include these more administrative steps within their overall action plans to track implementation progress as well as inform implementation modifications that may arise throughout the intervention period.

The final step in the generalized model is evaluating the results. While evaluation will be discussed in chapter 6, it is important to note that evaluation measures and methodology should be decided upon during the early phases of the project, and specifically during the development of goals, objectives, and the project logic model, which is discussed in more detail in the following section.

Logic Models

Logic models are used in program planning and design to illustrate or create a "picture" of your entire project. Logic models are often presented sequentially to show how program activities can create change within communities or among individuals.[9] Most logic models use four primary categories: inputs, activities, outputs, and outcomes (short term, intermediate, and long term).[14] Although some models will expand on the four primary categories, for example by including more descriptive categories to discuss program participants within the activities category, the basic design follows these four primary categories (figure 5.1).

Inputs are resources or assets you have within your organization or agency to complete your program. These include financial resources, staff, volunteers, and partners. It is more visually appealing to present the inputs in separate categories to easily identify the materials, resources, and human capital available for your program.

All major activities within your program should be listed within the activities category in a logic model. Activities should be written so that they are specific and measurable. This will make it easier for development of the outputs—which are a direct result of your program activities. For example, a program activity might be, "Provide training to 100 teachers on nutrition education curriculum." An **output** or a direct result of this activity would then be, "100 teachers trained on nutrition education curriculum." Sometimes program planners will add a timeline to their activities. This timeline should also be reflected in the outputs. Using our same example from before, one

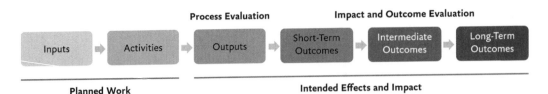

Figure 5.1. Basic logic model structure with examples.

activity might read, "Provide training to 100 teachers on nutrition education curriculum by month three." In addition, the output would also be revised to state, "Provided training to 100 teachers on nutrition education curriculum by month three."

As shown in figure 5.1, the inputs and activities are the planned components or resources available to deliver your program. The outputs and outcomes are the result or impact your program will have on your target population. It is usually best to create logic models in conjunction with the development of program evaluation plans.[14] Logic models can assist program planning staff and evaluators in identifying the key process evaluation measures needed for the program (listed in the outputs) as well as the impact or outcome evaluation measures (listed in the outcomes). Process evaluation is used to assess the degree to which the program was implemented as designed as well as to gather information about the quality of and satisfaction with the program among participants and program staff. Impact evaluation is completed to assess changes in participant determinants of health behavior change, such as increased knowledge and skills around healthy cooking and food purchasing or motivations to improve health behaviors (e.g., confidence in eating five fruits and vegetables per day). Outcome evaluation is completed to assess health impact changes within the program participants, including behavior change and changes in health status. For example, these could include increasing daily intake of fruits and vegetables or reductions in chronic disease incidence, such as diabetes.

Similar to program goals and objectives, when describing outcomes within logic models, program planners use the SMART format as discussed above: **S**pecific, **M**easurable, **A**ttainable, **R**ealistic, and **T**imed.[9] Again, outcomes should answer *how many* participants are *changing* (increasing or decreasing) health outcomes by a *certain rate* and by a given *date or time*. Outcomes are usually presented within three separate categories within logic models, including short term, intermediate, and long term. With respect to logic model development, short-term outcomes include changes in populations that can be realized within zero to three months post-program implementation. These include changes in knowledge, attitudes, beliefs, and skills. Intermediate outcomes include changes in populations that can be achieved within six months to one or two years post-program implementation. These outcomes usually include behavior changes, such as changes in fruit and vegetable consumption, and some skills, such as cooking meals from home more than three times per week. Long-term outcomes are changes achieved in populations five or more years post-program implementation. These include changes in rates of morbidity, mortality, and quality of life, such as a reduction in the incidence of obesity, diabetes, or other chronic disease as a result of program implementation.

Using Logic Models in Nutrition Programs

Logic models are used often in planning nutrition programs to create a roadmap of the intervention as well as to help assess the measures needed for program evaluation. For example, figure 5.2 illustrates a logic model of nutrition interventions located within food retail settings.[15] As this model was included within a review article of several food retail interventions, the inputs were not included within their illustration. The activities, outputs, and outcomes are listed, however, and help describe the expected changes to be realized within each target population. These include intermediate behavior change outcomes, such as increased purchasing and consumption of healthy foods, and long-term outcomes of improvements in health status.

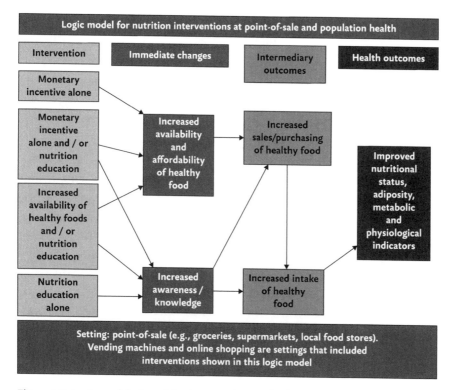

Figure 5.2. Logic model of nutrition interventions in food retail settings. *Source:* Adapted from Liberato, S., R. Bailie, and J. Brimblecombe. 2014. "Nutrition Interventions at Point-of-Sale to Encourage Healthier Food Purchasing: A Systematic Review." *BMC Public Health* 14:919. doi:10.1186/1471-2458-14-919.

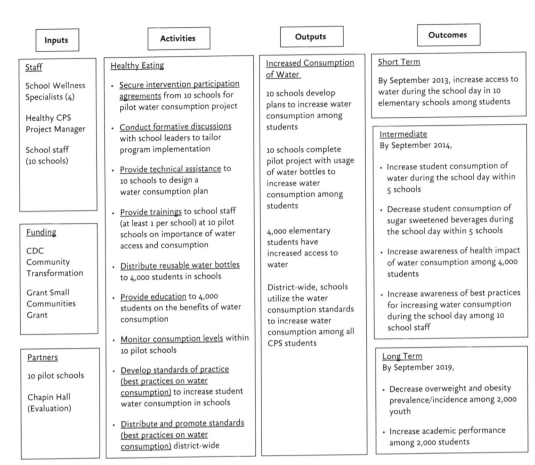

Inputs	Activities	Outputs	Outcomes
<u>Staff</u> School Wellness Specialists (4) Healthy CPS Project Manager School staff (10 schools) <u>Funding</u> CDC Community Transformation Grant Small Communities Grant <u>Partners</u> 10 pilot schools Chapin Hall (Evaluation)	<u>Healthy Eating</u> • <u>Secure intervention participation agreements</u> from 10 schools for pilot water consumption project • <u>Conduct formative discussions</u> with school leaders to tailor program implementation • <u>Provide technical assistance</u> to 10 schools to design a water consumption plan • <u>Provide trainings</u> to school staff (at least 1 per school) at 10 pilot schools on importance of water access and consumption • <u>Distribute reusable water bottles</u> to 4,000 students in schools • <u>Provide education</u> to 4,000 students on the benefits of water consumption • <u>Monitor consumption levels</u> within 10 pilot schools • <u>Develop standards of practice (best practices on water consumption)</u> to increase student water consumption in schools • <u>Distribute and promote standards (best practices on water consumption)</u> district-wide	<u>Increased Consumption of Water</u> 10 schools develop plans to increase water consumption among students 10 schools complete pilot project with usage of water bottles to increase water consumption among students 4,000 elementary students have increased access to water District-wide, schools utilize the water consumption standards to increase water consumption among all CPS students	<u>Short Term</u> By September 2013, increase access to water during the school day in 10 elementary schools among students <u>Intermediate</u> By September 2014, • Increase student consumption of water during the school day within 5 schools • Decrease student consumption of sugar sweetened beverages during the school day within 5 schools • Increase awareness of health impact of water consumption among 4,000 students • Increase awareness of best practices for increasing water consumption during the school day among 10 school staff <u>Long Term</u> By September 2019, • Decrease overweight and obesity prevalence/incidence among 2,000 youth • Increase academic performance among 2,000 students

Figure 5.3. Logic model of the Healthy Chicago Public Schools water pilot project. *Source:* Adapted from Chicago Public Schools, Office of Student Health and Wellness. 2013. Water Access Pilot Project. Program records.

Other nutrition programs, such as those within school-based settings, have used logic models for specific components of a complex intervention, such as the Healthy Chicago Public Schools (Healthy CPS) water consumption intervention described at the beginning of this chapter. This work, in addition to several other interventions—which together were called "Healthy CPS"—was funded by the Centers for Disease Control and Prevention (CDC)[16] (Grant Number: 1H75DP004181-01) from 2012-2014 and helped to launch the Healthy CPS initiative for the district, which still exists today.[17] As a component of the initial Healthy CPS work, a pilot program in 10 schools was initiated to increase water intake among elementary-aged youth. The logic model for this program is listed in figure 5.3. As the logic model illustrates, an increase in water intake and a decrease in sugary drink consumption was expected among half of the student participants as a result of this intervention. Unfortunately, these objectives were not realized due to the complex nature of delivering a "water bottle" intervention within schools during the school day. These complexities and overall outcomes are discussed further within the case study at the beginning of this chapter.

Using Theory in Nutrition Program Planning

Broadly, **theory** is defined as the evidenced guidelines or principles used to develop an understanding of an unknown set of circumstances.[18] In the public health domain, theory is utilized to guide the understanding of health-related behaviors both on an individual as well as a community and population level. Through the utilization of theory, program planners and other health researchers employ a systematic method of understanding health and the factors driving health outcomes. This is especially relevant to the planning, development, and implementation of nutrition interventions because nutrition-related behaviors are influenced by personal, social, and environmental factors. When theory is applied thoughtfully and appropriately, it has the capacity to guide nutrition intervention work. As such, the goal of this section is to orient the reader to the broad and overarching goals and components of theory, provide an overview of the types of theoretical frameworks available, illustrate the value of different theoretical approaches, and provide examples of informative and successful uses of theory in nutrition intervention work.

What Is Theory?

Theory can get a bad reputation as it is often depicted as abstract and hard to grasp, but when it is broken down it becomes more relatable and easier to understand. Broadly, theory can be likened to a lighthouse, guiding people to an ideal endpoint. However, to get to a desired endpoint or outcome, one must break down the theoretical process into the components of concepts, constructs, and variables. **Concepts** are the overarching vision or big idea that the theory postulates. **Constructs** are the road map or the guiding force directing the overarching concept, whereas **variables** are the checks and balance or the quantifiable factors that reveal the significance of each part of the theory. All of these components work together within the boundaries of the theory, providing the space in which to work.

Theoretical Approaches and Their Value

Theory can be conceptualized and applied in a variety of ways, including the individual or intrapersonal level, the social or interpersonal level, as well as at a community or environmental level. All of these conceptualizations are important and meaningful, yet they must be carefully chosen based on the scope of work one sets out to accomplish. Individual-level health theories, such as the health belief model, the theory of reasoned action, and the transtheoretical model, focus on the behaviors manifested within people and are also referred to as the intrapersonal level. Considering health at the intrapersonal level can be critical because health is a complex and ever-changing state that can vary and present in different ways across different individuals. **Self-efficacy**, a personal and individual belief in one's own ability to be successful with the task at hand (e.g., an individual's confidence in their ability to prepare vegetables or make a healthy eating choice in the cafeteria at school), is a common construct that intrapersonal theories set out to intervene on and enhance. Additionally, **intrapersonal theories** aim to guide the consideration of individual characteristics including knowledge, beliefs, cognitions, motivations, and perceptions. When applied to nutritional intervention work, intrapersonal theories often seek to identify effective ways to increase an individual's knowledge about healthy eating behaviors, increase self-efficacy toward the adoption of healthy eating practices, as well as positively shape individual beliefs and perceptions about healthy food choices.[19,20]

Theoretical Application in Nutrition Interventions

At the intrapersonal level, the theory of reasoned action and planned behavior are excellent examples of theory application within nutrition interventions. Oftentimes thought of in conjunction with one another, the theory of planned behavior is an enhancement of the theory of reasoned action.

Both theories take the premise that all personal health behavior changes are based on intention—the degree to which someone is ready to engage in a given behavior. The theories expand on this concept, finding that one's degree of intention toward a behavior change is influenced by attitudes, subjective norms, and control. That is, one's individual intention to engage in a health behavior is influenced by their deep-rooted beliefs, their social network's reactions, and their perceived control over the behavior. Both the theory of reasoned action and the theory of planned behavior are heavily represented in nutrition literature where they have been largely utilized to inform dietary changes[21,22] as well as to predict and intervene on breastfeeding intentions.[23,24]

The transtheoretical model is also well-established in nutritional intervention work because it identifies changes to health behavior through stepwise stages. By conceptualizing it as these stages of change, the focus becomes more about the process rather than attempting to identify one pinnacle event. Further, the transtheoretical model asserts that the process to health behavior change is largely influenced by an individual's motivation or readiness for change.[25] Constructs included in this model are indicative of the stepwise stages of change and include precontemplation, contemplation, preparation, action, and maintenance. By targeting these constructs, the model asserts that successful and sustainable health behavior change is achieved.[26] The transtheoretical model has been utilized successfully for healthy eating interventions aimed at reducing fast-food consumption[27] as well as increasing healthy eating through targeted nutrition counseling.[28]

Further, this model has also been utilized to intervene on healthy eating and literacy in special populations such as individuals diagnosed with type 2 diabetes.[29]

Interpersonal-level theories seek to encourage healthy eating and enhanced nutrition through the provision of social support.[30] One of the most heavily utilized **interpersonal theories** within nutrition-based work is the SCT, which broadly asserts that there is a dynamic and reciprocal interaction between one's health behaviors, their personal factors, as well as their proximal environment.[31] Consideration of personal factors such as self-regulation and outcome expectations as well as the support and resources that an environment offers are considered as critical contributors to the dynamic interplay this theory represents. Yet, this theory prioritizes the consideration for efficacy, both of the self as well as from a collective or group capacity.[32] Many family- and community-focused nutrition interventions have been guided by the tenets of SCT aimed at healthy familial cooking,[33,34] frequency and healthiness of family meals,[35] and preventing childhood obesity through community-conscious nutrition efforts.[36] Recently, technology and Internet-based health behavior interventions have also utilized SCT to improve healthy eating behaviors.[37,38] In sum, the SCT provides a useful framework that considers not only the individual influences on health behavior but also the interrelated social supports and environmental influences that shape behavior, such as an individuals' diet.

Social Ecological Models

In addition to theoretical considerations that account for intra- and interpersonal levels, a broader and more inclusive understanding has emerged that encourages health experts to consider the factors influencing health at multiple levels. Ecological models are broadly utilized among behavioral scientists and are operationalized differently based on the behavioral influences of interest. As a result, ecological models can be thought of as adaptable as they have the capacity to capture and inform numerous behaviors.

The basic underpinnings of historical models have informed today's contemporary frameworks. Bronfenbrenner first described ecological theory and the social ecological framework as multiple contexts in which health behavior occurs.[39] These include the micro-, meso-, exo-, and macrosystems, which constitute interdependent, active structures, ranging from influences most proximal at the microsystem level (e.g., parent–child interaction) to influences more distal and outside of immediate overt experience (e.g., societal norms).[39] The **microsystem** is the immediate physical and social environment in which the individual interacts and functions and includes the most proximal level of influence on an individual. The **mesosystem** reflects the interrelationships between microsystems, in that issues in one microsystem (e.g., family conflict, food insecurity, consumption of unhealthy foods) can affect how one functions in another (e.g., behavioral or academic difficulties at school). At the **exosystem** level, the individual is indirectly affected by social settings that he or she does not directly experience (e.g., parents' issues at work or loss of a job carry over into interactions with a child at home— including eating behaviors). Finally, the larger cultural context in which these first three systems sit is conceptualized as the **macrosystem** and involves culture and all related constructs within "culture" (beliefs, values, traditions, etc.). There is also an underlying chronosystem that reflects patterns of events within these four systems over time. McLeroy and colleagues[40] further adopted Bronfenbrenner's original model for health promotion programs to illustrate a health-specific and multilevel approach. He and colleagues identified intrapersonal factors, interpersonal processes and groups, institutional factors, community factors, and public policy as the specific sources influencing health behaviors. McLeroy's work spurred an ongoing conversation and consideration for the multilevel factors influencing health behaviors that has contributed to outcome-specific models targeting the development of holistic school environments where healthy school cafeterias, nutrition education, and nutrition-based school policies are used to ignite positive and sustainable nutrition change in students. Box 5.1 describes how public health nutrition researchers have applied and tailored ecological and socioecological models.[41-43]

Health Impact Pyramid

The **Health Impact Pyramid** is a public health–specific representation of ecologically based models in that it comprehensively considers the societal factors that are in most urgent need of intervention and illustrates how program planners can have the greatest impact on large numbers of the population.[44] This is especially relevant to nutrition-related work given the known associations between unhealthy eating behaviors and low socioeconomic status, urban environments, and race.[45-47] Conceptualized as a pyramid, the factors with high capacity to impact population-level health are at the base or largest area of the framework (socioeconomic and contextual changes), building up to the smallest areas relatable to more individual-level health (one-to-one counseling and clinical interventions) (figure 5.4). The Health Impact Pyramid identifies socioeconomic factors as the foundational and therefore most impactful factor of nutrition-related health, followed by environmental context, protective interventions, clinical interventions, and counseling or educational interventions.[44,48] It is important to understand that, although the model illustrates factors according to their hypothesized magnitude, it is not intended to suggest that interventions only work on the foundational or largest components of the pyramid; rather, research should work across the pyramid levels to create dynamic

Box 5.1. Nutrition-Specific Ecological and Socioecological Models

Several nutrition-specific, ecological and socioecological models of eating behavior have been developed to conceptualize the multilevel determinants of eating behavior and nutrition-related health outcomes and to guide interventions.

One of the first nutrition-specific models to formalize the idea that there are multiple levels of influence on eating behavior was developed by Karen Glantz and colleagues.[1] Glantz and colleagues put forth their model in 2005, motivated by the idea that environmental and policy solutions would be required to thwart the epidemic of obesity and suboptimal diet quality in the United States and other high-income countries. The model was based on early literature suggesting that aspects of our nutrition environment, including the cost of food and the availability of healthy and unhealthy food in the local neighborhood food environment was associated with dietary outcomes. They proposed multiple "environments" of influence on eating behavior. Namely, the Community Nutrition Environment, including the types and locations of food outlets, the Organizational Nutrition Environment, including home, school, work, and other institutions, and the Consumer Nutrition Environment, including the price, promotion and placement of items in store, the availability of healthy options, and nutrition information, and the Information Environment, including media and advertising. Government and industry policies influence all of these environments and, in turn, these environments influence eating patterns directly and through their impact on individual factors, such as psychosocial factors and perceptions of the nutrition environment.

In 2008, a paper by Mary Story and colleagues[2] further developed the ideas of multiple, layered influences on eating behaviors. They use the socioecological model as a starting place and depict the model using the commonly applied image of concentric circles, with the individual factors at the center, followed by social environments, physical environments, and macro-level environments. This model expands factors described as influencing eating behavior at each level, with cognitions, skills and behaviors, biological factors, and demographic factors recognized as playing a role at the individual level, and family, friends, and peers playing a role at the

social level. The physical environments layer includes institutions such as work and schools, and also includes home, neighborhood, and food outlets. The macro-level environments include societal and cultural norms, food and beverage industry, food marketing and media, food and agricultural policy, economic systems, food production and distribution systems, government and political structures and policies, health care systems, and land use and transportation.

In essence, the model built out the multitude of factors that influence eating behaviors, categorizing them by levels, with indication that the higher levels (i.e., macro-level environments) can influence all the lower levels (i.e., physical environments, social environments, and individual factors). Other scholars have added to these foundational, nutrition-specific theoretical models by adding directionality to indicate which factors are thought to influence each other and indicating at what levels interventions are needed to affect change (e.g., see Swinburn model as discussed in chapter 8 and Bleich et al.[3] and the health impact model discussed in this chapter), and introducing feedback loops among the multiple levels of influence and more fully acknowledging the role of biology (e.g., see Glass and McAttee[4]).

References

1. Glanz, K., J. F. Sallis, B. E. Saelens, and L. D. Frank. 2005. Healthy Nutrition Environments: Concepts and Measures. *American Journal of Health Promotion*. https://doi.org/10.4278/0890-1171-19.5 .330.

2. Story, M., K. M. Kaphingst, R. Robinson-O'Brien, and K. Glanz. 2008. "Creating Healthy Food and Eating Environments: Policy and Environmental Approaches." *Annual Review of Public Health*. https://doi.org/10.1146/annurev.publhealth .29.020907.090926.

3. Bleich, S. N., J. Jones-Smith, J. A. Wolfson, X. Zhu, and M. Story. 2015. "The Complex Relationship between Diet and Health." *Health Affairs* 34 (11). https://doi.org/10.1377/hlthaff.2015.0606.

4. Glass, T. A., & M. J. McAtee. 2006. "Behavioral Science at the Crossroads in Public Health: Extending Horizons, Envisioning the Future." *Social Science and Medicine*. https://doi.org/10.1016/j .socscimed.2005.08.044.

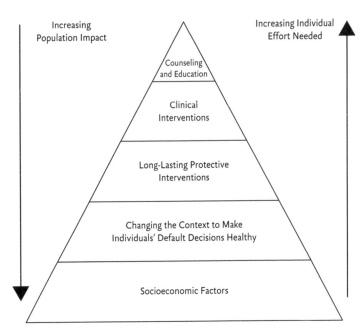

Figure 5.4. The Health Impact Pyramid. *Source:* Frieden, T. R. 2010. "A Framework for Public Health Action: The Health Impact Pyramid." *American Journal of Public Health* 100 (4): 590–595. http://doi.org/10.2105 /AJPH.2009.185652.

multilevel investigations that can offer useful guidance for a variety of public health concerns.

The Health Impact Pyramid offers breadth in that it provides a framework for a variety of nutrition-based outcomes, yet it also offers in-depth space and guidance to drill down on complex issues related to healthy eating. For example, vulnerable populations including low-income people and children have been targeted for sugar-sweetened beverage consumption, a significant factor in obesity, due to its low cost in comparison to its healthy whole-fruit and vegetable counterparts. Brownell and Frieden, utilizing the health impact lens, asserted that the most effective means for diminishing such consumption was to decrease the affordability of these drinks through local, state, and national beverage taxes. As these findings indicate, it may not just be the individual on which we intervene, rather the environmental forces driving individual and population behaviors.[49]

There are a number of different theoretical approaches that can guide and inform the development, implementation, and sustainability of nutrition-specific program planning. Theory has been developed to offer support in a multitude of different situations and across multiple levels including intrapersonal, interpersonal, and environmental. Intrapersonal theories inform personal health issues, offering contemplation of an individual's unique characteristics such as knowledge, attitude, and self-efficacy. Interpersonal theories hinge on the consideration of social norms and social support, offering consideration into how relationships and other collective perceptions can influence health behaviors. However, perhaps the most comprehensive theoretical approaches utilize an ecological framework allowing for consideration within and across the intra- and interpersonal levels and beyond. Social ecological frameworks, such as the Health Impact Pyramid, challenge researchers to think about health-related issues across a multitude of settings and circumstances, offering both breadth and depth to nutritional program planning and development.

Conclusion

Thoughtful and thorough program planning is essential for programs aimed at producing health behavior change. This chapter introduced the generalized model for program planning, which follows five steps: assessing needs; setting goals and objectives; developing an intervention; implementing the intervention; and evaluating the results. Logic models as vital planning tools for program and intervention design were considered. Finally, the importance of theory for guiding the development of programs and interventions was reviewed, and prominent intrapersonal and interpersonal theories applied to health and nutrition behavior were discussed.

Review Questions

1. What are the advantages of using a program planning model in designing nutrition interventions?
2. How do the components of the generalized model for program planning inform each other?
3. What are the components of the SMART format for writing goals and objectives?
4. What is the purpose of using logic models in planning nutrition programs?
5. Why is it important to use behavior change theory in the program planning process?

References

1. James, Janet, Peter Thomas, David Cavan, and David Kerr. 2004. "Preventing Childhood Obesity by Reducing Consumption of Carbonated Drinks: Cluster Randomised Controlled Trial." *British Medical Journal* 328 (7450): 1237. https://doi.org/10.1136/bmj.38077.458438.EE.

2. Muckelbauer, Rebecca, Steven L. Gortmaker, Lars Libuda, Mathilde Kersting, Kerstin Clausen, Bettina Adelberger, and Jacqueline Müller-Nordhorn. 2016. "Changes in Water and Sugar-Containing Beverage Consumption and Body Weight Outcomes in Children." *British Journal of Nutrition* 115 (11): 2057–66. https://doi.org/10.1017/S0007114516001136.

3. Chicago Public Schools, and Office of Student Health and Wellness. 2013. "Water Access Pilot Program."

4. "Healthy Snack and Beverage." Board Report 12-1114-PO1. 407.3. 2012. Chicago Public Schools.

5. "Local School Wellness Policy for Students." Board Report 12-1024-PO1. 704.7. 2012. Chicago Public Schools.

6. Food and Nutrition Service. 2011. "SP 28-2011—Revised, Child Nutrition Reauthorization 2010: Water Availability During National School Lunch Program Meal Service." Alexandria, VA: United States Department of Agriculture.

7. Hunnicutt, David. 2007. "The Power of Planning: A Good Plan Today Is Better than a Perfect Plan Tomorrow." Wellness Councils of America: www.welcoa.org. 2007. http://www.ndworksitewellness.org/docs/step4-power-of-planning.pdf.

8. McKenzie, James F., Brad L. Neiger, and Rosemary Thackeray. 2016. *Planning, Implementing, & Evaluating Health Promotion Programs: A Primer.* 7th ed. San Francisco, CA: Pearson.

9. *Logic Model Development Guide: Using Logic Models to Bring Together Planning, Evaluation, and Action.* 2004. Battle Creek, MI: W. K. Kellogg Foundation. https://www.bttop.org/sites/default/files/public/W.K.KelloggLogicModel.pdf.

10. World Health Organization. n.d. "E-Library of Evidence for Nutrition Actions (ELENA)." http://www.who.int/elena/en/.

11. Office of Disease Prevention and Health Promotion. 2020. "Nutrition and Weight Status: Interventions & Resources." Healthy People 2020. https://www.healthypeople.gov/2020/topics-objectives/topic/nutrition-and-weight-status/ebrs#ebr_header.

12. Missouri Department of Health and Senior Services. n.d. "Example Evidence-Based Interventions at a Glance." Community Health Improvement Resources. https://health.mo.gov/data/interventionmica/Nutrition/index_5.html.

13. Hawe, Penelope, Alan Shiell, and Therese Riley. 2009. "Theorising Interventions as Events in Systems." *American Journal of Community Psychology* 43 (3-4): 267-76. https://doi.org/10.1007/s10464-009-9229-9.

14. Centers for Disease Control and Prevention. 2013. "Community Needs Assessment: Participant Workbook." Atlanta, GA. https://www.cdc.gov/globalhealth/healthprotection/fetp/training_modules/15/community-needs_pw_final_9252013.pdf.

15. Liberato, Selma C., Ross Bailie, and Julie Brimblecombe. 2014. "Nutrition Interventions at Point-of-Sale to Encourage Healthier Food Purchasing: A Systematic Review." *BMC Public Health* 14 (1): 919. https://doi.org/10.1186/1471-2458-14-919.

16. Centers for Disease Control and Prevention. 1999. "Framework for Program Evaluation in Public Health." *MMWR Recommendations and Reports* 48 (RR-11): 1-40.

17. Office of Student Health and Wellness. 2016. "Healthy CPS." Chicago Public Schools. 2016. https://cps.edu/Programs/HealthyCPS/Pages/HealthyCPS.aspx.

18. Glanz, K., B. K. Rimer, and K. Viswanath, eds. 2008. *Health Behavior and Health Education: Theory, Research, and Practice.* 4th ed. San Francisco, CA: John Wiley and Sons.

19. Duyn, Mary Ann S. Van, Alan R. Kristal, Kevin Dodd, Marci K. Campbell, Amy F. Subar, Gloria Stables, Linda Nebeling, and Karen Glanz. 2001. "Association of Awareness, Intrapersonal and Interpersonal Factors, and Stage of Dietary

Change with Fruit and Vegetable Consumption: A National Survey." *American Journal of Health Promotion* 16 (2): 69-78. https://doi.org/10.4278/0890-1171-16.2.69.

20. Raynor, Hollie A., and Catherine M. Champagne. 2016. "Position of the Academy of Nutrition and Dietetics: Interventions for the Treatment of Overweight and Obesity in Adults." *Journal of the Academy of Nutrition and Dietetics* 116 (1): 129-47. https://doi.org/10.1016/j.jand.2015.10.031.

21. Conner, Mark, Paul Norman, and Russell Bell. 2002. "The Theory of Planned Behavior and Healthy Eating." *Health Psychology* 21 (2): 194-201. http://www.ncbi.nlm.nih.gov/pubmed/11950110.

22. Lautenschlager, Lauren, and Chery Smith. 2007. "Understanding Gardening and Dietary Habits among Youth Garden Program Participants Using the Theory of Planned Behavior." *Appetite* 49 (1): 122-30. https://doi.org/10.1016/j.appet.2007.01.002.

23. Guo, J. L., T. F. Wang, J. Y. Liao, and C. M. Huang. 2016. "Efficacy of the Theory of Planned Behavior in Predicting Breastfeeding: Meta-Analysis and Structural Equation Modeling." *Applied Nursing Research* 29 (February): 37-42. https://doi.org/10.1016/j.apnr.2015.03.016.

24. Zhu, Yu, Zhihong Zhang, Yun Ling, and Hongwei Wan. 2017. "Impact of Intervention on Breastfeeding Outcomes and Determinants Based on Theory of Planned Behavior." *Women and Birth* 30 (2): 146-52. https://doi.org/10.1016/j.wombi.2016.09.011.

25. Prochaska, James O., and Carlo C. DiClemente. 1982. "Transtheoretical Therapy: Toward a More Integrative Model of Change." *Psychotherapy: Theory, Research & Practice* 19 (3): 276-88. https://doi.org/10.1037/h0088437.

26. Prochaska, James O., and Wayne F. Velicer. 1997. "The Transtheoretical Model of Health Behavior Change." *American Journal of Health Promotion* 12 (1): 38-48. https://doi.org/10.4278/0890-1171-12.1.38.

27. Jalambadani, Zeinab, Gholamreza Garmarodi, Mehdi Yaseri, Mahmood Tavousi, and Korush Jafarian. 2017. "The Effect of Education on Reducing Fast Food Consumption in Obese Iranian Female Adolescents: An Application of the Transtheoretical Model and the Theory of Planned Behaviour." *Iranian Red Crescent Medical Journal* 19 (10). https://doi.org/10.5812/ircmj.13017.

28. Karintrakul, Sasipha, and Jongjit Angkatavanich. 2017. "A Randomized Controlled Trial of an Individualized Nutrition Counseling Program Matched with a Transtheoretical Model for Overweight and Obese Females in Thailand." *Nutrition Research and Practice* 11 (4): 319. https://doi.org/10.4162/nrp.2017.11.4.319.

29. Tseng, Hsu-Min, Shu-Fen Liao, Yu-Ping Wen, and Yuh-Jue Chuang. 2017. "Stages of Change Concept of the Transtheoretical Model for Healthy Eating Links Health Literacy and Diabetes Knowledge to Glycemic Control in People with Type 2 Diabetes." *Primary Care Diabetes* 11 (1): 29-36. https://doi.org/10.1016/j.pcd.2016.08.005.

30. Cruwys, Tegan, Kirsten E. Bevelander, and Roel C. J. Hermans. 2015. "Social Modeling of Eating: A Review of When and Why Social Influence Affects Food Intake and Choice." *Appetite* 86 (March): 3-18. https://doi.org/10.1016/j.appet.2014.08.035.

31. Bandura, A. 1986. *Social Foundations of Thought and Action: A Social Cognitive Theory.* Englewood Cliffs, NJ: Prentice-Hall, Inc.

32. Bandura, A. 1997. *Self-Efficacy: The Exercise of Control.* New York: W. H. Freeman and Company.

33. Cunningham-Sabo, Leslie, Barbara Lohse, Stephanie Smith, Ray Browning, Erin Strutz, Claudio Nigg, Meena Balgopal, Kathleen Kelly, and Elizabeth Ruder. 2016. "Fuel for Fun: A Cluster-Randomized Controlled Study of Cooking Skills, Eating Behaviors, and Physical Activity of 4th Graders and Their Families." *BMC Public Health* 16 (1): 444. https://doi.org/10.1186/s12889-016-3118-6.

34. Muzaffar, Henna, Jessica J. Metcalfe, and Barbara Fiese. 2018. "Narrative Review of Culinary Interventions with Children in Schools to Promote Healthy Eating: Directions for Future Research and Practice." *Current Developments in Nutrition* 2 (6). https://doi.org/10.1093/cdn/nzy016.

35. Flattum, Colleen, Michelle Draxten, Melissa Horning, Jayne A. Fulkerson, Dianne Neumark-Sztainer, Ann Garwick, Martha Y. Kubik, and Mary Story. 2015. "HOME Plus: Program Design and Implementation of a Family-Focused, Community-Based Intervention to Promote the Frequency and Healthfulness of Family Meals, Reduce Children's Sedentary Behavior, and Prevent Obesity." *International Journal of Behavioral Nutrition and Physical Activity* 12 (1): 53. https://doi.org/10.1186/s12966-015-0211-7.

36. Knol, Linda L., Harriet H. Myers, Sheila Black, Darlene Robinson, Yawah Awololo, Debra Clark, Carson L. Parker, Joy W. Douglas, and John C. Higginbotham. 2016. "Development and Feasibility of a Childhood Obesity Prevention Program for Rural Families: Application of the Social Cognitive Theory." *American Journal of Health Education* 47 (4): 204-14. https://doi.org/10.1080/19325037.2016.1179607.

37. Bandura, A. 2009. "Social Cognitive Theory of Mass Communication." In *Media Effects: Advances in Theory and Research,* edited by Jennings Bryant and Mary Beth Oliver, 3rd ed., 110-40. New York: Routledge, Taylor & Francis Group.

38. DiFilippo, K. N., J. E. Andrade, W. Huang, and K. M. Chapman-Novakofski. 2015. "Development of a Tool to Evaluate the Quality of Nutrition Apps." *Journal of the Academy of Nutrition and Dietetics* 115 (9): A15. https://doi.org/10.1016/j.jand.2015.06.039.

39. Bronfenbrenner, Urie. 1977. "Toward an Experimental Ecology of Human Development." *American Psychologist* 32 (7): 513-31. https://doi.org/10.1037/0003-066X.32.7.513.

40. McLeroy, K. R., D. Bibeau, A. Steckler, and K. Glanz. 1988. "An Ecological Perspective on Health Promotion Programs." *Health Education Quarterly* 15 (4): 351-77. http://www.ncbi.nlm.nih.gov/pubmed/3068205.

41. Gutuskey, Lila, Nate McCaughtry, Bo Shen, Erin Centeio, and Alex Garn. 2016. "The Role and Impact of Student Leadership on Participants in a Healthy Eating and Physical Activity Programme." *Health Education Journal* 75 (1): 27-37. https://doi.org/10.1177/0017896914561878.

42. Lewallen, Theresa C., Holly Hunt, William Potts-Datema, Stephanie Zaza, and Wayne Giles. 2015. "The Whole School, Whole Community, Whole Child Model: A New Approach for Improving Educational Attainment and Healthy Development for Students." *Journal of School Health* 85 (11): 729-39. https://doi.org/10.1111/josh.12310.

43. Murray, Sharon D., James Hurley, and Shannon R. Ahmed. 2015. "Supporting the Whole Child Through Coordinated Policies, Processes, and Practices." *Journal of School Health* 85 (11): 795-801. https://doi.org/10.1111/josh.12306.

44. Frieden, Thomas R. 2010. "A Framework for Public Health Action: The Health Impact Pyramid." *American Journal of Public Health* 100 (4): 590-95. https://doi.org/10.2105/AJPH.2009.185652.

45. Cassady, Diana L., Karen Liaw, and Lisa M. Soederberg Miller. 2015. "Disparities in Obesity-Related Outdoor Advertising by Neighborhood Income and Race." *Journal of Urban Health* 92 (5): 835-42. https://doi.org/10.1007/s11524-015 -9980-1.

46. Richardson, Andrea S., Joanne E. Arsenault, Sheryl C. Cates, and Mary K. Muth. 2015. "Perceived Stress, Unhealthy Eating Behaviors, and Severe Obesity in Low-Income Women." *Nutrition Journal* 14 (1): 122. https://doi.org/10.1186/s12937 -015-0110-4.

47. Vilaro, Melissa J., Tracey E. Barnett, Anne Mathews, Jamie Pomeranz, and Barbara Curbow. 2016. "Income Differences in Social Control of Eating Behaviors and Food Choice Priorities among Southern Rural Women in the US: A Qualitative Study." *Appetite* 107 (December): 604-12. https://doi.org/10.1016/j.appet.2016.09 .003.

48. Thornton, Rachel L. J., Crystal M. Glover, Crystal W. Cené, Deborah C. Glik, Jeffrey A. Henderson, and David R. Williams. 2016. "Evaluating Strategies for Reducing Health Disparities By Addressing the Social Determinants of Health." *Health Affairs* 35 (8): 1416-23. https://doi.org/10.1377/hlthaff.2015.1357.

49. Brownell, Kelly D., and Thomas R. Frieden. 2009. "Ounces of Prevention— The Public Policy Case for Taxes on Sugared Beverages." *New England Journal of Medicine* 360 (18): 1805-8. https://doi.org/10.1056/NEJMp0902392.

6

Monitoring and Evaluation in Nutrition Programs

Julie C. Ruel-Bergeron, Andrew L. Thorne-Lyman, and Marie Ruel

LEARNING OBJECTIVES

- Explain the role and value of program monitoring and evaluation in public health nutrition programming
- Articulate the differences between program monitoring, process evaluation, program evaluation, and nutrition surveillance, and how they collectively contribute to improved public health nutrition programming and policy making
- Describe the various types of data sources, methods used, and challenges faced in the collection and analysis of monitoring and evaluation data
- Critically assess monitoring and evaluation designs in published studies
- Demonstrate skill in the principles of designing a rigorous and useful evaluation plan
- Understand the role of nutrition surveillance in program monitoring and evaluation

Case Study: Monitoring and Evaluation Design of a Large-Scale Nutrition Program in Malawi

In 2010, 47% of the Malawian population under the age of 5 were stunted.[1] In 2011, Malawi was among the first countries to join the Scaling Up Nutrition (SUN) movement,[2] a global initiative that countries can join to commit to ending malnutrition in all its forms. In 2014, Malawi demonstrated its commitment to nutrition through the implementation of a district-wide nutrition program that aimed to reduce stunting among children under 2 years of age. The program, *Right Foods at the Right Time: Targeting Nutrition of Children under Two*, delivered a package of interventions aimed to improve maternal and child nutrition during the first 1,000 days (from conception to the child's second birthday) that included: (1) monthly small-quantity lipid-based nutrient supplements to all children 6-23 months of age; (2) social and behavior change communication to improve maternal diets and infant and young child feeding (IYCF) and hygiene practices; (3) scale-up of community-based management of acute malnutrition to 100%; and (4) nutrition-sensitive agriculture actions such as promotion of small livestock rearing and home gardens. The program was led by the Government of Malawi, with technical, logistical, and financial support from the World Food Programme, World Vision Malawi, and the Children's Investment Fund Foundation, respectively. Johns Hopkins University led the impact evaluation of the program to measure the three-year impact on child stunting and anemia, as well as intermediate outcomes such as infant and young child feeding practices.

The *Right Foods at the Right Time* monitoring and evaluation (M&E) framework that was developed in partnership between the multiple stakeholders involved in the program (Government of Malawi, World Food Programme, World Vision Malawi, Children's Investment Fund Foundation, and Johns Hopkins University) included a combination of comprehensive and repeated surveys and studies that generated both immediate and longer-term program feedback and evidence that was used for course correction and continued learning about the feasibility and effectiveness of delivering the selected package of interventions at scale (figure 6.1). Three program monitoring systems were designed and established with technical and logistical support from World Food Programme and World Vision Malawi:

1. Participant tracking and registration through an electronic and mobile platform (SCOPE). This platform was used to enroll beneficiaries and track their monthly attendance at small-quantity lipid-based nutrient supplement distributions during the period of the child's eligibility. Data from SCOPE were uploaded in real time to a business intelligence dashboard and enabled analysis of participation trends over the project period.
2. Quarterly post-distribution monitoring surveys, which were used to monitor output and outcome indicators, such as IYCF knowledge and practices and receipt of program services. Each of these surveys enrolled new, randomly selected cohorts of mothers of eligible children and pregnant women.
3. Routine monthly monitoring of input and output indicators related to the implementation of the social and behavior change communication activities such as worker performance and delivery of interventions, collected and compiled by World Vision Malawi and submitted to the Government of Malawi and World Food Program for review and analysis.

Alongside the routine monitoring activities described, Johns Hopkins University led a quasi-experimental impact evaluation that included a combination of the following research activities:

1. Three cross-sectional surveys (base-, mid-, and end-line) conducted in the program and a neighboring comparison district to assess program impact on primary outcomes of interest, which included child height-for-age z-score, stunting, and anemia.
2. Two longitudinal cohorts of children followed in 6-month intervals from 6 to 24 months of age to measure differences in child growth patterns in the program and comparison districts.

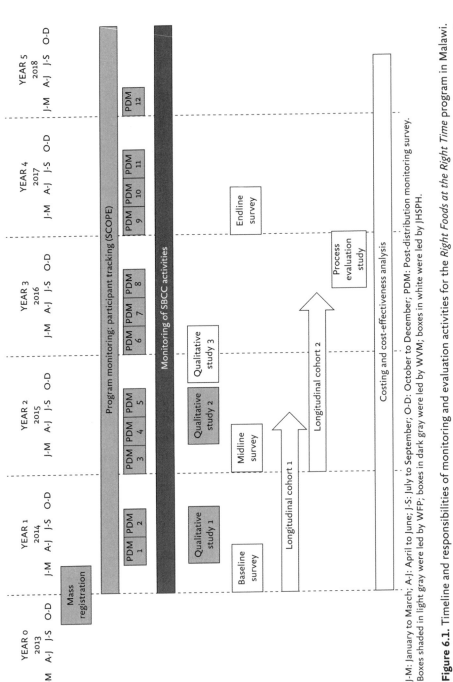

Figure 6.1. Timeline and responsibilities of monitoring and evaluation activities for the *Right Foods at the Right Time* program in Malawi.

Source: Ruel-Bergeron, J., et al. 2019. "Monitoring and Evaluation Design of Malawi's Right Foods at the Right Time Nutrition Program." *Evaluation and Program Planning* 73: 4.

J-M: January to March; A-J: April to June; J-S: July to September; O-D: October to December; PDM: Post-distribution monitoring survey. Boxes shaded in light gray were led by WFP; boxes in dark gray were led by WVM; boxes in white were led by JHSPH.

3. A process evaluation study in the program district to measure program fidelity, with a focus on quality of implementation of interventions.
4. A qualitative study in the program district to measure facilitators and barriers to program access and use.
5. A costing and cost-effectiveness analysis to quantify implementation costs of the nutrition program and to measure the cost-consequences (savings from preventing chronic and acute malnutrition) of the interventions vis-à-vis the primary program outcomes and impact.

The Malawi program M&E framework represents a comprehensive set of research activities, which were instrumental for understanding the context in which the program was implemented, the reasons underlying caregiver and community member decisions and behaviors related to the use of the program and adoption of recommended practices, the quality of implementation of various program activities, and why and how impacts were achieved (or not) with the selected interventions. Importantly, the strategic use of incoming data from the comprehensive monitoring system was instrumental for program course correction and service delivery improvements to maximize impact.

Program monitoring and evaluation (M&E) are a set of complementary yet distinct research activities that measure the design, implementation, and effect of projects and programs on targeted populations.[3] **Program monitoring** is a process of setting and tracking goals, indicators, and targets that represent program operations and progress in implementation.[4] Program evaluation, on the other hand, is the systematic and rigorous assessment of the results achieved by a program and its interventions.[4] M&E, though separate, should ideally be planned and designed in tandem but conducted by different teams or types of practitioners.[3] For instance, monitoring should be done by program planners who have an in-depth understanding of program design and implementation that researchers do not have. Conversely, researchers should design and conduct the evaluation, which requires a set of research and analytical skills that program implementation teams often lack. The overall goal is to bring findings together at the analysis stage to fully comprehend whether and how a program produced the intended impact; whether program implementation, quality of service delivery, and utilization by targeted beneficiaries were optimal; and document the cost-effectiveness of the program.

Program evaluation is a broad term that comprises M&E activities and is an essential organizational practice in public health that promotes the systematic improvement and accountability for public health and nutrition interventions.[3,5] The careful design and use of M&E systems to evaluate nutrition programs is increasingly recognized as essential for strengthening

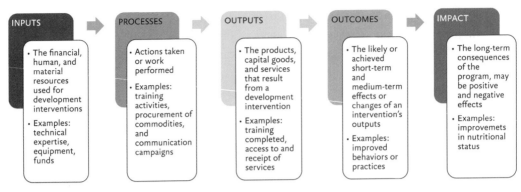

Figure 6.2. Elements and definitions of a program logic model.

program implementation and delivery and maximizing impact and cost-effectiveness.[6] Learning from program evaluation supports evidence-based policy making, which is needed for replication and scale up, and ultimately, for marked and sustained health and nutrition improvements.[6,7]

Given the central role of M&E to program improvement and results measurement, M&E systems and associated data collection activities should always be considered and integrated at the earliest stages of program planning. The development of a program logic model that clearly illustrates program inputs, processes, outputs, outcomes, and impact is an invaluable tool that guides the selection of indicators used in M&E systems.[4] Measurement of each of these types of indicators (described in figure 6.2) is, of course, dependent on what they are and represent, but is most comprehensively addressed using both qualitative and quantitative methodologies, each of which can be conducted repeatedly and at various stages of program implementation.

M&E strategies can include program monitoring, operational or process evaluations, cost-effectiveness analyses, nutrition surveillance, and impact evaluation.[4] Data for each of these processes can and should be collected using a **stepwise approach** to evaluation (figure 6.3), which involves the collection and use of data from design, to implementation process, utilization and coverage of the program (monitoring), and impact and cost-effectiveness (evaluation). The stepwise approach is also used to understand and measure program implementation details that are then used to attribute impact (or lack of) to the program's implementation. Lastly, note the feedback loops within the stepwise approach, which highlight how each research or information-gathering process feeds into the next, with the ultimate goal of informing future scale up, programming, and policy making.[8]

In this chapter, we unpack the main elements of program M&E, including program monitoring, **process evaluation**, and program evaluation. We begin with a brief overview of program logic models (described in detail in

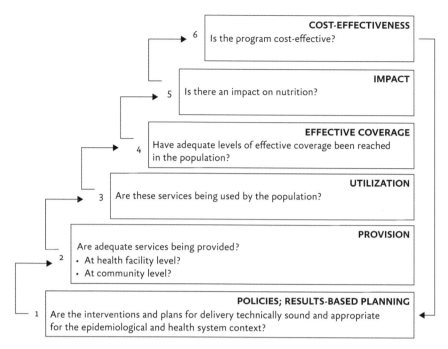

Figure 6.3. Stepwise approach to program monitoring and evaluation. *Source:* Adapted from Victora C. G., D. Walker, B. Johns, and J. Bryce. 2012. "Evaluations of Large-Scale Health Programs." In M. Merson, R. E. Black, and A. J. Mills, editors. *Global Health: Diseases, Programs, Systems, and Policies*, pp. 815–51. Burlington, MA: Jones & Bartlett Learning.

chapter 5) as the basis for the development of M&E frameworks, and then dive into program monitoring, with definitions of the types of indicators and their respective purposes in measuring program implementation and progress. We then describe process evaluation, with an emphasis on the objectives, terminology, and categories of indicators that can be used to best unpack the "black box" of program implementation. We then delve into **impact evaluation** and the objective and scope of the different types of evaluation(s), purposes, and study designs. Lastly, we include a presentation of nutrition surveillance and its applications in program M&E, with an illustrative example from Bangladesh.

Program Logic Models

Also referred to as logframes, logical frameworks, impact models, and results frameworks, program logic models are essential, multipurpose visual tools used to guide program planning and management.[9] Despite the wide variation in terminologies, philosophies, approaches, and applications used for these tools today, their primary purpose remains to illustrate the logical sequence of how a program progresses from inputs, processes, outputs, and outcomes, to bring about the intended impact (figure 6.2).[5,9] Visualizing a program in such a way clarifies how and whether—with the inputs provided, their distribution, and uptake—the program will be sufficient to achieve its goals. This in turn sets realistic expectations for program planners and developers, aids in the definition of evaluation questions and measurements, and guides analysis and interpretation of results. Logic models are often displayed in a flow chart, map, or table and can go beyond the program's overall structure and operation plan to include the infrastructure needed to support program operations.[5] Perhaps most importantly, the program logic model highlights assumptions underlying the conditions needed to bring about change in outcomes and thus strengthens claims of causality for endpoints that are not directly measured but linked in a causal chain supported by prior research.[10]

Although much more can be said about program logic models (see chapter 5), we discuss them here simply to create a link to their use in program M&E. Definitions of inputs, processes, outputs, outcomes, and impact are presented in figure 6.2 and reflect the Organization for Economic Cooperation and Development's definitions of these key terms.[11]

In this chapter, we present monitoring as covering both implementation and performance indicators that are measured by program inputs, processes and outputs, and evaluation as covering outcomes and impact.[4]

Program Monitoring

Data and information collected through monitoring activities is ongoing, and its main purpose is to track how implementation is proceeding on a regular basis while the program is being implemented. As discussed in the introduction and given its purpose, program monitoring should be designed and carried out by program planners and implementers, who will also be the primary users of the incoming information. For example, monitoring data can be used to adapt the program to better reach and respond to the evolving needs of the target population.[4,6]

Since the primary focus of monitoring is to track the operational aspects of programs, indicators included in monitoring frameworks typically measure inputs, processes, and outputs. Examples of program monitoring indicators that have been used in nutrition programming are outlined in table 6.1. Indicators included in program monitoring systems are often assessed using administrative or routine information data systems, such as health management information systems,[12] which can be used to summarize information in an easy-to-use format to keep track of project activities, budget, and personnel.[3] The innovative use of information technology, such as mobile technology to track program coverage, participation, and utilization of services, can greatly improve the efficiency of monitoring systems both in terms

Table 6.1. Sample Information Collected by Nutrition Program Monitoring Systems to Measure Program Inputs, Processes, and Outputs

Category of indicator	Types of information collected by nutrition program monitoring system
Inputs	▪ Program funding ▪ Presence of a nutrition policy ▪ Availability of frontline workers to implement program activities ▪ Nutrition commodities and supplies (e.g., micronutrient supplements, ready-to-use supplementary or therapeutic foods)
Process	▪ Training activities delivered to frontline workers ▪ Procurement and availability of supplies needed to conduct program activities (e.g., scale, length board, communication materials, growth charts, child health cards) ▪ Procurement of nutrition commodities
Output	▪ Completion of training protocol by frontline workers ▪ Program coverage of each intervention

of their data capture as well as processing and analysis for timely data-driven program adaptations.

In some instances, monitoring systems may also include periodic and repeated measurement of outcome indicators by use of a population-based survey, such as in the Malawi example, maintaining the purpose of using this data to feed back into and strengthen program operations. The measurement of outcome indicators, however, almost always requires field data collection (surveys) and thus holds important cost implications.[12]

Perhaps the most important contribution of program monitoring is its provision of valuable insights as to where program implementation problems or bottlenecks may be arising, why interventions may be failing or succeeding, and which aspects of the implementation should be adjusted to improve targeting and coverage of interventions.[3] Also, since information is collected and reviewed repeatedly, areas of concern can be addressed and/or the program can be course corrected or adapted to changing needs of the target population. The term *adaptive programming* is often used to reflect this information feedback mechanism wherein data is collected and used to improve and adapt program implementation so that it can more effectively achieve its goals.

In the context of evaluation, program monitoring data provides contextual information, especially as it relates to the types of inferences that can be made about any observed program impact. For example, if the monitoring data indicates that the program's implementation was fraught with unsolved process and delivery problems, findings of lack of impact on key outcomes may be attributed—at least in part—to poor implementation rather than inadequate

Box 6.1. How Process Evaluation Was Used to Disentangle Impact Evaluation Results of the Homestead Food Production Program in Cambodia

Homestead food production programs are typically directed at women and smallholder farmers to provide them with the tools and skills needed to cultivate home gardens and raise small livestock that can be used for home consumption and to increase family income that is used to further purchase micronutrient-rich foods such as meat, eggs, and others. Ideally, the foods cultivated or purchased are consumed by nutritionally vulnerable groups within the household (pregnant and lactating women and young children). Such programs are often complemented by behavior change communication interventions aimed to improve maternal nutrition and health knowledge and behaviors related to infant and young child feeding practices. Between 2005 and 2007, an impact evaluation of a homestead food production program in Cambodia that aimed to increase the production and consumption of diverse and nutritious foods year-round as a means of improving maternal and child nutrition outcomes was conducted.[37] The results of the impact evaluation indicated that although production of nutritious foods and dietary diversity among target beneficiaries increased, there was no improvement in child anthropometry or anemia.[37] To better understand why the program was unsuccessful in improving

child growth and anemia despite positive impacts on production and consumption diversity, a process evaluation was conducted to assess whether program components along three hypothesized pathways of impact (see figure) were implemented and utilized as planned.[38] The comprehensive data collection, gathering, and analysis along each of these pathways revealed challenges in relation to the knowledge, motivation, and compensation of village health volunteers who assisted in the delivery of the educational intervention, as well as explicit gaps between the production and consumption of certain nutrient-rich foods (eggs).[38] The use of program impact pathways provided insights into which areas of implementation (the production-income pathways rather than the production-consumption pathway) were more likely to yield changes in dietary behaviors among the target population. Most importantly, this work highlighted that despite identified necessary tweaks to the implementation process, it was unlikely that without additional program components and inputs, for example, access to water, distribution or sale of micronutrient supplements, or the addition of small-animal-source production activities (e.g., ducks, pigs, fish), the program could not have realized its expected impacts on child nutrition outcomes.[38]

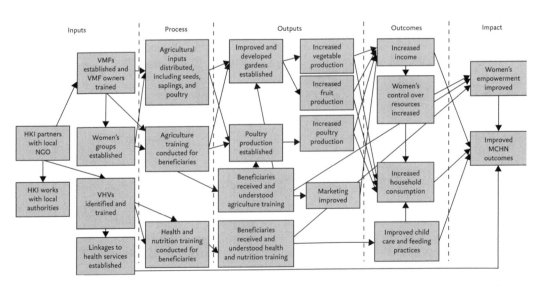

Program impact pathways for the Cambodia homestead food production program. HKI: Helen Keller International; VMF: Village model farms; VHV: Village health volunteer. *Source:* Olney, D. K., S. Vicheka, M. Kro, et al. 2013. "Using Program Impact Pathways to Understand and Improve Program Delivery, Utilization, and Potential for Impact of Helen Keller International's Homestead Food Production Program in Cambodia." *Food Nutrition Bulletin* 34 (2): 169–84.

design or poor choice of interventions. Alternatively, monitoring data showing a well-implemented, high-coverage, high-quality program can help support the plausibility of positive impact results.[3]

Process Evaluation

Very closely tied to program monitoring is **process evaluation**, which has been deemed an essential component of impact evaluation since the 1960s.[13] Although many of the same types of indicators are collected and analyzed for both program monitoring and process evaluation, they serve vastly different purposes. As opposed to program monitoring whose main role is to support day-to-day program-related decisions, process evaluation is an integral part of a program's overall evaluation plan and its main purpose is to assess *how* programs achieve their impacts (or why they fail to achieve them). Process evaluations should be rooted in "program theory"[14] and include an initial step consisting of engaging all relevant stakeholders to develop theory-based program impact pathways (PIP).[15] Theory-driven program impact pathways involve specifying the causal pathways through which each intervention component will contribute to the overall impacts of the program.[15] Importantly, the program impact pathways specify the conditions that are needed to drive intended impacts, as well as the assumptions that are made regarding how the program will achieve them.[15] Please refer to the example provided in box 6.1, which presents the process evaluation of a program in Cambodia that used program impact pathways to make conclusions about why the program did not achieve its intended impacts.

Process evaluation is thus used to test the program's implementation theory, defined as the details of how a program is implemented "to bring about the desired interactions with the target population and provide the planned services."[16] Process evaluation is a common tool used to test **implementation theory**, as it allows for the systematic study and understanding of program delivery and constraints, why they arise, and how they might influence program outcomes.[13] This, again, is different from program monitoring where the same type of information is collected, but with the goal of identifying and implementing immediate course correction so that the program operates as intended to reach targeted delivery and coverage levels. Process evaluation is thus an important component of program impact evaluation, which can answer questions about how a program works and can help open the so-called black box of program implementation.[15,17] This is particularly important in nutrition programming, where interventions are complex and may have several interacting components.[15] Knowing the extent to which all intervention components were actually implemented, often at multiple locations, is critical for disentangling their effects at the evaluation stage.[13]

Using process evaluation to tease out the implementation-related pathways of impact also reduces the likelihood of making a Type III error, which results from evaluating a program that has not been adequately implemented and can lead to drawing false conclusions about the effectiveness of an intervention (or lack thereof).[13,18] Process evaluation strengthens the internal and external validity of the impact evaluation's results: internal validity refers to the extent that the impact seen is truly a result of the program, and external validity refers to the extent to which such a program is generalizable to other populations,[19] such that the processes that lead to impact are thoroughly documented, including the successes, failures, and inefficiencies that may arise in similar or other environments, and how they were or can be addressed.[6]

Process evaluation typically uses mixed methods including both qualitative and quantitative approaches to understand specific implementation components, such as program recruitment, maintenance, context, and barriers to implementation, among others.[13] The specific set of implementation components assessed through process evaluation varies,[13,20,21] with the most commonly used being Linnan and Steckler's,[13] but the most recent and comprehensive being Proctor and colleagues'.[21] The components of process evaluation outlined by Proctor and colleagues include acceptability, adoption, appropriateness, feasibility, fidelity (including elements of program quality), penetration, and sustainability; their definitions and types of measurements are outlined in table 6.2. The selection of the research method and/or tools used to assess program components is highly dependent on the program and what is being measured, but it can range from quantitative surveys, checklists, and review of attendance logs and project archives to more qualitative in-depth interviews, focus groups, and observation.

Program Evaluation

The evaluation component of M&E measures outcomes and impact indicators laid out in the program's **logic model**, which are most often collected using surveys. Evaluations should be conducted externally,[22] can be formative or summative,[12,22] and can be set up to measure the efficacy or effectiveness of interventions.[23] Depending on the degree of certainty desired with regard to being able to attribute observed impacts to the program activities, various types of evaluation designs are available and include adequacy, plausibility, and probability designs.[12] All of these terminologies are expanded upon in this chapter.

External evaluations are those that are conducted by an independent research team that is not involved in the program implementation process.[22] Despite the need to maintain a certain level of independence between the evaluation and programmatic entities, close collaboration between the two is critical for providing contextual and programmatic experience and expertise that the evaluators need to design their evaluation plan. Moreover, the evaluators need a clear picture of program activities and interventions (which can be derived from the program impact pathways developed jointly with

Table 6.2. Key Process Evaluation Components, Terminologies, and Measurement Methods

Process evaluation component	Description	Other terms in literature	Available measurement
Acceptability	The perception among implementation stakeholders that a given treatment, service, practice, or innovation is agreeable, palatable, or satisfactory.	Satisfaction with various aspects of the innovation (e.g., content, complexity, comfort, delivery, and credibility)	■ Survey ■ Qualitative or semi-structured interviews ■ Administrative data
Adoption	The intention, initial decision, or action to try or employ an innovation or evidence-based practice. Adoption can be measured from the perspective of the provider or organization.	Uptake; utilization; initial implementation; intention to try	■ Administrative data ■ Observation ■ Qualitative or semi-structured interviews
Appropriateness	The perceived fit, relevance, or compatibility of the innovation or evidence-based practice for a given practice setting, provider, or consumer; and/or the perceived fit of the innovation to address a particular issue or problem.	Perceived fit; relevance; compatibility; suitability; usefulness; practicability	■ Survey ■ Qualitative or semi-structured interviews ■ Focus groups
Feasibility	The extent to which a new treatment or innovation can be successfully used or carried out within a given agency or setting. The concept of feasibility is typically invoked retrospectively as a potential explanation of an initiative's success or failure, as reflected in poor recruitment, retention, or participation rates. Feasibility may also refer to the complexity of the program's interventions or activities and whether these can be delivered in a given context. For instance, is the program feasible given how it is designed and staffed?	Actual fit or utility; suitability for everyday use; practicability	■ Survey ■ Administrative data
Fidelity (including elements of program quality)	The degree to which an intervention was implemented as it was prescribed in the original protocol or as it was intended by the program developers. Typically measured as: (1) adherence to the program protocol, (2) dose delivered, and (3) quality of delivery.	Delivered as intended; adherence; integrity; quality of program delivery	■ Observation ■ Checklists ■ Self-report

(continued)

Table 6.2 (continued)

Process evaluation component	Description	Other terms in literature	Available measurement
Penetration	The integration of a practice within a service setting and its subsystems. Calculated as the number of eligible persons who use a service, divided by the total number of persons eligible for the service.	Coverage; reach; level of institutionalization; spread; service access	▪ Case audit ▪ Checklists
Sustainability	The extent to which a newly implemented treatment is maintained or institutionalized within a service setting's ongoing, stable operations.	Maintenance; continuation; durability; incorporation; integration; institution-alization; sustained use; routinization	▪ Case audit ▪ Semi-structured interviews ▪ Questionnaire ▪ Checklist

Source: Adapted from Proctor E., H. Silmere, R. Raghavan, et al. 2011. "Outcomes for Implementation Research: Conceptual Distinctions, Measurement Challenges, and Research Agenda." *Administration and Policy in Mental Health and Mental Health Services Research* 38 (2): 65–76.

program implementers) so that they can develop their evaluation tools in such a way that they correctly capture the information needed to make conclusions about program impact.

Program evaluation is most often equated with ***summative* evaluations**, which are those that are used to make decisions about the program being evaluated.[12] For example, the results of a summative evaluation may be used by a decision maker, funder, or program planner to decide whether to continue, change, expand, or end a project or intervention.[12] ***Formative* evaluations**, also referred to as needs assessment, preprogram research, and development research, are aimed at improving program design prior to program development and implementation.[8,24] In formative evaluations, various research methods are used prior to the program design phase to understand and inform program planners on (1) the context in which the intervention(s) will take place, (2) specific behaviors of concern, (3) determinants of those behaviors, and (4) resources that are available to the program.[24] Information collected during formative assessments may therefore include, for example, determinants of behavior, access to communication channels, policies that might affect the intervention, and community attitudes that could inhibit or promote the use of the program or adoption of the behavior(s) of interest.[24] And, as with most other M&E activities described in this chapter, formative assessment is most effective when conducted using mixed methods combining quantitative and qualitative tools. In this chapter and in our discussion about evaluation, we are referring to summative evaluations unless otherwise noted.

Another important concept in program evaluation design and decision-making is whether the evaluation will measure **program efficacy** or **program effectiveness**. Before diving into the difference between those is the difference between efficacy and program efficacy. Efficacy of an intervention or treatment is usually tested through clinical trials that by default impose strictly controlled environments. The objective of assessing an intervention's efficacy is to determine whether the intervention actually works to achieve the intended outcome; for example, an efficacy study might involve testing the impact of giving different doses of vitamin A on vitamin A status. It is important to establish the biological efficacy of interventions before rolling them out or scaling up their delivery through public health programs. Evaluations of program efficacy, on the other hand, are those that seek to understand whether an intervention or a package of interventions have an impact when implemented under ideal or strict conditions or circumstances of implementation, within the context of a public health program (i.e., field conditions).[23] Program efficacy evaluations require much stricter control and close supervision of the conditions of implementation than usual programs so that they represent an ideal delivery system and are as standardized as possible across all program intervention sites. An example of program efficacy are the International Lipid-Based Nutrient Supplements (iLiNS) Project[25] trials done in Burkina Faso,[26] Ghana,[27] and Malawi,[28,29] which were conducted in field conditions but involved very close monitoring of the provision and consumption of supplements, which represented conditions that would not be realistic in most programmatic contexts. Another example of program efficacy would be to evaluate whether vitamin A supplementation of children aged 6 to 59 months improved vitamin A status and/or reduced vitamin A deficiency in that target population.

Program effectiveness measures whether the intervention or set of interventions have an effect under "real-life" conditions or circumstances, such as in the context of ongoing nutrition programs implemented by governmental or nongovernmental organizations.[23] In the measurement of program effectiveness, the evaluators usually have less control over the delivery of the interventions and of their uptake and use/adoption by targeted beneficiaries than in program efficacy trials. The fact that implementation is less controlled in effectiveness compared to efficacy trials highlights the importance of conducting comprehensive process evaluations to help understand potential implementation or utilization bottlenecks that may impede the program's ability to deliver on expected impacts. The Malawi vignette provided at the beginning of this chapter is an example of an evaluation of program effectiveness. Continuing with the series of vitamin A examples, the Devta trial, which was implemented under field conditions without necessarily achieving high coverage, would constitute a program effectiveness evaluation. Despite the distinctions presented here between program efficacy and effectiveness, Bryce and colleagues highlight the difficulty in conducting evaluations that are entirely *efficacy* or entirely *effectiveness* evaluations given the nature of public health program implementation.[23] Thus, this dimension of program evaluation should be thought of as more of a continuum than a clear demarcation of one versus the other.[23]

Additional considerations in program evaluation include which type of design to use: adequacy, plausibility, or probability design. This decision is hinged on a number of factors, most importantly the level of certainty and degree of attribution of any impact to the program that is desired; the decision should also be based on specific study objectives, funding envelope, program design, and government or donor preferences on ethical and other evaluation-related matters. Therefore the study design that is to be used is often not solely in the control of the evaluator. Regarding the degree of certainty (or ability to claim causality between intervention/program and impact measures) that each of these designs provide, an adequacy design would provide the lowest degree of confidence while a probability design would represent high confidence, with plausibility somewhere in between the two. Nevertheless, both plausibility and probability designs can be used to attribute program impact to program activities. The basics of adequacy, plausibility, and probability designs are presented in table 6.3 and discussed below; the publication by Habicht et al., titled *Evaluation Designs for Adequacy, Plausibility, and Probability of Public Health Programme Performance*, is an excellent resource on the topic and the basis for what is presented here.

Adequacy **assessments** answer the question about whether expected changes occurred in indicators of interest as compared to previously established adequacy criteria.[12] Adequacy designs can measure absolute numbers, for instance, the number of micronutrient powders delivered to children aged 6 to 23 months, or reflect a change over a given time period, such as a decrease in the proportion of children under 5 years who are stunted. Although adequacy designs do not causally link program activities to measured changes in target indicators, they can provide reassurance that the expected goals are being met, which can be important for program continuation.[12] Additionally, if the adequacy design finds that program targets are not being reached, it may open the door for another study design to be conducted to identify the causes of failure and/or to guide course correction.

Plausibility **assessments** go a few steps beyond adequacy assessments to provide more certainty regarding whether the impacts observed are due to the program rather than to other external influences.[12] Plausibility designs require the inclusion of a control group against which external factors, or confounding factors, can be ruled out as reasons for observed effects;[12] the control group can be chosen before the evaluation is begun or afterwards, during the analysis of data.[12] Habicht and colleagues provide examples of the types of control groups, which include (1) historical controls, which en-

Table 6.3. Types of Designs Used in Summative Program Effectiveness Evaluations

Type of evaluation	Research question answered	Possible study designs	Control group needed?
Adequacy	Are the expected changes occurring?	Descriptive studies • Cross-sectional • Longitudinal	No
Plausibility	Do the observed changes seem to be due to the program?	Quasi-experimental observational studies • Cross-sectional • Longitudinal • Longitudinal-control • Case-control	Yes
Probability	Does the program have a statistically significant impact on nutrition outcomes?	Randomized controlled trials	Yes

tails a pre- and post-program comparison of change within one population; (2) internal controls, which is either a subgroup of the target population that received either a limited or no intervention because they refused services or were not reached, or a case-control design that compares previous exposure to the program among those with and without the disease; and (3) external controls, which are entire populations (typically based on geography) who have not received the program. The biggest value of the control group is its ability to measure and later control for potentially confounding factors, so that the intervention and control groups are as similar in all relevant characteristics except exposure to the intervention.[12] With this type of evaluation, the plausibility that the program is "causally" associated with the impacts documented increases with the quality of selection of the control group and with the level of rigor in analytical methods that control for potentially confounding factors. Analyses of dose response (e.g., whether improvements in impact indicators increases with greater exposure to the program) is another important analytical approach that can be used to strengthen the plausibility that the impact identified is due to the program.

Probability **assessments** are designed to provide a high level of certainty that the changes observed in the target population are due to the program's interventions (i.e., causal relationship).[12] Although probability designs are the gold standard of academic efficacy research, they require randomized assignment of treatment and control activities, which often does not make them suitable or viable options in the context of complex public health nutrition programs. First, significant efforts may need to be made to facilitate randomization in the context of a community-based nutrition program: all eligible services, communities, and sometimes individuals need to be listed well before program implementation to carry out the randomization process. The randomization also needs to be planned for before the program is implemented, which may be difficult to achieve. For example, program planners and/or decision makers may have already chosen a location for the program to be implemented, which can inherently limit the number of units eligible for community or cluster randomization and consequently make it difficult to achieve balance in treatment and control groups. Often, decision makers also find it unethical to withhold an intervention that is likely to be beneficial, for the sake of having a comparison (control) group. Aside from these logistical and political challenges, it is important to recognize the stringency required of randomized controlled trials, which, in turn, may result in programmatic conditions that more closely resemble program efficacy, as opposed to a program effectiveness assessment.[12] Habicht and colleagues posit that the gains from a probability assessment in increasing internal validity (showing that the results observed are directly attributable to the program) must be weighed against the losses in external validity (applicability to other contexts).[12]

Other considerations for program evaluation planning include the timeline of the evaluation and whether repeated measurements are desired or required. If repeat measurements are to be conducted, some thought will need to go into whether these should be done on the same (i.e., longitudinal design) or different (i.e., cross-sectional design) individuals or populations. The program design and associated research questions will inform this decision, but ideally, the program's evaluation component is planned as early as possible and alongside program and monitoring systems development. This allows for the collection of baseline data prior to the start of program implementation, as well as for a thorough and continued documentation of program processes as they evolve over time. The number—and timing—of follow-up assessments are also dependent on a number of factors, such as the amount of time required for the program to reach full scale and high coverage, and the time required for the biological effect of the interventions to take place in the target population.[22] For example, child stunting is often the impact indicator used in nutrition evaluations conducted in low- and middle-income contexts, but it is an indicator that may take, at minimum, 12 to 24 months to respond to interventions. Therefore, the timing between evaluation measurements (baseline and end line) should take this into account if using child stunting as the main impact indicator.

Surveillance as an Aid to Impact Evaluation

The French origins of the word **surveillance** (*sur* [over] and *veiller* [watch]) suggest that surveillance is similar in concept to monitoring. Nutrition surveillance systems come in many forms and vary in content, design, and implementation (see chapter 2 for more detail on types of nutrition surveillance), but a fundamental aspect of all nutrition surveillance is that it involves the repeated collection or collation of nutrition-related data with the purpose of detecting trends that can (and should) be used to trigger action to improve nutrition.[30]

A simple example of **nutrition surveillance** comes from humanitarian emergencies, where nongovernmental organizations (NGOs) and the United Nations often collaborate to develop systems that monitor the number of new admissions of acutely malnourished children to treatment centers. When consolidated across centers and regions, and tracked over time, this type of information is often used as a crude indicator to track whether an emergency situation is improving or worsening, and it may also be used to allocate resources to centers with a growing caseload. However, this type of data is limited by uncertain generalizability to the broader catchment population due to potential selection bias; many factors may influence the treatment-seeking behavior for malnutrition, including population proximity to the treatment center, perceptions of the severity of malnutrition, or the value of seeking treatment, for example. A classic paper from Malawi noted that "cross-sectional clinic-based data should be assumed invalid for targeting purposes unless proved otherwise" yet few follow-up studies have tested this hypothesis.[31]

Another type of surveillance, consisting of repeated population-based sample surveys, addresses this limitation. In Bangladesh and Indonesia, large systems developed by Helen Keller International (HKI) in the 1990s and implemented for many years with government and NGO collaboration were designed to track multiple indicators of nutritional status (child stunting, wasting, being underweight, night blindness, anemia, and maternal body mass index) along with determinants of malnutrition such as child and maternal dietary quality, food prices, infectious disease prevalence, and agricultural production.[32-34] Unlike previous surveillance efforts, which operated under the concept of "the simpler, the better," one of the goals of these systems was to understand the multicausal etiology of malnutrition and provide information to inform action in different sectors.

Data were collected multiple times over the calendar year. For example, in Bangladesh, data were collected six times per year corresponding to different seasons, from about 10,000 rural and 1,300 urban children each round.[32] The sampling approach for the system was designed to focus on sentinel sites in different parts of the country to provide representative pictures of different regions of the country as well as the country as a whole. Although not initially designed as a tool to monitor impact of programs, over time, these systems were used to help assess and enhance the impact of many programs including the national preschool vitamin A program in Bangladesh[35] (see box

6.2) and Indonesia,[36] the National Nutrition Program in Bangladesh, and a social marketing campaign promoting dark-green leafy vegetables and eggs in Indonesia.[34]

For purposes of program evaluation, having data from an independent surveillance system may be valuable for a number of reasons. First, it can provide an independent picture of changes in key indicators related to exposure to intervention coverage and/or outcomes, which may be viewed by policy makers as more trustworthy than internal data systems. The repeated and frequent nature of data collection in a system can also allow for a more granular understanding of change (for example, understanding seasonal swings in malnutrition) that may not be possible using a standard pre- and post-evaluation approach. Such systems may be particularly useful in situations where emergencies (floods, rising food prices, or droughts) disrupt programs, as they can help evaluators understand the potential impact of such events when M&E systems are not set up to capture such unanticipated occurrences. Additionally, not all programs can afford to put in place rigorous systems to capture outcome-level indicators, and having at least some indication of trends in outcomes can be valuable. However, unless there is purposive oversampling in program areas (as was done in Bangladesh for the National Nutrition Program, for example), the sample sizes of children/households living in areas exposed to programs may not be adequately powered from a statistical perspective to capture change.

Conclusion

In this chapter, we presented a broad overview of M&E. We used the logic model as the starting point for the development of an M&E framework and under which a stepwise program evaluation can be conducted. We teased out the main purposes of each of the components of M&E, namely, the use of

- monitoring for continuous, repeated, and timely programmatic feedback that can and should be used for course correction and program adaptation throughout the life of the program;
- process evaluation to unpack the black box of program implementation, document program impact pathways, and use the findings to support interpretation of the program impact results;
- impact evaluation to systematically measure the impact of nutrition programs and respective interventions on nutrition outcomes; and
- surveillance as a tool that can help track outcomes and coverage of programs and to understand contextual factors that may influence program impact.

The terminologies and considerations outlined in this chapter and within each of the broad domains of M&E in the context of nutrition programming were not exhaustive but were meant to provide a foundation for the principles that underlie these essential program processes. We also aimed to highlight the importance of a well-functioning and comprehensive M&E framework for evidence-based decision-making and scale-up of nutrition programming.

Review Questions

1. What are some of the main challenges associated with implementing a comprehensive monitoring and evaluation framework in the context of a nutrition program? Some bullets to guide your thinking:
   a. Internal vs. external evaluators
   b. Data quality
   c. Priorities of the various stakeholders involved in program evaluation (program recipients, planners, implementers, and evaluators)
   d. Ethical concerns
   e. Financial concerns
2. Discuss the differences between intervention or treatment efficacy, program efficacy, and program effectiveness and why the three are needed in the context of public health.

3. Pretend that you are a program planner and have contributed to the design and implementation of a large public health nutrition program in your country. Think about and discuss some of the reasons for which you should not be in charge of evaluating that program.

4. Think about the three types of program evaluation designs presented in this chapter: adequacy, plausibility, and probability. Discuss scenarios in which you would use each of these designs and why.

5. Review the opening vignette that highlights the Malawi program M&E framework and activities. Discuss what you would do differently if you were designing either the program monitoring system or evaluation activities and defend your reasoning.

References

1. National Statistical Office, and ICF Macro. 2011. "Malawi Demographic and Health Survey 2010." Zomba, Malawi, and Calverton, Maryland: NSO and ICF Macro.

2. Scaling Up Nutrition. 2011. "Scaling Up Nutrition." Washington, DC.

3. Levinson, F. James, Beatrice Lorge Rogers, Kristin M. Hicks, Thomas Schaetzel, Lisa Troy, and Collette Young. 1999. "Monitoring and Evaluation of Nutrition Programs in Developing Countries." *Nutrition Reviews* 57 (5): 157-64. https://doi.org/10.1111/j.1753-4887.1999.tb01797.x.

4. Khandker, Shahidur R., G. B Koolwal, and Hussian A. Samad. 2010. *Handbook on Impact Evaluation: Quantitative Methods and Practices*. Washington, DC: The World Bank. https://doi.org/10.1596/978-0-8213-8028-4.

5. Centers for Disease Control and Prevention. 1999. "Framework for Program Evaluation in Public Health." *MMWR Recommendations and Reports* 48 (RR11): 1-40.

6. Gertler, Paul J., Sebastian Martinez, Patrick Premand, Laura B. Rawlings, and Christel M. J. Vermeersch. 2011. *Impact Evaluation in Practice*. Washington, DC: The World Bank.

7. Sera, Yumi, and Susan Beaudry. 2007. "Monitoring & Evaluation." Washington, DC: The World Bank.

8. Victora, Cesar G., Damian Walker, Benjamin Johns, and Jennifer Bryce. 2012. "Evaluations of Large-Scale Health Programs." In *Global Health: Diseases, Programs, Systems, and Policies*, edited by Michael Merson, Robert E. Black, and Anne J. Mills, 3rd ed., 815-51. Burlington, MA: Jones & Bartlett Learning.

9. Kim, Sunny S., Jean-Pierre Habicht, Purnima Menon, and Rebecca J. Stoltzfus. 2011. "How Do Programs Work to Improve Child Nutrition? Program Impact Pathways of Three Nongovernmental Organizations Intervention Projects in the Peruvian Highlands." *IFPRI Discussion Paper*. Washington, DC.

10. Lipsey, Mark W. 1993. "Theory as Method: Small Theories of Treatment." *New Directions for Program Evaluation* 57: 5-38.

11. OECD. 2010. "Glossary of Key Terms in Evaluation and Results Based Management." *Evaluation and Aid Effectiveness*, no. 6: 38.

12. Habicht, J. P., C. G. Victora, and J. P. Vaughn. 1999. "Evaluation Designs for Adequacy, Plausibility and Probability of Public Health Programme Performance and Impact." *International Journal of Epidemiology* 28 (1): 10-18. https://doi.org/10.1093/ije/28.1.10.

13. Linnan, Laura, and Allan Steckler. 2002. "Process Evaluation for Public Health Interventions and Research: An Overview." Edited by Laura Linnan and Allan Steckler. https://doi.org/10.1016/j.evalprogplan.2003.09.006.

14. Rossi, Peter H., Mark W. Lipsey, and Howard E. Freeman. 2004. *Evaluation: A Systematic Approach.* 7th edition. Thousand Oaks, CA: Sage.

15. Rawat, Rahul, Phuong H. Nguyen, Disha Ali, Kuntal Saha, Silvia Alayon, Sunny S. Kim, Marie Ruel, and Purnima Menon. 2013. "Learning How Programs Achieve Their Impact: Embedding Theory-Driven Process Evaluation and Other Program Learning Mechanisms in Alive & Thrive." *Food and Nutrition Bulletin* 34 (3 Suppl): S212-25. https://doi.org/10.1177/15648265130343S207.

16. Rossi, Peter H., Mark W. Lipsey, and Howard E. Freeman. 2004. "Expressing and Assessing Program Theory." In *Evaluation: A Systematic Approach*, 7th ed., 155-88. Thousand Oaks: Sage.

17. Wilson, Dawn K, Sarah Griffin, Ruth P Saunders, Heather Kitzman-Ulrich, Duncan C Meyers, and Leslie Mansard. 2009. "Using Process Evaluation for Program Improvement in Dose, Fidelity and Reach: The ACT Trial Experience." *The International Journal of Behavioral Nutrition and Physical Activity* 6: 79. https://doi.org/10.1186/1479-5868-6-79.

18. Basch, Charles E., Elena M. Sliepcevich, Robert S. Gold, David F. Duncan, and Lloyd J. Kolbe. 1985. "Avoiding Type III Errors in Health Education Program Evaluations: A Case Study." *Health Education Quarterly* 12 (4): 315-31. http://www.ncbi.nlm.nih.gov/pubmed/4077544.

19. Habicht, Jean-pierre, and Gretel Pelto. 2014. "From Biological to Program Efficacy: Promoting Dialogue among the Research, Policy, and Program Communities." *Advances in Nutrition* 5: 27-34. https://doi.org/10.3945/an.113.004689.nutrition.

20. Baranowski, Tom, and Gloria Stables. 2000. "Process Evaluations of the 5-a-Day Projects." *Health Education & Behavior* 27 (2): 157-66. https://doi.org/10.1177/109019810002700202.

21. Proctor, Enola, Hiie Silmere, Ramesh Raghavan, Peter Hovmand, Greg Aarons, Alicia Bunger, Richard Griffey, and Melissa Hensley. 2011. "Outcomes for Implementation Research: Conceptual Distinctions, Measurement Challenges, and Research Agenda." *Administration and Policy in Mental Health and Mental Health Services Research* 38 (2): 65-76. https://doi.org/10.1007/s10488-010-0319-7.

22. Victora, Cesar G., Damian Walker, Benjamin Johns, and Jennifer Bryce. 2012. "Evaluations of Large Scale Health Programs." In *Global Health: Disease, Programs, Systems, and Policies,* edited by Michael H. Merson, Robert E. Black, and Ann J. Mills, 3rd ed., pp. 815-51. Burlington, MA: Jones & Bartlett Learning.

23. Bryce, Jennifer, Cesar G. Victora, Jean-Pierre Habicht, J. Patrick Vaughan, and Robert E. Black. 2004. "The Multi-Country Evaluation of the Integrated Management of Childhood Illness Strategy: Lessons for the Evaluation of Public Health Interventions." *American Journal of Public HealthAm J Public Health* 9494 (3): 406-15. https://doi.org/10.2105/AJPH.94.3.406.

24. Gittelsohn, Joel, Marguerite Evans, Mary Story, Sally M. Davis, Lauve Metcalfe, Devorah L. Helitzer, and Theresa E. Clay. 1999. "Multisite Formative Assessment for the Pathways Study to Prevent Obesity in American Indian

Schoolchildren." *American Journal of Clinical* 69 (4): 767S-772S. https://doi.org/10 .1097/OGX.0000000000000256.Prenatal.

25. "The ILiNS Project." 2017. University of California-Davis. https://ilins. ucdavis.edu/.

26. Hess, Sonja Y., Souheila Abbeddou, Elizabeth Yakes Jimenez, Jérôme W Somé, Stephen A. Vosti, Zinéwendé P. Ouédraogo, Rosemonde M. Guissou, Jean-Bosco Ouédraogo, and Kenneth H. Brown. 2015. "Small-Quantity Lipid-Based Nutrient Supplements, Regardless of Their Zinc Content, Increase Growth and Reduce the Prevalence of Stunting and Wasting in Young Burkinabe Children: A Cluster-Randomized Trial." Edited by James G. Beeson. *PLoS One* 10 (3): e0122242. https://doi.org/10.1371/journal.pone.0122242.

27. Adu-afarwuah, Seth, Anna Lartey, Kenneth H. Brown, Stanley Zlotkin, André Briend, and Kathryn G. Dewey. 2007. "Randomized Comparison of 3 Types of Micronutrient Supplements for Home Fortification of Complementary Foods in Ghana: Effects on Growth and Motor Development." *The American Journal of Clinical Nutrition* 86 (2): 412-20.

28. Pulakka, Anna, Per Ashorn, Yin B. Cheung, Kathryn G. Dewey, Ken Maleta, S. Vosti, and Ulla Ashorn. 2015. "Effect of 12-Month Intervention with Lipid-Based Nutrient Supplements on Physical Activity of 18-Month-Old Malawian Children: A Randomised, Controlled Trial." *European Journal of Clinical Nutrition* 69 (2): 173-78. https://doi.org/10.1038/ejcn.2014.138.

29. Ashorn, Per, Lotta Alho, Ulla Ashorn, Yin Bun Cheung, Kathryn G Dewey, Ulla Harjunmaa, Anna Lartey, et al. 2015. "The Impact of Lipid-Based Nutrient Supplement Provision to Pregnant Women on Newborn Size in Rural Malawi: A Randomized Controlled Trial 1-4." *The American Journal of Clinical Nutrition* 101: 387-97. https://doi.org/10.3945/ajcn.114.088617.1.

30. United Nations Children's Fund (UNICEF). 1976. "Methodology of Nutrition Surveillance: Report of a Joint FAO/UNICEF/WHO Expert Committee." New York, NY.

31. Pelletier, David L., and Catherine F. Johnson. 1994. "The Validity of Clinic-Based Nutrition Surveillance Data: A Study from Selected Sites in Northern Malawi." *Food and Nutrition Bulletin* 15 (4): 308-19.

32. McClure, K., and E. Haytmanek. 2010. *Mitigating the Nutritional Impacts of the Global Food Price Crisis*. Washington, DC: National Academies Press. https://doi.org /10.17226/12698.

33. Thorne-Lyman, Andrew L., Natalie Valpiani, Kai Sun, Richard D. Semba, Christine L. Klotz, and Klaus Kraemer. 2010. "Household Dietary Diversity and Food Expenditures Are Closely Linked in Rural Bangladesh, Increasing the Risk of Malnutrition Due to the Financial Crisis." *The Journal of Nutrition* 140 (1): 182s-8s. https://doi.org/10.3945/jn.109.110809.

34. Pee, Saskia de, Martin W. Bloem, Satoto, Ray Yip, Asmira Sukaton, Roy Tjiong, Roger Shrimpton, Muhilal, and Benny Kodyat. 1998. "Impact of a Social Marketing Campaign Promoting Dark-Green Leafy Vegetables and Eggs in Central Java, Indonesia." *International Journal of Vitamin Nutrition Research* 68 (6): 389-98. http://www.ncbi.nlm.nih.gov/pubmed/9857267.

35. Akhter, N., C. Witten, G. Stallkamp, V. Anderson, S. de Pee, and N. Haselow. 2008. "Children Aged 12-59 Months Missed through the National Surveillance Project." *The Journal of Field Actions* 1.

36. Berger, Sarah G., Saskia de Pee, Martin W. Bloem, Siti Halati, and Richard D. Semba. 2007. "Malnutrition and Morbidity Are Higher in Children Who Are Missed by Periodic Vitamin A Capsule Distribution for Child Survival in Rural Indonesia." *The Journal of Nutrition* 137 (5): 1328-33. https://doi.org/10.1093/jn/137.5.1328.

37. Olney, Deanna K., Aminuzzaman Talukder, Lora L. Iannotti, Marie T. Ruel, and Victoria Quinn. 2009. "Assessing Impact and Impact Pathways of a Homestead Food Production Program on Household and Child Nutrition in Cambodia." *Food and Nutrition Bulletin* 30 (4): 355-69. https://doi.org/10.1177/156482650903000407.

38. Olney, Deanna K., Sao Vicheka, Meng Kro, Chhom Chakriya, Hou Kroeun, Ly Sok Hoing, Aminzzaman Talukder, et al. 2013. "Using Program Impact Pathways to Understand and Improve Program Delivery, Utilization, and Potential for Impact of Helen Keller International's Homestead Food Production Program in Cambodia." *Food and Nutrition Bulletin* 34 (2): 169-84. https://doi.org/10.1177/156482651303400206.

PART TWO

Major Nutrition-Related Disease Burdens

7

Nutrition-Related Disease Burdens in High-Income Countries

Colin D. Rehm

LEARNING OBJECTIVES

- Describe the role of the demographic, epidemiologic, and nutrition transitions in shaping the leading causes of disease in countries
- List the leading nutrition-related diseases and the dietary risk factors responsible for these diseases in high-income countries
- Describe general methods used to estimate the disease burden due to suboptimal diet

Case Study: The Science and History of *Trans* Fat and Cardiovascular Disease

Artificial **trans fat** were first introduced in the early 1900s after being invented by a German chemist named Wilhelm Normann. *Trans* fats are created by adding hydrogen to liquid vegetable oils to create a solid or semisolid fat. *Trans* fats had numerous advantages over other fats, specifically butter and lard: they did not require refrigeration, had a much longer shelf life, and were cheaper and easier to use in food production. In the United States, the rights to the technique were obtained by Procter & Gamble, who began marketing Crisco as the first hydrogenated shortening. Common forms of *trans* fats include margarine, shortening, and frying oils. One particularly problematic source of *trans* fat, particularly from the 1950s onward, was margarines, which were often used by consumers trying to avoid saturated fats found in butter. At the time, saturated fats were an oft-cited cause of heart disease.[1,2] In addition to artificial *trans* fats, there are also naturally occurring *trans* fats, mostly found in red meat and dairy products, though this section will refer to artificial *trans* fats as just *trans* fats for simplicity.

As early as the 1970s there was limited scientific evidence that *trans* fats were not a healthful alternative to other fats, though this research did not impact regulation in the United States.[3,4] By the early 1990s and the emergence of additional evidence, particularly from large prospective cohort studies, it became more and more clear that *trans* fats likely caused an increased risk of heart disease. Specifically, a 1993 paper out of the Nurses' Health Study published in *The Lancet*, found that women in the highest quintile of *trans* fat intake had a 50% increased risk of heart disease.[5] While no paper can singly lead to policy change, additional evidence was found of an association with heart disease and a general consensus emerged in the scientific community.[6-11] The mechanism by which *trans* fat increases heart disease risk is through increasing levels of low-density lipoprotein (LDL), while also lowering high-density lipoprotein (HDL), thereby increasing the risk of heart disease. As compared to saturated fats, which only increase LDL, *trans* fats were particularly risky because of their parallel impact on HDL.[12,13] Furthermore, there is evidence that *trans* fat consumption increases systemic inflammation and endothelial dysfunction, both of which are independent risk factors of heart disease.[14]

As with any purported health risk, there is considerable uncertainty as to when science should be translated to policy. In retrospect, it can be all too easy to ridicule or apply judgment regarding perceived inaction when we later learn "we" were correct (or to criticize action when "we" may have been wrong [e.g., beta-carotene and vitamin A and lung cancer]).[15] With that in mind, given new evidence regarding the harms of *trans* fat, policy efforts to reduce intake of *trans* fat were explored throughout the world. In the United States, this approach started with a Food and Drug Administration (FDA) proposal to add *trans* fat content to the Nutrition Facts Panel in 1999, a decision not fully realized until 2008.[16] Even after the label was implemented in the United States it was still criticized as any amount of *trans* fat less than 0.5 grams per serving could be labeled as containing zero *trans* fats. Consumers were educated to assess the ingredients for key terms like *hydrogenated* to identify foods that contain *trans* fat. The addition of a *trans* fat label did lead some food producers to reformulate products.[17]

While the United States spent considerable time implementing the *trans* fat label, one country was particularly aggressive in eliminating *trans* fats in the food supply. Denmark implemented a policy seriously limiting the use of *trans* in 2003. Details on the policy making process are described in detail elsewhere, but the highlights are provided here.[18,19] In brief, a professional advocacy organization called the Danish Nutrition Council played a critical role by producing a scientific report on the health effects of *trans* fat. Other organizations in the region argued that *trans* fat was no more harmful than saturated fat and should not be the target of extra intervention. Through a series of reports (1994, 2001, 2003) spearheaded by the Danish Nutrition Council, food manufacturers, mainly the margarine industry, began to voluntarily reduce the use of *trans* fats as a response to these reports and the connected media campaigns. One notable aspect of the Danish experience was that food manufacturers began voluntarily reducing *trans* fat. In addition, strong support from the Ministers of Food and Agriculture is cited as an important aspect of the process.

In 2003 the policy was formally implemented, which required the content of *trans* fats to not exceed 2 grams per 100 grams of oil or solid fat. For comparison, partially hydrogenated shortening has about 43% (or 43 grams per 100 grams) of the total fat content from *trans* fat. This policy therefore banned *trans* fats above the set level of 2 grams per 100 grams. After the policy was implemented, one area of pushback was whether the proposed *trans* fat ban violated European Union free trade agreements, though the case was ultimately dropped. It is not terribly surprising that Denmark was the first country to ban *trans* fat as it is a socially progressive country (Denmark ranks number 1 on the Social Progress Index), whose residents are generally more accepting of government intervention,[20] as opposed to high-income countries with somewhat more libertarian leanings, such as the United States.

Later evaluations examining the impact of the ban found that rates of decline in coronary heart disease (CHD) mortality was the highest in Denmark as compared to other EU members,[21] though this study was not able to control well for other factors that may have contributed to this reduction. A later, more sophisticated evaluation comparing mortality rates as observed in Denmark to a "synthetic" Denmark where no policy was implemented found that the ban reduced cardiovascular disease mortality in Denmark by 22 deaths per 100,000 people per year, or about 5.5% per year.[22] To put this effect size in context, in Denmark in 2016, the mortality rate from unintentional injuries (e.g., falls, drowning, motor vehicle collisions) was 20 per 100,000, meaning that the *trans* fat ban was roughly equivalent to eliminating all mortality from unintentional injuries.

Bans on *trans* fat followed throughout other high-income countries, including Austria, Switzerland, Iceland, and Sweden, among others. In the United States, local jurisdictions and states, such as New York City, Montgomery County (MD), and California, among many others, implemented *trans* fat bans. In 2013 the US FDA announced a preliminary determination that partially hydrogenated oils are no longer "generally regarded as safe," a critical decision that would eventually lead to gradual implementation of widespread reformulation and elimination of artificial *trans* fats in the US food supply. An evaluation from New York found that early *trans* fat bans in New York counties were associated with a substantial decrease in heart attacks (7.8% decline), thus adding to growing evidence that policies to ban *trans* fats resulted in significant public health benefits.[23]

Although the leading causes of death and disease for **high-income countries** and low-income countries (see box 7.1 for definitions of high- and low-income countries) are different, in both cases, many of the leading causes of death and disease in the United States and other high-income countries are nutrition-related diseases, meaning that specific foods, nutrients, dietary patterns, or weight status are implicated as causes of these diseases. For instance, the leading causes of death in the United States include ischemic heart disease, diabetes, and stroke, which have been linked to high body mass index (BMI) and suboptimal diet. In fact, current research suggests that dietary

Box 7.1. Defining High-Income Countries

There are a number of methods that can be used to define countries as *high-income*. The current chapter uses definitions produced by the World Bank are based on the **gross national income (GNI)**.[24] Gross National Income is the gross domestic product plus the value from resident wages received abroad, property income and taxes and subsidies received from abroad. For the current chapter we defined **high-income countries** as those with a gross national income between $3,956 and $12,235 (upper-middle income) and a GNI ≥$12,236 (high income). Lower-income and lower-middle income countries are discussed in chapter 9. Almost half (49.4%) of the world population reside in high- (15.5%) and upper-middle-income countries (33.9%). The six most populous high-income countries include the United States, Japan, Germany, France,

the United Kingdom, and Italy. The most populous upper-middle-income countries include China, Brazil, Russia, Mexico, Iran, and Turkey. There is substantial variation in gross national income for high-income countries, ranging 20-fold from $82,390 (Norway) to $4,060 (Tonga). See figure showing the high-income countries.

Beyond the World Bank income-based grouping, perhaps the most commonly used measure is the **Human Development Index (HDI)**, produced by the United Nations Development Programme.[25] The HDI combines data on life expectancy, education, and GNI to create a summary measure not driven entirely by income. Given that GNI is one component of the HDI, there is a very strong exponential correlation between HDI and GNI (r = 0.89).

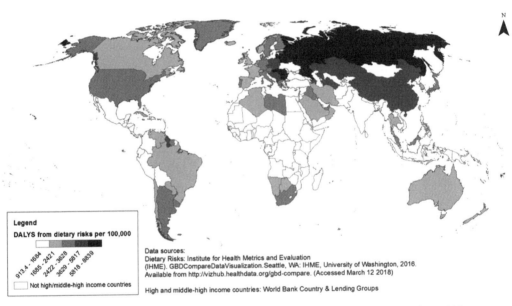

Legend

DALYS from dietary risks per 100,000

913.4 - 1684   1685 - 2421   2422 - 3628   3629 - 5817   5818 - 8839

Not high/middle-high income countries

Data sources:
Dietary Risks: Institute for Health Metrics and Evaluation (IHME). GBDCompareDataVisualization.Seattle, WA: IHME, University of Washington, 2016. Available from http://vizhub.healthdata.org/gbd-compare. (Accessed March 12 2018)

High and middle-high income countries: World Bank Country & Lending Groups

Map of high- and middle-high income countries per World Bank criteria and disability-adjusted life years (DALYs) per 100,000 from dietary risks (2016). *Source:* Institute for Health Metrics and Evaluation (IHME). GBD Compare. Seattle, WA: IHME, University of Washington, 2017. http://vizhub.healthdata.org/gbd-compare.

factors may be responsible for up to 45% of cardiometabolic deaths in the United States.[26]

This chapter will introduce the concepts of the population-level **disease burdens**. We will briefly discuss how the demographic, epidemiologic, and nutrition transitions influence the population-level disease burdens and discuss the leading causes of death in high-income countries. We will then take a closer look at how public health researchers estimate the degree to which nutritional factors contribute to the risk for various diseases and ultimately the population-level disease burdens. This task of estimating the degree to which nutritional factors are related to leading diseases and causes of death is a multistep process that requires many inputs. We will examine the basic inputs required and the process for determining disease and death burdens and for attributing these diseases and deaths to risk factors, such as dietary factors.

Disease Burdens and the Epidemiologic, Demographic, and Nutrition Transitions

The disease burden in high-income countries is typified by a relatively higher burden of **noncommunicable disease** and a relatively lower burden related to **communicable disease**, undernutrition, and injuries. This contrasts with the disease burden in low-income countries, which is typified by a relatively higher burden of communicable diseases, undernutrition, and injury and a relatively lower burden of noncommunicable diseases. Typically, as countries experience economic development, the disease burden distribution changes, with a shift away from communicable disease and undernutrition towards noncommunicable diseases. The differences in the relative contribution of these different types of diseases in countries across the income spectrum can be seen in box 7.1.

Figure 7.1 provides details on which diseases contribute the most to the total disease burden for the United States, China, India, and Ethiopia, the most populous high-, upper-middle, low-middle, and low-income countries, respectively, based on World Bank cutoffs. The left-hand side of each graph refers to noncommunicable disease; top right, infectious diseases and nutritional deficiencies; and lower right, injuries.

The term **epidemiologic transition** is used to describe this shift in the disease burden from communicable disease, undernutrition and injuries (resulting in high infant, under 5, and maternal mortality, and low life expectancy) to noncommunicable disease. The epidemiologic transition is a gradual process that takes many decades. It is difficult to put an exact date on when a country or region has undergone the epidemiologic transition, but in the United States, the epidemiologic transition appeared to begin around the turn of the 20th century and was complete around the time of World War II.[27,28] The epidemiologic transition is accompanied by a demographic transition

A

United States
Both sexes, All ages, 2016, DALYs

Annual % change
1990 ▸ to 2017 ▸
DALYs/100,000

B

China
Both sexes, All ages, 2016, DALYs

Annual % change
1990 ▸ to 2017 ▸
DALYs/100,000

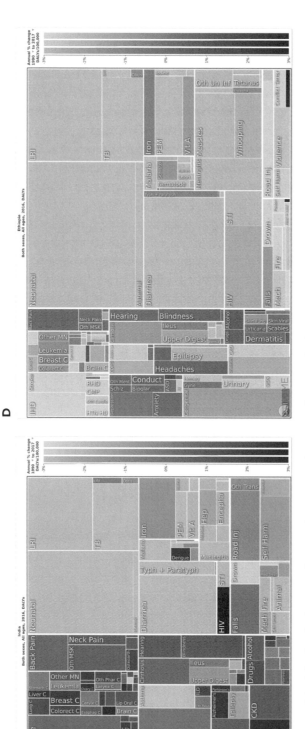

Figure 7.1. Comparison of disability burden by cause for United States (A), China (B), India (C), and Ethiopia (D). *Source:* 2016 Global Burden of Disease Study. Institute for Health Metrics and Evaluation (IHME). GBD Compare. Seattle, WA: IHME, University of Washington, 2017. http://vizhub.healthdata.org/gbd-compare.

where mortality rates and fertility rates decline, resulting in lower natural population growth and a gradual aging of the population (according to the US Census, the median age increased from 29 to 37.2 from 1940-2010). At the population level, both the epidemiologic and demographic transition are proceeded or accompanied by rising incomes and urbanization,[29] and improvements to public health infrastructure and health care.

Related to the epidemiologic and demographic transition is the **nutrition transition**. The nutrition transition is typically characterized by a shift away from a traditional plant- and cereal-based diet to a more "Western" diet, characterized by increasing consumption of sugar, fat, and animal protein, as well as more calories in general.[30-32] The nutrition transition is directly linked to the epidemiologic transition in that changes in the dietary patterns of the population and increased availability of adequate amounts and specific types (e.g., animal protein) of food result in a lower burden of undernutrition, protein energy malnutrition, and related outcomes, but an increased burden in obesity, diabetes, some cancers, and other cardiovascular risk factors. These three "transitions" each collectively contribute to changes in the risk factor distribution of the population (e.g., increases in protein intake) and changes in the burden of disease (e.g., decreasing burden related to child growth problems due to protein energy malnutrition).[33] Low- and middle-income countries are actively undergoing these three transitions, and in many areas they are simultaneously experiencing a high burden of communicable and noncommunicable diseases.[34] This double burden of disease or dual-nutrition burden (both terms are used) poses a major public health challenge. The nutrition transition and the double burden of disease are both discussed in more depth in chapter 10.

Overview of Dietary Risks as a Contributor to the Disease Burden

Table 7.1 presents the top 10 leading causes of death, morbidity, and disability (death plus disability) for high-income countries. The impact of a cause (e.g., cardiovascular disease) or a risk factor (e.g., smoking) on the combined concepts of morbidity and mortality is referred to as the disease burden. As such, the disease burden can be measured for direct causes of ill health, such as cancer or heart disease, or for risk factors, which can be thought of as the causes of the causes, and would include behavioral, environmental, or metabolic risk factors, such as smoking, air pollution, or elevated body mass index. Details on estimating the disease burden are described below, with special consideration of how dietary risk factors are assessed. For high-income countries, the leading causes of death were ischemic heart disease, stroke, and Alzheimer's disease and dementia. The leading causes of morbidity were low back and neck pain, sense organ disease, and diabetes. The leading causes of disability overall were ischemic heart disease, stroke, and diabetes. In general terms, the leading causes of disability overall are a com-

Table 7.1. Top 10 Causes of Deaths, Morbidity, and Disability in High-Income Countries from the 2016 Global Burden of Disease Study

Leading causes of deaths (rank)	Leading causes of morbidity[a] (rank)	Leading causes of disability[b] (rank)
Ischemic heart disease (1)	Low back and neck pain (1)	Ischemic heart disease (1)
Stroke (2)	Sense organ diseases (2)	Stroke (2)
Alzheimer's disease and other dementias (3)	Diabetes, urogenital, blood and endocrine diseases (3)	Diabetes, urogenital, blood and endocrine diseases (3)
Diabetes, urogenital, blood and endocrine diseases (4)	Skin and subcutaneous diseases (4)	Low back and neck pain (4)
Chronic obstructive pulmonary disease (5)	Depressive disorders (5)	Road injuries (5)
Lung cancer (6)	Migraine (6)	Sense organ diseases (6)
Road injuries (7)	Anxiety disorders (7)	Lung cancer (7)
Chronic kidney disease (8)	Other musculoskeletal disorders (8)	Chronic obstructive pulmonary disease (8)
Liver cancer (9)	Falls (9)	Skin and subcutaneous diseases (9)
Colon and rectum cancer (10)	Oral disorders (10)	Depressive disorders (10)

[a] Morbidity refers to nonfatal health events.
[b] Disability refers to the combined contribution of morbidity and mortality.

bination of the leading causes of death and morbidity. Poor diet and elevated BMI have been associated with many of the leading causes of death and disability, so public health nutrition practitioners working in many high-income countries will focus on improving diet or weight status with the end goal of preventing these outcomes.

As noncommunicable diseases have become the primary public health threat in high-income countries in the postwar period, biomedical and public health research has shifted attention to identifying the behavioral and dietary contributors to disease.[1,2] Until the late 1990s, the focus of dietary risk factor research was typically focused on identifying single macronutrients (e.g., saturated fat) or micronutrients vitamins (e.g., vitamin C, sodium, or potassium)[35] that might play a role in disease risk. More recently, there has been a shift to focus on the contribution of foods and dietary patterns, as opposed to individual nutrients,[36,37] as risk factors in disease risk. The rationale for the more recent focus on foods and dietary patterns is described in chapter 10. To this end, dietary guidelines in multiple countries now embrace

Table 7.2. Relative Risks Associated with Dietary Factors among 40- to 44-Year-Olds from the 2016 Global Burden of Disease Study

	Units of relative risk interpretation	Cardiometabolic outcomes[a]				Lung cancer	Cancers[b]	
		Ischemic heart disease	Ischemic stroke	Hemorrhagic stroke	Diabetes		Colorectal cancer	Esophageal cancer
Dietary risk factor with direct association								
Low fruit	100 g/d	1.131	1.48	1.365	1.113	1.076	—	1.153
Low whole grains	50 g/d	1.228	1.466	1.276	1.208	—	—	—
Low vegetables	100 g/d	1.126	1.132	1.102	—	—	—	—
High processed meat	50 g/d	1.545	—	—	1.824	—	1.179	—
Low nuts & seeds	4.05 g/d	1.084	—	—	1.045	—	—	—
High red meat	100 g/d	—	—	—	1.288	—	1.167	—
Low fiber	20 g/d	1.45	—	—	—	—	1.236	—
Low omega-3	100 mg/d	1.173	—	—	—	—	—	—
Low PUFA	5% energy/d	1.114	—	—	—	—	—	—
High *trans* fat	2% energy/d	1.517	—	—	—	—	—	—
Low milk	226.8 g/d	—	—	—	—	—	1.113	—
Low calcium	1000 mg/d	—	—	—	—	—	1.372	—
Low legumes	50 g/d	1.332	—	—	—	—	—	—
Dietary risk factor with mediated association								
High sugar-sweetened beverages	Per 5 kg/m²	1.599	1.826	2.389	3.16	—	M: 1.177 / F: 1.059	M: 1.391 / F: 1.351
High sodium	Per 10 mmHg systolic BP	1.568	1.628	1.874	—	—	—	—

[a] Relative risks for only a select number of cancers with the highest burden of disease attribute to diet are presented here. Additionally, there are summary relative risks for fruit related to lip and oral cavity cancer, nasopharynx cancer, other pharynx cancer, and larynx cancer. For sodium there are additional relative risks for rheumatic heart disease, hypertensive heart disease, other cardiomyopathy, atrial fibrillation and flutter, peripheral vascular disease, endocarditis, chronic kidney disease (CKD) due to diabetes, CKD due to hypertension, CKD due to glomerulonephritis, and CKD due to other causes.

[b] Data presented for males as there is effect.

a diet pattern approach as opposed to focusing on single nutrients[38-40] (see chapter 14 for a comparison of different countries' dietary guidelines).

In terms of attributing population-level disease burdens to different dietary factors, given the methodological constraints of disease burden work, most research to date has focused on individual foods/food groups or nutrients, having not yet extended to dietary patterns. For instance, table 7.2 displays a summary of relative risks of leading causes of ill health associated with 10 different dietary factors.

The relative risks displayed in table 7.2 were used by the 2016 Global Burden of Disease project (described in further detail later in this chapter) to estimate the contribution of each of these factors to the population burden of disease and are presented for the 40- to 44-year-old age group for illustrative purposes. For older ages, the relative risks are typically smaller and vice versa for younger. It is important to remember that the interpretation of these relative risks depends on the units in which they are parameterized. While some of these relative risks may appear quite small, they are for more modest amounts of intake (e.g., 4.05 g/d of nuts/seeds = 4 almonds). If we converted this to equal a common serving of nuts (e.g., 28 grams), the relative risk would be about 1.75 (for those interested, the details of the calculation are provided here: take the natural log of 1.084, multiply by 6.92 [28 / 4.05] and exponentiate to get the relative risk for a 28 g/d decrease).

Numerous dietary factors are thought to have a causal relationship with adverse outcomes, namely cardiometabolic outcomes (cardiovascular disease plus diabetes) and some cancers. The primary cardiometabolic outcomes of interest are ischemic heart disease, ischemic stroke, hemorrhagic stroke, and diabetes. For diabetes, established dietary risk factors include processed meats, red meat, and sugar-sweetened beverages (SSB, mediated through impact of SSBs on BMI), and protective factors include fruit, whole grains, and nuts and seeds.[41-44] For both ischemic and hemorrhagic stroke, sodium and SSBs are thought to be causally associated risk factors and fruit, whole grains, and vegetables are thought to be protective factors.[45,46] Processed meat, *trans* fat, SSBs, and sodium are all risk factors for ischemic heart disease. Fruit, whole grains, vegetables, nuts and seeds, fiber, omega-3 fats, polyunsaturated fats, and legumes all have a protective association with ischemic heart disease.[42,44,45,47,48] For cancer, there is a modest protective association between fruit consumption and lung cancer.[49] Colorectal cancer is the cancer outcome with the strongest links to diet. Processed meat, red meat, and SSBs are all risk factors for colorectal cancer, and fiber, milk, and calcium are thought to be protective factors.[49,50] For esophageal cancer, fruit is a protective factor and SSBs are a risk factor.[51,52]

Tables such as table. 7.2 are summaries of an immense amount of scientific data. There can be disagreement as to the inclusion/exclusion of a specific risk factor–outcome pair. The Continuous Update Project (CUP) out of the World Cancer Research Fund (WCRF) and American Institute for Cancer Research (AICR) produces detailed reports summarizing the association between diet and cancer outcomes.[50] In most cases, these reports align with others, though differential interpretation of the evidence can occur. For colorectal cancer, the CUP indicates that there is evidence that whole grains reduce the risk of colorectal cancer, but the Global Burden of Disease study does not include a relative risk for this diet-disease relationship. However, the two projects do agree on processed meat, red meat, dietary fiber, and dairy products.[52] Similarly, there is typically agreement on the lack of convincing or probable associations. The CUP includes no dietary factors as probable or convincing risk factors for breast cancer or prostate cancer, consistent with the relative risks used by the Global Burden of Disease (GBD) project.[50,52] Some potential dietary risk factors for cardiometabolic disease that were not included in the 2016 GBD study but for which there could be some argument about their inclusion include yogurt (diabetes), glycemic load (ischemic heart disease, stroke, and diabetes), and potassium (stroke).[53] For readers interested in exploring the leading causes of death and disability in different countries or regions on their own, I recommend visiting the Global Burden of Disease Compare tool available online (https://vizhub.healthdata.org/gbd-compare/).[54] This tool is updated with each cycle of the Global Burden of Disease report and can be used to estimate disease and risk factor burdens by location (e.g., country, sub-national area for some countries or regional aggregations), time, sex, and age group.

Overview of Methods to Assess Disease Burden

The statement at the beginning of this chapter that "45% of cardiometabolic deaths are thought to be attributed to suboptimal dietary intake" is deceptively simple.[26] In fact, formally characterizing the burden of disease is a time- and methodologically intensive process. Prior to the 1990s there was no cohesive framework for assessing the burden of disease and the contribution of specific risk factors to the disease burden. Lacking such a framework, stakeholders could select the estimates that put their topic in the best (or worst) light depending on their interests. As an illustrative, fictitious example, a diabetes advocacy group interested in building a case that diabetes is a leading contributor to death rates could count all diabetes deaths and a subset of ischemic heart disease and stroke deaths (given the well-established association between diabetes and these outcomes). At the same time, a heart disease organization could count all cardiovascular deaths and some diabetes deaths. All of a sudden you could have a single death counted multiple times by a handful of organizations. In addition, due to data limitations on nonfatal health states, prior to the 1990s, there tended to be undue focus on the causes of death (e.g., heart disease and cancer), as opposed to the causes of disability and general ill health (e.g., mental health or joint pain). The advent of the comparative risk assessment (CRA) framework by Murray and Lopez for the 1990 Global Burden of Disease (GBD) study funded by the World Bank in collaboration with Harvard University and the World Health Organization substantially increased the rigor of disease burden work, sidestepping the problem described above. Specific improvements included the use of comparable methods for all calculations, incorporating data on nonfatal health status, and adjusting for known biases in the data.

Among the key findings from the 1990 Global Burden of Disease study were that noncommunicable diseases were significant causes in all regions (not just high-income countries) and that mental health disorders were major causes of disability that were previously underappreciated. In addition, the study found that noncommunicable disease were a leading cause of ill health throughout the world, including lower-income regions. With new iterations of the Global Burden of Disease study every few years (and annually in recent years), the methods have undergone substantial improvements and inputs have become increasingly complex and sophisticated.

Briefly, the CRA framework allows for the estimation of the burden of disease to be attributed to a specific cause of risk factor in a manner that is completely internally consistent. The availability of internally consistent data is a critical step in using data to inform program and policy development. Comparative risk assessment (CRA) work allows us to ask the important conceptual, albeit simplified, question: if we can intervene in one area, assuming all interventions are equally effective, where should we intervene? Unfortunately, the real world is messy in that some interventions are much more effective, some are effective but costly, and so on. These methods can also be adapted to compare the impact of potential policies and for determining the cost-effectiveness of potential interventions.

This section briefly summarizes the key inputs into the CRA framework and describes the practical assumptions required to systematically assess the burden of disease. This sort of work requires an immense amount of data and calculations. The 2016 Global Burden of Disease risk factor report alone includes more than 400 pages of methodological details and 3,500 pages of formatted output.[54] Additional publications highlight the causes of death and disability.[55-57]

Summarizing Exposure-Disease Relationships

One necessary input to the comparative risk assessment model is an estimate of the degree to which exposure to a risk factor (i.e., *trans* fat) increases risk of disease (i.e. ischemic heart disease). We call these **exposure–disease relationships**. This section provides a brief overview of the steps taken to estimate exposure-disease relationships. The first step in summarizing the impact of an exposure-disease relationship is determining if a potential risk factor is an actual cause of ill health or disease. In some cases, establishing such an association is relatively straightforward (e.g., smoking is causally re-lated to lung cancer), but for other risk factors, particularly for those that are behavioral in nature (such as dietary intake), inferring causation is difficult and can often lead to controversy and disagreement. In biomedical research, often the randomized controlled trial is hailed as the best study design for determining whether a risk factor causes a disease. However, randomized controlled trials are often not feasible for studying diet-disease relationships due to the fact that many noncommunicable diseases develop over a lifetime and it is unrealistic to randomize individuals to a specific diet for a long enough period of time to influence the development of disease endpoints (this is discussed more in chapter 3).

Instead, other approaches must be used to weigh the evidence for or against a particular risk factor being a causal agent in disease. One common framework for evaluating whether an association is likely causal is the Brad-ford Hill approach.[58] Sir (Austin) Bradford Hill was an influential epidemi-ologist, who, with Richard Doll, led some of the earliest investigations into smoking as a cause of lung cancer.[59] While his approach is often referred to as a "criteria," an exposure-disease relationship may not meet all "criteria" but still be determined to be likely to be "causal."[60] The criteria include the strength of the association (usually assessed by the size of the relative risk), the consistency of the exposure-disease association (is the same association observed in other studies conducted in other populations?), the specificity of the association (is the association strongest when we expect it to be the strongest?), the temporal relationship between exposure and outcome (does the exposure proceed the outcome?), the biological gradient or dose response (do higher amounts of exposure lead to increased/decreased risk?), coherence (are laboratory studies consistent with epidemiologic studies?), analogy (does a comparable risk factor have an impact on a comparable outcome?), the bi-ological plausibility, and experimental evidence (are randomized controlled trials available?). The trump card in the Bradford Hill approach is the pres-ence of experimental evidence, which is quite challenging in the nutritional context given the practical challenges in changing individuals' dietary hab-its over the long term as noted above. However, some nutritional questions, particularly those looking at short-term outcomes (e.g., change in blood pres-sure) or where the intervention is relatively straightforward (e.g., use olive oil or eat nuts) are more suited to experiments[61-63] but can still be difficult to implement in practice.[64]

Nevertheless, for most exposure-disease relationships adequate experi-mental evidence is lacking, so observational studies must be used. **Prospec-tive cohort studies** are the most common source of information about poten-tial diet-disease relationships. Traditional case-control studies are of limited use in nutritional epidemiology given concerns about retrospectively assessing dietary intakes and reverse causation, though nested case-control studies are frequently used when biomarkers of dietary intake are available.[65,66]

Researchers often use an approach called **meta-analysis** to combine the results of numerous observational studies (or randomized controlled trials) to come up with a single combined estimate of the association between a dietary factor and a health outcome based on the weight of the published science. Originally created to pool data from randomized controlled trials of drugs, which often had small sample sizes, meta-analyses have been widely used for observational studies on various population health topics, including nutrition.[41-44,47,48,53,66] While a powerful tool to combine scientific data, the use of meta-analyses in nutritional epidemiology has been critiqued due to differences in dietary assessment methods and baseline exposure distributions, for lacking consistent comparators, and most importantly, differences in study quality.[67] Furthermore, simply combining error-prone or confounded estimates of exposure–disease relationships does nothing to eliminate these biases or strengthen causal inference.

Table 7.2 is an example of summary estimates of diet-disease relationships for which evidence was compelling enough to consider these factors causally related to disease risk.

Characterizing Risk Factor Distributions

After deciding what dietary risk factors are "causes" of disease, data summarizing the extent to which the population is exposed or not exposed to that risk factor is needed. This is sometimes referred to as assessing the distribution of the risk factor. Taking the example of fruit, an established risk factor for heart disease, diabetes, and lung cancer among others, we need to understand how much fruit the population consumes (e.g., the distribution of intake). In practice, this is done by combining numerous data sources to develop age, sex, time, and country distributions for each risk factor. In other words, what was the distribution of fruit intake among women 40-44 years of age in the United States in 2016? These data inputs are then repeated for all the strata or groups of interest. Using group-level data is critical, as risk factor distributions can vary dramatically by age, sex, geography, and so on.

Data from nationally representative surveys are a key source of data on risk factor distributions. The prevalence of smoking, for example, can be reasonably well estimated from population-based surveys, with some adjustments for potential underreporting to correct for known biases. For other factors, including dietary factors, deriving high-quality estimates of risk factor distributions is more complex. Chapter 3 describes the primary approaches to assessing diets, including the food frequency questionnaire (FFQ) and 24-hour dietary recall (24H). FFQs are typically used in large nutritional epidemiology observational studies that require a fast and relatively low-cost method for assessing the habitual dietary intakes of a large population in epidemiologic studies[68] but are not the primary tool used for population-based dietary surveillance. For dietary surveillance (as described further in chapter 2), methods like 24H recalls or food records, which attempt to capture all foods/beverages consumed (as opposed to a sample of foods), are used. While FFQs can be used to rank individual intakes, they are not the best tool to address nutrient (in)sufficiency, an important historical and current use of dietary surveillance surveys. Statistical models can be built that combine data from various data sources (e.g., combine data from FFQs and food disappearance data) and correct for differences in modalities of data collection across time and geography.

The measurement characteristics of different dietary instruments differ from instrument-to-instrument and from dietary factor to dietary factor (e.g., vitamin C measurements tend to be more valid than sodium).[69] In limited cases, biomarkers can be used to estimate exposure distributions.[68] For dietary factors relevant to high-income countries, urinary sodium is the only biomarker of nutritional intake used in burden of disease work.[70,71]

The Potential Impact Fraction and the Theoretical Minimum Risk Exposure Level

After determining the distribution of current intakes of each dietary factor, the next step in determining the population-level disease burden is to measure the distance between current intakes and optimal intakes. The potential impact fraction is the proportion of risk out of the total risk for a particular outcome or cluster of outcomes (e.g., ischemic heart disease) that can be eliminated by changing the current level of the risk factor distribution (e.g., sodium intake) to some counterfactual (e.g., alternative or hypothetical) distribution (i.e., reducing sodium intake to recommended levels or the lowest observed levels in the population).[72] The population impact fraction is an expansion of the epidemiologic concept of the population attributable fraction, which is just a population impact fraction that completely eliminates the exposure.[60] Using the example of sugar-sweetened beverages (SSBs), a population attributable fraction could be easily calculated if the counterfactual for SSBs was no consumption, but a population impact fraction would be needed if we reduced the consumption in the population by one-third. Readers interested in the calculation details of both the population impact and attributable fractions can find this information elsewhere.[72,73]

Calculating the population impact fraction requires the creation of a meaningful counterfactual or hypothetical exposure distribution. Some options for this counterfactual include the plausible minimum, a feasible minimum, or a cost-effect minimum. Current comparative risk assessment work generally uses something called the theoretical minimum risk exposure level (TMREL), which refers to "the level of risk exposure that leads to minimum risk for individuals."[54] For some behavioral and environmental risk factors this value equates to no exposure. However, for dietary factors, creating the TMREL is more difficult. For dietary factors associated with increased disease risk, zero intake may or may not be theoretically possible (e.g., for *trans* fat or red meat). For dietary factors associated with a decreased disease risk, infinitely high intake is a problematic notion. In most cases, the theoretical minimum risk exposure level is based on the lowest risk observed exposure distribution in some population. The TMREL by its very name is a "theoretical" distribution; it does not mean that the optimal value can feasibly be achieved given the current food environment—rather, it has been observed in some population and is therefore theoretically possible. In many cases, environmental constraints may limit the level. For example, low omega-3 intake may be difficult to bring to optimum levels in regions where seafood is not widely available or accessible (e.g., consider Sudan as compared to Japan). Different studies use different theoretical minimum risk exposure levels, but examples used in the 2016 GBD study include between zero and 1% for energy from *trans* fat, energy from polyunsaturated fatty acids (PUFA) between 9% and 13%, and consumption of nuts and seeds between 16 and 25 g/d.[54]

Disability-Adjusted Life Years (DALYs)

Thus far we have discussed the inputs needed to understand how risk factors may impact population health. These inputs are combined to produce something called a **disability-adjusted life year (DALY)**, which is a combined metric that includes data on both fatal events and nonfatal disease states (described below) in an effort to provide a single measure that strives to measure population health. Earlier in the chapter we discussed the disease burden, which is typically measured using the DALY. The DALY was first developed as part of the 1993 World Development Report.[73] A DALY measures the number of years of life lost due to morbidity/disability or death using data from three common inputs: mortality, epidemiologic data on health states that are nonfatal, and estimates of the value of health states relative to ideal health. At the very least, these inputs are needed by age and sex, but if the interest is in estimating differences in health status by other individual factors (e.g., race/ethnicity or education) or for specific geographies (e.g., county or state) the data need to be available for each of these populations, just like when determining the risk factor distributions.

There are two primary inputs to the DALY—the years lived with disability (YLD) and the years of life lost (YLL)—and the sum of these two components is the DALY (see figure 7.2).

Prior to its advent, health policy discussions tended to focus on causes of death, as these were most readily measured. This led to more public health resources devoted to leading causes of death (e.g., cancer or heart disease) as opposed to disability (e.g., depression or back pain).[73]

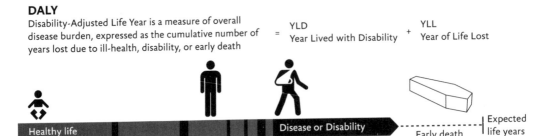

DALY
Disability-Adjusted Life Year is a measure of overall
disease burden, expressed as the cumulative number of
years lost due to ill-health, disability, or early death

= YLD
Year Lived with Disability

+ YLL
Year of Life Lost

Healthy life

Disease or Disability

Early death

Expected
life years

Figure 7.2. Conceptual description of disability-adjusted life year (DALY) for a hypothetical person. *Source:* Planemad (CC BY-SA [https://creativecommons.org/licenses /by-sa/3.0)]). https://commons.wikimedia.org/wiki/File:DALY_disability_affected_life _year_infographic.png.

Years of life lost (YLL) is the number of years that a life was cut short due to a disease and is generally straightforward to calculate for a given population. Assuming that death data are accurate (this is not always the case), YLL is the number of years of life lost before a prespecified "anchor point" for a given population. Anchor points can vary from study to study, but recently, the life expectancy of Japanese women (~88 years) has been used as this is the highest observed life expectancy by age, sex, and country strata. If a person dies before this age, the difference between their age at death and this anchor point are used to calculate the YLL. Deaths happening after the anchor point contribute no data.

Years lived with disability (YLD) is the second component of the DALY calculation and is based on nonfatal disease states (e.g., loss of limb, moderate depression, or loss of function due to a stroke). For each health state a **disability weight (DW)** is assigned that ranges, in theory, from 0 to <1.0 (a DW of 1.0 would be the equivalent of death).[74] Higher disability weights equate to more severe disability and those closer to 0 represent less severe disability. Table 7.3 provides some examples of DW for diabetes complications. Having controlled diabetes leads to a DW of 0.03 as compared to end-stage renal disease requiring dialysis, which has a DW of 0.57. In a hypothetical population of 100,000, where 5% of the population has uncomplicated diabetes, there would be 150 years lived with disability due to this health state (or 150 YLD per 100,000). If 0.25% of the population is estimated to have end-stage renal disease with dialysis due to diabetes, there were 142.5 YLD due to this health state (or 142.5 per 100,000). An advantage of the YLD is that it accounts for both the severity and the prevalence of disease, as opposed to relying on simple prevalence estimates.

With the YLL and YLD, DALYs are calculated by adding these two values together. Like any epidemiologic summary measure, DALYs can be presented as an absolute number, rate, or proportion (of total DALYs). The absolute number of DALYs gives an idea of the absolute burden of disease

Table 7.3. Example of Disability Weights Associated with Selected Diabetes Complications

Sequela/health state	Description	Disability weight (DW)
End-stage renal disease on dialysis due to diabetes mellitus	Is tired and has itching, cramps, headache, joint pains, and shortness of breath. The person needs intensive medical care every other day, lasting about half a day.	0.57
Diabetic neuropathy	Has pain, tingling, and numbness in the arms, legs, hands, and feet. The person sometimes gets cramps and muscle weakness.	0.13
Uncomplicated diabetes mellitus	Has a chronic disease that requires medication every day and causes some worry but minimal interference with daily activities.	0.03

but is impacted by the underlying population size (e.g., China experienced 347,655,394 DALYs in 2016 while Fiji experienced 346,175 DALYs). Perhaps a more useful metric for the DALY is the DALY rate (e.g., DALYs per 100,000) (China, 25,431 DALYs per 100,000; Fiji, 40,166). The DALY rate is particularly helpful for comparing the absolute burden of disease between two places (e.g., is China healthier than Fiji? Yes, it appears that this is the case based on these data). However, because DALYs are a somewhat difficult construct to interpret (unlike deaths or cancer cases), their interpretation as a rate is not terribly straightforward. A more intuitive presentation of DALYs can be the proportion of total DALYs attributed to a specific cause of disease or risk factor. An important limitation of this approach is that the proportion is inherently impacted by the total number of DALYs. In this sense, two countries can experience the same burden estimated as a DALY rate due to a risk factor but the proportions may vary because the number of DALYs (e.g., the absolute health status) of the two countries differ. This approach is best limited to comparing the burden in a specific country or region at a fixed time point, as opposed to across different geographies or time points that have a different denominator, when the DALY rate is preferred.

Modeling Policy Approaches

Given that dietary risks in high-income countries have the highest proportional impact on the disease burden among risk factors, there has been considerable interest in developing policy approaches to improve dietary intakes and reduce the burden of disease.[75] Commonly proposed policies include, but are not limited to the following: menu labeling in fast-food restaurants, improving school lunches, changing rules around what foods can and cannot be obtained by individuals using food assistance programs, taxing unhealthful foods, subsidizing healthful foods, changing school and day care food regulations, mass media campaigns, restricting advertising of foods to children, banning specific nutrients, mandates and bans requiring reformulation (e.g., for sodium or *trans* fat), and changing food labels.[76] Modifications to the approach described above can be used to compare the impact of various policy proposals, assuming that data on the policy effects or impacts are available.[77-82] Such studies can be used to determine the policy efforts that will have the biggest bang for the buck in terms of improving population health and reducing health disparities.

Overview of Risk-Factor Burden

As discussed in the section on quantifying the disease and risk factor burden, some of the disease burden may be unattributedthis may be due to gaps in our understanding of etiology (e.g., Alzheimer's disease or migraine) or genetic conditions where risk factors are obviously not modifiable (e.g., congenital birth defects). Globally, approximately 55% of the disease burden is unattributed to risk factors. Outcomes commonly linked to dietary risk factors, such as ischemic heart disease, stroke, diabetes, and colorectal cancer, have an attributable burden of 94% (i.e., 94% of ischemic disease can be attributed to known risk factors), 89%, 100%, and 53%, respectively. With this in mind, the leading risk factors for disability among high-income countries include diet (12.3%), high systolic blood pressure (11.2%), tobacco (10.4%), high BMI (8.2%), alcohol and drug use (8.2%), and elevated fasting plasma glucose (7.4%). These proportions cannot simply be added together due to correlations between them, but they still serve as a useful guide as to the relative ranking of different risk factors.

The countries with the highest and lowest burden attributable to each of these dietary factors are presented in table 7.4. There is substantial heterogeneity in the contribution of these risk factors to disease at the national level. For all dietary risks combined, Qatar and Peru have the fewest DALYs per 100,000 attributable to suboptimal diet, while the burden is highest in Bulgaria, Belarus, Russia, and Fiji. For most dietary factors, former Soviet Republics and Eastern Bloc countries have the highest disease burden attributable to dietary factors. For sodium, China has a high burden due to sodium (1,536 DALYs per 100,000), and for processed meat the United States has the highest burden (388 DALYs per 100,000). For sugar-sweetened beverages, Mexico stands out as having the highest attributable burden (132 DALYs per 100,000).

The countries with the lowest attributable burden also merit some attention. For all dietary risks, Qatar, Peru, Equatorial Guinea, Ecuador, and Israel have the lowest attributable burden due to diet. For whole grains, a number of Latin American countries have the lowest attributable burden, while

Table 7.4. Top Five and Bottom Five Countries by Risk Factor Burden for Each Dietary Factor in the Global Burden of Disease 2016, in DALYs per 100,000

Top 5		Bottom 5		Top 5		Bottom 5	
All dietary risks				**Whole grains**			
Bulgaria	8,839	Qatar	913	Fiji	3,690	Venezuela	2
Belarus	8,542	Peru	983	Belarus	2,833	Colombia	10
Russia	8,123	Equatorial Guinea	1,097	Bulgaria	2,790	Costa Rica	11
Fiji	8,056	Ecuador	1,193	Russia	2,780	Mexico	12
Latvia	7,782	Israel	1,222	Latvia	2,409	Panama	21
Vegetables				**Fruit**			
Fiji	1,366	Qatar	6	Fiji	2,427	Qatar	72
Russia	1,311	Israel	28	Bulgaria	2,180	Oman	76
Latvia	1,056	Turkey	38	Russia	2,042	Dominican Republic	91
Lithuania	1,021	Bahrain	67	Latvia	1,948	The Bahamas	122
Croatia	909	Iran	77	Belarus	1,920	Equatorial Guinea	140
Legumes				**Nuts/seeds**			
Belarus	1,158	United Arab Emirates	0	Fiji	2,508	Qatar	92
Russia	849	Cuba	1	Belarus	2,176	Equatorial Guinea	208
Latvia	844	Brazil	6	Russia	1,811	Israel	225
Azerbaijan	808	Costa Rica	7	Bulgaria	1,776	Maldives	242
Bulgaria	724	Turkey	9	Lithuania	1,691	Peru	284
Sodium				**Seafood omega-3 fats**			
Bulgaria	2,209	Samoa	70	Belarus	1,337	Japan	2
Romania	1,719	American Samoa	75	Bulgaria	1,207	Qatar	74
Hungary	1,567	Maldives	105	Russia	1,092	Israel	98
China	1,536	Turkey	113	Azerbaijan	1,022	Equatorial Guinea	103
Macedonia	1,416	United Kingdom	116	Fiji	952	Bermuda	111
Fiber				**Processed meat**			
Bulgaria	862	Equatorial Guinea	49	United States	388	Thailand	1
Russia	704	Qatar	53	Lithuania	334	Peru	1
Hungary	679	Mexico	61	Latvia	313	Ecuador	2
Latvia	654	Peru	79	Norway	312	Saudi Arabia	3
Slovakia	605	Israel	92	United Kingdom	267	Turkey	3
Red meat				**Milk**			
Taiwan	114	Iraq	0	Hungary	133	Qatar	8
Austria	79	Guyana	0	Bulgaria	118	Oman	10
Argentina	77	Maldives	0	Serbia	112	Maldives	11
Bulgaria	77	Iran	0	Slovakia	111	Kuwait	11
Portugal	70	Jamaica	0	Croatia	107	Turkmenistan	11
Calcium				**Trans fat**			
Hungary	200	Qatar	7	Latvia	924	Lebanon	1
Slovakia	154	Oman	12	Azerbaijan	337	Israel	3
Serbia	136	Kuwait	13	Estonia	218	Namibia	3
Croatia	135	Albania	14	Lithuania	213	Spain	3
Hungary	133	Maldives	14	Iran	207	Italy	3

(continued)

Table 7.4 (continued)

Top 5		Bottom 5			Top 5		Bottom 5	
PUFA				**Sugar-sweetened beverages**				
Belarus	791	Fiji	1		Mexico	132	Maldives	4
Estonia	467	Iceland	2		Brazil	45	Namibia	4
Turkmenistan	441	Ecuador	2		Trinidad and Tobago	42	China	5
Poland	406	Taiwan	2		Qatar	41	Tonga	6
Russia	381	Turkey	3		Virgin Islands, US	38	Algeria	6

Note: Top 5 countries are high risk. DALY = disability-adjusted life year; PUFA = polyunsaturated fatty acids.

for vegetables countries with the lowest burden tend to be in the Middle East. For legumes, three Latin American and two Middle Eastern countries have the lowest attributable burden. Japan, not surprisingly, has an exceptionally low burden due to insufficient seafood omega-3 fat intake. The burden attributable to specific dietary factors is primarily driven by differences in intake compared to optimal levels. In the examples above, each of the countries with the lowest/highest burden tend to have amongst the lowest/highest intake for that dietary factor.

In general terms, the burden of BMI is typically highest in Oceania and Pacific Islands (e.g., Fiji, American Samoa), as is the burden of elevated fasting plasma glucose. Elevated blood pressure (e.g., Bulgaria, Belarus, Romania) and alcohol and drugs (e.g., Russia, Belarus, and Romania) follow a similar geographic pattern.[83]

While looking at the cumulative impact of dietary risks is helpful, it fails to tell us what specific dietary factors are responsible for more ill health than others, which has important implications for the development of population-based interventions (e.g., should we focus on policies around sodium or *trans* fat reduction, given limited public health resources?). Among high-income countries, the relative burden attributable to the 15 dietary factors is as follows: whole grain (3.5% of DALYs), sodium (3.3%), fruit (2.9%), nuts/seeds (2.3%), vegetables (1.4%), seafood omega-3 fats (1.4%), fiber (0.9%), legumes (0.8%), PUFA (0.4%), processed meat (0.3%), calcium (0.2%), milk (0.2%), *trans* fat (0.2%), red meat (0.1%), and sugar-sweetened beverages (0.1%). Like the other risk factors, these proportions are not additive; but the relative ranking is illustrative. Assuming no heterogeneity across countries and the availability of equally effective interventions, we would be best off, from a population health shifting intakes toward whole grains, followed by reducing sodium and increasing fruit intakes. Based on this data alone, we would not choose to prioritize strategies around red meat or sugar-sweetened beverages.

The dietary risks for the most populous high- and middle-high-income countries are provided in table 7.5. Among the most populous high-income

Table 7.5. Dietary Risk in DALYs per 100,000 for Five Most Populous High-Income and Middle-High-Income Countries

	All dietary risks	Vegetables	Legumes	Sodium	Fiber	Red meat	Calcium	PUFA	Whole grains	Fruit	Nuts/ seeds	Seafood omega-3 fats	Processed meat	Milk	Trans fat	SSB
Five most populous high-income countries																
United States	3,143	426	259	635	212	62	54	35	961	641	412	304	388	51	202	36
Japan	2,540	98	21	930	144	9	126	37	652	561	410	2	132	96	10	8
Germany	3,436	539	332	510	320	48	70	155	927	719	665	417	212	70	61	22
United Kingdom	2,340	338	184	116	243	24	75	135	670	560	476	262	267	55	42	33
France	2,006	299	154	258	204	39	70	42	565	527	349	177	73	65	13	10
Five most populous middle-high-income countries																
China	4,023	331	240	1,536	246	32	63	166	1,136	1,077	631	425	6	49	13	5
Brazil	1,960	493	6	330	195	51	39	31	196	382	592	220	19	31	24	45
Russia	8,123	1,311	849	1,202	704	17	91	381	2,780	2,042	1,811	1,092	265	82	72	16
Mexico	1,679	286	24	186	61	42	26	44	12	356	587	203	121	19	167	132
Iran	2,169	77	108	397	174	0	27	20	848	271	477	412	4	19	207	8

Note: DALY = disability-adjusted life year; PUFA = polyunsaturated fatty acids; SSB = sugar-sweetened beverage.

countries, Germany and the United States have the highest diet burden while France and the United Kingdom have the lowest. The United States jumps out for a high burden due to whole grain, seafood omega-3, processed meat, red meat, and *trans* fat consumption compared to the other high-income countries. Japan has a very low burden for vegetables, legumes, SSBs, and seafood omega-3s but has a somewhat higher burden due to sodium than other high-income countries. Germany stands out for a high whole grain, fruit, vegetable, legume, nuts/seeds, and seafood omega-3 burden compared to others. The United Kingdom has a lower sodium burden than other countries, due, likely in part, to aggressive sodium reduction efforts.[84] Lastly, France has the lowest burden among the five most populous high-income countries and doesn't stand out as having any exceedingly high burdens as compared to the other populous high-income countries.

For middle-high-income countries, Russia has the worst burden attributable to suboptimal diet, followed by China and Iran. Among middle-high-income countries, Mexico and Brazil have the lowest burden. Russia has the highest burden for most important dietary risk factors, particularly whole grains, fruit, vegetables, and nuts/seeds. China has a very high sodium burden, and Iran has the highest *trans* fat burden. Brazil and Mexico have similar distributions, but both have higher than average burdens due to SSBs despite having a low dietary burden overall.

Changes in Risks from 1990–2016

Across all high-income countries assessed here, DALYs attributable to dietary factors declined by about 12%, from 3,757 DALYs per 100,000 to 3,318 per 100,000, as shown in table 7.6. For each dietary risk factor, the decline was most dramatic for fruit (–26%), sodium (–22%), processed meat (–26%), red meat (–65%) and PUFA (–18%). The burden attributable to SSBs and milk both increased by more than 25%, and changes for other dietary risk factors were more modest. These declines may be driven by changes in the risk factor distribution (e.g., changes in dietary intake) or by other changes such as population aging. For other cardiometabolic risk factors, both BMI and high fasting plasma glucose have increased by more than 25% while the burden attributable to systolic blood pressure has modestly declined (–5%). Figure 7.3 shows the change in DALYs per dietary risks for the high-income countries with a population greater than 5 million in 2016. Most countries experienced a decline or very modest increase; Libya, Paraguay, the United Arab Emirates, Saudi Arabia, Mexico, South Africa, and Iran experienced the greatest proportional increase in DALYs attributable to dietary risks. Proportional declines were most dramatic in Denmark, Israel, Norway, United Kingdom, Czech Republic, Australia, and Sweden.

Table 7.6. Change in DALYs per 100,000 Attributable to Dietary Factors and Cardiometabolic Risk Factors from 1990 to 2016 in High-Income Countries

Dietary factor and cardiometabolic risk factors	DALYs per 100,000		Percentage change (%)
	1990	2016	
All dietary risks	3,757	3,319	−11.7
High sodium	1,134	880	−22.4
Low fruit	1,063	790	−25.7
Low whole grains	1,023	954	−6.8
Low nuts & seeds	678	633	−6.6
Low vegetables	464	470	1.2
Low seafood omega-3 fats	411	371	−9.7
Low fiber	269	243	−9.5
Low legumes	199	218	9.8
Low PUFA	148	121	−18.1
High processed meat	109	80	−26.3
Low calcium	55	61	10.9
High red meat	40	14	−64.5
Low milk	39	50	27.1
High sugar-sweetened beverages	11	19	68.1
High systolic blood pressure	3,182	3,025	−4.9
High BMI	1,636	2,221	35.7
High fasting plasma glucose	1,589	1,997	25.6

Note: PUFA = polyunsaturated fatty acids.

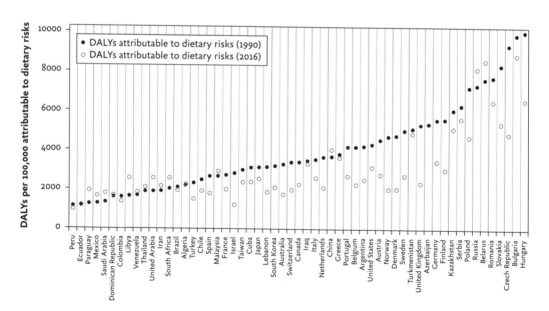

Figure 7.3. Change in DALYs per 100,000 attributable to dietary risks among high-income countries with a population greater than 5,000,000 in 2016, sorted by DALYs attributable to diet risks in 1990.

Socio-demographic Disparities, Differences, and Subnational Data

Thus far we have focused exclusively on national estimates, which may mask differences and disparities within countries by population subgroups or geography. The burden of disease attributable to diet is almost always substantially higher among men as opposed to women. This higher burden is driven by two factors: first, men tend to have poorer dietary intakes than women, and second, men are more impacted by the outcomes that are related to dietary risks. While dietary intakes tend to improve among older adults, the absolute burden attributable to dietary factors (e.g., DALYs per 100,000) increases monotonically with age, while the proportion of DALYs attributable to diet generally peaks around 55–59 years of age, decreasing thereafter due to the emergence of additional health risks.

Not included in the GBD studies is information on how the burden of disease and risk factors may differ by other population subgroups, including race/ethnicity or socioeconomic status (e.g., income, education, or social class). The exclusion of this data from the GBD is primarily due to major data gaps, and it would be a substantial undertaking to add this information to the project. In addition, the choice of additional stratifications is highly context dependent. In the United States, stratification by race/ethnicity or some measure of socioeconomic status would be most interesting, but in other places other stratifications may be of greater interest. In the United States, we found that the proportion of diet-related cardiometabolic mortality was higher among non-Hispanic blacks and Hispanic adults, as compared to non-Hispanic white adults, and lowest among those with a college degree as opposed to those lacking a high school degree.[26] These disparities were particularly strong for sugar-sweetened beverages and low nuts/seeds consumption, though they were also apparent for fruits, vegetables, and whole grains—an unsurprising result given the gradient in intake of these food groups.[85] Given the small number of studies that have engaged this topic, this is an area of future research.

Beyond gender, age, race/ethnicity, and socioeconomic status, there may also be interest in subnational data on health risks. This information can be highly valuable when there are substantial differences in health status or risk factors by geography, if the country is exceedingly large, and/or the responsibility to health is operationalized at a nonnational level (e.g., state health departments in the United States). Within the GBD study, as of 2018, publicly available subnational data is available for US States (n = 51), Mexican states (n = 32), English regions (n = 9), Japanese prefectures (n = 47), and Indian states and union territories (n = 36).[86,87] Within the United States, there is substantial heterogeneity in DALYs attributable to suboptimal diet at the state level, with risk greatest in West Virginia (5,094 DALYs per 100,000), Mississippi (5,063), and Alabama (4,616), and lowest in Utah (1,958), Colorado (2,099), and California (2,278).[87] State-level data on specific dietary factors driving ill health may be informative for developing population-specific interventions, though as is always the case state-level data may also mask local differences and disparities. With that said, the absence of data for a specific geography of interest should not impede disease prevention activities; it is important to use the best available data to guide such work but not let the lack of data act as a firewall. Readers are encouraged to explore these data using the GBD Compare tool. As new iterations of the project are updated, more subnational data become will become available.

Conclusion

Understanding the contribution of dietary factors to ill health is essential to inform the creation of programs and policies to improve diet. In high-income countries, based on currently available data, whole grains, sodium, fruit, and nuts/seeds are the leading dietary factors associated with adverse health outcomes. Dietary factors primarily influence heart disease, stroke, and diabetes, but also some cancers. Despite modest improvements in the disease burden attributable to dietary factors over the past few decades, dietary factors will remain among the leading causes of ill health in high-income countries. In addition to identifying the dietary factors best suited for population-based improvements, the approaches described here can be used to model the impact that policy changes may have on improving population health.

Review Questions

1. What are the leading causes of death and disability in high-income countries? Why is it important to look at both death and disability?
2. Describe the key inputs needed to estimate the contribution of a specific dietary factor to the disease burden.
3. What dietary factors have the greatest impact on the disease burden in high-income countries? What dietary factors have the smallest burden?
4. What is the most likely reason why a country may have a high or low disease burden due to a particular dietary factor?
5. What component of the Bradford-Hill "criteria" is most often lacking in the nutritional epidemiology literature and why?
6. If you are a health planner in a specific country, would you want to use DALYs or deaths to determine the leading causes of ill health? What would be the main limitation of using the other approach?
7. True or false: You can always infer causality from meta-analyses because they combine multiple studies.
8. What were some of the main improvements made upon the advent of the comparative risk assessment framework for measuring population health upon past work?
9. According to the Global Burden of Disease project, Mexico has amongst the highest burden of disease attributable to sugar-sweetened beverages among all

countries. Does this mean that Mexico should prioritize policy and program approaches to reduce consumption of sugar-sweetened beverages as opposed to other dietary factors?

References

1. Keys, A.B. 1980. *Seven Countries: A Multivariate Analysis of Death and Coronary Heart Disease*. Cambridge, MA: Harvard University Press.

2. Hjermann, I., K. Velve Byre, I. Holme, and P. Leren. 1981. "Effect of Diet and Smoking Intervention on the Incidence of Coronary Heart Disease. Report from the Oslo Study Group of a Randomised Trial in Healthy Men." *The Lancet* 2 (8259): 1303-10. http://www.ncbi.nlm.nih.gov/pubmed/6118715.

3. Jackson, R.L., J.D. Morrisett, H.J. Pownall, A.M. Gotto, A. Kamio, H. Imai, R. Tracy, and F.A. Kummerow. 1977. "Influence of Dietary Trans-Fatty Acids on Swine Lipoprotein Composition and Structure." *Journal of Lipid Research* 18 (2): 182-90.

4. Mattson, F. H., E. J. Hollenbach, and A. M. Kligman. 1975. "Effect of Hydrogenated Fat on the Plasma Cholesterol and Triglyceride Levels of Man." *The American Journal of Clinical Nutrition* 28 (7): 726-31. https://doi.org/10.1093/ajcn/28.7.726.

5. Willett, W. C., M. J. Stampfer, J. E. Manson, G. A. Colditz, F. E. Speizer, B. A. Rosner, L. A. Sampson, and C. H. Hennekens. 1993. "Intake of Trans Fatty Acids and Risk of Coronary Heart Disease among Women." *The Lancet* 341 (8845): 581-85. http://www.ncbi.nlm.nih.gov/pubmed/8094827.

6. Gillman, M.W., L.A. Cupples, D. Gagnon, B.E. Millen, R.C. Ellison, and W.P. Castelli. 1997. "Margarine Intake and Subsequent Coronary Heart Disease in Men." *Epidemiology* 8 (2): 144-49.

7. Ascherio, A., and W.C. Willett. 1997. "Health Effects of Trans Fatty Acids." *American Journal of Clinical Nutrition* 66 (4 Suppl): 1006s-1010s.

8. Pietinen, P., A. Ascherio, P. Korhonen, A. M. Hartman, W. C. Willett, D. Albanes, and J. Virtamo. 1997. "Intake of Fatty Acids and Risk of Coronary Heart Disease in a Cohort of Finnish Men. The Alpha-Tocopherol, Beta-Carotene Cancer Prevention Study." *American Journal of Epidemiology* 145 (10): 876-87. http://www.ncbi.nlm.nih.gov/pubmed/9149659.

9. Hu, F.B., M.J. Stampfer, J.E. Manson, E. Rimm, G.A. Colditz, B.A. Rosner, C.H. Hennekens, and W.C. Willett. 1997. "Dietary Fat Intake and the Risk of Coronary Heart Disease in Women." *New England Journal of Medicine* 337 (21): 1491-99. https://doi.org/10.1056/NEJM199711203372102.

10. Bolton-Smith, C., M. Woodward, S. Fenton, and C. A. Brown. 1996. "Does Dietary Trans Fatty Acid Intake Relate to the Prevalence of Coronary Heart Disease in Scotland?" *European Heart Journal* 17 (6): 837-45. http://www.ncbi.nlm.nih.gov/pubmed/8781822.

11. Ascherio, A., C.H. Hennekens, J.E. Buring, C. Master, M.J. Stampfer, and W.C. Willett. 1994. "Trans-Fatty Acids Intake and Risk of Myocardial Infarction." *Circulation* 89 (1): 94-101.

12. Lichtenstein, A.H., L.M. Ausman, S.M. Jalbert, and E.J. Schaefer. 1999. "Effects of Different Forms of Dietary Hydrogenated Fats on Serum Lipoprotein

Cholesterol Levels." *New England Journal of Medicine* 340 (25): 1933–40. https://doi .org/10.1056/NEJM199906243402501.

13. Mensink, R.P., and M.B. Katan. 1990. "Effect of Dietary Trans Fatty Acids on High-Density and Low-Density Lipoprotein Cholesterol Levels in Healthy Subjects." *New England Journal of Medicine* 323 (7): 439–45. https://doi.org/10.1056 /NEJM199008163230703.

14. Lopez-Garcia, E., M.B. Schulze, J.B. Meigs, J.E. Manson, N. Rifai, M.J. Stampfer, W.C. Willett, and F.B. Hu. 2005. "Consumption of Trans Fatty Acids Is Related to Plasma Biomarkers of Inflammation and Endothelial Dysfunction." *The Journal of Nutrition* 135 (3): 562–66. https://doi.org/10.1093/jn/135.3 .562.

15. Goodman, G. E., M. D. Thornquist, J. Balmes, M. R. Cullen, F. L. Meyskens, G. S. Omenn, B. Valanis, and J. H. Williams. 2004. "The Beta-Carotene and Retinol Efficacy Trial: Incidence of Lung Cancer and Cardiovascular Disease Mortality During 6-Year Follow-up After Stopping Carotene and Retinol Supplements." *JNCI Journal of the National Cancer Institute* 96 (23): 1743–50. https://doi.org/10.1093/jnci /djh320.

16. Food and Drug Administration, and HHS. 2003. "Food Labeling: Trans Fatty Acids in Nutrition Labeling, Nutrient Content Claims, and Health Claims. Final Rule." *Federal Register* 68 (133): 41433–506. http://www.ncbi.nlm.nih.gov /pubmed/12856667.

17. Mozaffarian, D., M.F. Jacobson, and J.S. Greenstein. 2010. "Food Reformulations to Reduce Trans Fatty Acids." *New England Journal of Medicine* 362 (21): 2037–39. https://doi.org/10.1056/NEJMc1001841.

18. Astrup, A. 2006. "The Trans Fatty Acid Story in Denmark." *Atherosclerosis Supplements* 7 (2): 43–46. https://doi.org/10.1016/j.atherosclerosissup.2006.04.010.

19. World Health Organization. Eliminating Trans Fats in Europe: A Policy Brief. Copenhagen: WHO Regional Office for Europe, 2015.

20. "Social Progress Index." n.d. http://www.socialprogressimperative.org/.

21. Nichols, M., N. Townsend, P. Scarborough, and M. Rayner. 2013. "Trends in Age-Specific Coronary Heart Disease Mortality in the European Union over Three Decades: 1980-2009." *European Heart Journal* 34 (39): 3017–27. https://doi.org /10.1093/eurheartj/eht159.

22. Restrepo, B.J., and M. Rieger. 2016. "Denmark's Policy on Artificial Trans Fat and Cardiovascular Disease." *American Journal of Preventive Medicine* 50 (1): 69–76. https://doi.org/10.1016/j.amepre.2015.06.018.

23. Brandt, E.J., R. Myerson, M.C. Perraillon, and T.S. Polonsky. 2017. "Hospital Admissions for Myocardial Infarction and Stroke Before and After the Trans-Fatty Acid Restrictions in New York." *JAMA Cardiology* 2 (6): 627–634.

24. "How Are the Income Group Thresholds Determined?" n.d. The World Bank. https://datahelpdesk.worldbank.org/knowledgebase/articles/378833-how -are-the-income-group-thresholds-determined.

25. "Human Development Index (HDI)." n.d. United Nations Development Reports. http://hdr.undp.org/en/content/human-development-index-hdi.

26. Micha, R., J.L. Peñalvo, F. Cudhea, F. Imamura, C.D. Rehm, and D. Mozaffarian. 2017. "Association Between Dietary Factors and Mortality From Heart

Disease, Stroke, and Type 2 Diabetes in the United States." *JAMA* 317 (9): 912. https://doi.org/10.1001/jama.2017.0947.

27. Preston, Samuel H. 1976. *Mortality Patterns in National Populations: With Special Reference to Recorded Causes of Death.* New York: Academic Press.

28. Omran, A. R. 1977. "Epidemiologic Transition in the United States: The Health Factor in Population Change." *Population Bulletin* 32 (2): 1-42. http://www.ncbi.nlm.nih.gov/pubmed/12335110.

29. Galor, O., and D.N. Weil. 2000. "Population, Technology, and Growth: From Malthusian Stagnation to the Demographic Transition and Beyond." *American Economic Review* 90 (4): 806-28. https://doi.org/doi: 10.1257/aer.90.4.806.

30. Popkin, B. M., and P. Gordon-Larsen. 2004. "The Nutrition Transition: Worldwide Obesity Dynamics and Their Determinants." *International Journal of Obesity* 28 (S3): S2-9. https://doi.org/10.1038/sj.ijo.0802804.

31. Pingali, P. 2007. "Westernization of Asian Diets and the Transformation of Food Systems: Implications for Research and Policy." *Food Policy* 32 (3): 281-98. https://doi.org/https://doi.org/10.1016/j.foodpol.2006.08.001.

32. Imamura, F., R. Micha, S. Khatibzadeh, S. Fahimi, P. Shi, J. Powles, D. Mozaffarian, and Global Burden of Diseases Nutrition and Chronic Diseases Expert Group (NutriCoDE). 2015. "Dietary Quality among Men and Women in 187 Countries in 1990 and 2010: A Systematic Assessment." *The Lancet Global Health* 3 (3): e132-42. https://doi.org/10.1016/S2214-109X(14)70381-X.

33. Hawkes, C. 2006. "Uneven Dietary Development: Linking the Policies and Processes of Globalization with the Nutrition Transition, Obesity and Diet-Related Chronic Diseases." *Global Health* 2: 4. https://doi.org/10.1186/1744-8603-2-4.

34. Tzioumis, E., and L.S. Adair. 2014. "Childhood Dual Burden of Under- and Overnutrition in Low- and Middle-Income Countries: A Critical Review." *Food and Nutrition Bulletin* 35 (2): 230-43. https://doi.org/10.1177/156482651403500210.

35. Garland, C., R. B. Shekelle, E. Barrett-Connor, M. H. Criqui, A. H. Rossof, and O. Paul. 1985. "Dietary Vitamin D and Calcium and Risk of Colorectal Cancer: A 19-Year Prospective Study in Men." *The Lancet* 1 (8424): 307-9.

36. Hu, F.B. 2002. "Dietary Pattern Analysis: A New Direction in Nutritional Epidemiology." *Current Opinion in Lipidology* 13 (1): 3-9.

37. Fung, T.T., E.B. Rimm, D. Spiegelman, N. Rifai, G.H. Tofler, W.C. Willett, and F.B. Hu. 2001. "Association between Dietary Patterns and Plasma Biomarkers of Obesity and Cardiovascular Disease Risk." *The American Journal of Clinical Nutrition* 73 (1): 61-67. https://doi.org/10.1093/ajcn/73.1.61.

38. Ministry of Food and Environment of Denmark. 2018. "The Official Dietary Guidelines." Danish Veterinary and Food Administration. 2018. https://www.foedevarestyrelsen.dk/english/Food/Nutrition/The_dietary_recommendations/Pages/default.aspx.

39. United States Department of Health and Human Services, United States Department of Agriculture, and United States Dietary Guidelines Advisory Committee. 2015. "Dietary Guidelines for Americans, 2015-2020." 8th ed. Washington, DC: US Department of Health and Human Services and US Department of Agriculture. http://health.gov/dietaryguidelines/2015/guidelines/.

40. Public Health England. 2018. "The UK Eatwell Guide." https://www.gov.uk/government/publications/the-eatwell-guide.

41. Aune, D., N. Keum, E. Giovannucci, L.T. Fadnes, P. Boffetta, D.C. Greenwood, S. Tonstad, L.J. Vatten, et al. 2016. "Whole Grain Consumption and Risk of Cardiovascular Disease, Cancer, and All Cause and Cause Specific Mortality: Systematic Review and Dose-Response Meta-Analysis of Prospective Studies." *BMJ* 353 (June): i2716. https://doi.org/10.1136/bmj.i2716.

42. Li, M., Y. Fan, X. Zhang, W. Hou, and Z. Tang. 2014. "Fruit and Vegetable Intake and Risk of Type 2 Diabetes Mellitus: Meta-Analysis of Prospective Cohort Studies." *BMJ* 4 (11): e005497. https://doi.org/10.1136/bmjopen-2014-005497.

43. Afshin, A., R. Micha, S. Khatibzadeh, and D. Mozaffarian. 2014. "Consumption of Nuts and Legumes and Risk of Incident Ischemic Heart Disease, Stroke, and Diabetes: A Systematic Review and Meta-Analysis." *The American Journal of Clinical Nutrition* 100 (1): 278–88. https://doi.org/10.3945/ajcn.113.076901.

44. Aune, D., T. Norat, P. Romundstad, and L.J. Vatten. 2013. "Whole Grain and Refined Grain Consumption and the Risk of Type 2 Diabetes: A Systematic Review and Dose-Response Meta-Analysis of Cohort Studies." *European Journal of Epidemiology* 28 (11): 845–58. https://doi.org/10.1007/s10654-013-9852-5.

45. Aburto, N.J, A. Ziolkovska, L. Hooper, P. Elliott, F.P. Cappuccio, and J.J. Meerpohl. 2013. "Effect of Lower Sodium Intake on Health: Systematic Review and Meta-analyses." *BMJ*, 346: 1326.

46. Hu, D., J. Huang, Y. Wang, D. Zhang, and Y. Qu, 2014. "Fruits and Vegetables Consumption and Risk of Stroke: A Meta-analysis of Prospective Cohort Studies." *Stroke* 45 (6), 1613–19.

47. Wang, X., Y. Ouyang, J. Liu, M. Zhu, G. Zhao, W. Bao, and F.B. Hu. 2014. "Fruit and Vegetable Consumption and Mortality from All Causes, Cardiovascular Disease, and Cancer: Systematic Review and Dose-response Meta-analysis of Prospective Cohort Studies." *BMJ* 349: 4490.

48. Micha, R.M., S.K. Wallace, and D. Mozaffarian. 2010. "Red and Processed Meat Consumption and Risk of Incident Coronary Heart Disease, Stroke, and Diabetes Mellitus: A Systematic Review and Meta-Analysis." *Circulation* 121 (21): 2271–83. https://doi.org/10.1161/CIRCULATIONAHA.109.924977.

49. Key, T.J. 2011. "Fruit and Vegetables and Cancer Risk." *British Journal of Cancer* 104 (1): 6–11.

50. Vieira, A. R., L. Abar, D. S. M. Chan, S. Vingeliene, E. Polemiti, C. Stevens, D. Greenwood, and T. Norat. 2017. "Foods and Beverages and Colorectal Cancer Risk: A Systematic Review and Meta-Analysis of Cohort Studies, an Update of the Evidence of the WCRF-AICR Continuous Update Project." *Annals of Oncology* 28 (8): 1788–1802. https://doi.org/10.1093/annonc/mdx171.

51. Liu, J., J. Wang, Y. Leng, and C. Lv. 2013. "Intake of Fruit and Vegetables and Risk of Esophageal Squamous Cell Carcinoma: A Meta-analysis of Observational Studies." *International Journal of Cancer* 133(2): 473–485.

52. World Cancer Research Fund and American Institute for Cancer Research. "Food, Nutrition, Physical Activity, and the Prevention of Cancer: A Global Perspective." 2018. https://www.wcrf.org/dietandcancer/about.

53. Micha, R., M. L. Shulkin, J. L. Penalvo, S. Khatibzadeh, G. M. Singh, M. Rao, S. Fahimi, J. Powles, et al. 2017. "Etiologic Effects and Optimal Intakes of Foods and Nutrients for Risk of Cardiovascular Diseases and Diabetes: Systematic Reviews and Meta-Analyses from the Nutrition and Chronic Diseases Expert Group (NutriCoDE)." *PLoS One* 12 (4): e0175149. https://doi.org/10.1371/journal .pone.0175149.

54. Gakidou, Emmanuela, Ashkan Afshin, Amanuel Alemu Abajobir, Kalkidan Hassen Abate, Cristiana Abbafati, Kaja M. Abbas, Foad Abd-Allah, et al. 2017. "Global, Regional, and National Comparative Risk Assessment of 84 Behavioural, Environmental and Occupational, and Metabolic Risks or Clusters of Risks, 1990–2016: A Systematic Analysis for the Global Burden of Disease Study 2016." *The Lancet* 390 (10100): 1345–1422. https://doi.org/10.1016/S0140-6736(17)32366-8.

55. "Global, Regional, and National Disability-Adjusted Life-Years (DALYs) for 333 Diseases and Injuries and Healthy Life Expectancy (HALE) for 195 Countries and Territories, 1990–2016: A Systematic Analysis for the Global Burden of Disease Study 2016." 2017. *The Lancet* 390 (10100): 1260–1344. https://doi.org/10.1016/s0140 -6736(17)32130-x.

56. Vos, Theo, Amanuel Alemu Abajobir, Kalkidan Hassen Abate, Cristiana Abbafati, Kaja M. Abbas, Foad Abd-Allah, Rizwan Suliankatchi Abdulkader, et al. 2017. "Global, Regional, and National Incidence, Prevalence, and Years Lived with Disability for 328 Diseases and Injuries for 195 Countries, 1990–2016: A Systematic Analysis for the Global Burden of Disease Study 2016." *The Lancet* 390 (10100): 1211–59. https://doi.org/10.1016/S0140-6736(17)32154-2.

57. Naghavi, Mohsen, Amanuel Alemu Abajobir, Cristiana Abbafati, Kaja M. Abbas, Foad Abd-Allah, Semaw Ferede Abera, Victor Aboyans, et al. 2017. "Global, Regional, and National Age-Sex Specific Mortality for 264 Causes of Death, 1980–2016: A Systematic Analysis for the Global Burden of Disease Study 2016." *The Lancet* 390 (10100): 1151–1210. https://doi.org/10.1016/S0140-6736(17)32152-9.

58. Hill, A. B. 1965. "The Environment and Disease: Association or Causation?" *Royal Society of Medicine* 58: 295–300. http://www.ncbi.nlm.nih.gov/pubmed/14283879.

59. Doll, R., and A. B. Hill. 1952. "A Study of the Aetiology of Carcinoma of the Lung." *British Medical Journal* 2 (4797): 1271–86. http://www.ncbi.nlm.nih.gov /pubmed/12997741.

60. Koepsell, Thomas D, and Noel S. Weiss. 2003. *Epidemiologic Methods: Studying the Occurrence of Illness.* Oxford/New York: Oxford University Press.

61. Estruch, Ramón, Emilio Ros, Jordi Salas-Salvadó, Maria-Isabel Covas, Dolores Corella, Fernando Arós, Enrique Gómez-Gracia, et al. 2013. "Primary Prevention of Cardiovascular Disease with a Mediterranean Diet." *New England Journal of Medicine* 368 (14): 1279–90. https://doi.org/10.1056/NEJMoa1200303.

62. Maruthur, Nisa M., Nae-Yuh Wang, and Lawrence J. Appel. 2009. "Lifestyle Interventions Reduce Coronary Heart Disease Risk: Results From the PREMIER Trial." *Circulation* 119 (15): 2026–31. https://doi.org/10.1161/CIRCULATIONAHA .108.809491.

63. Obarzanek, Eva, Frank M. Sacks, William M. Vollmer, George A. Bray, Edgar R. Miller, Pao-Hwa Lin, Njeri M Karanja, et al. 2001. "Effects on Blood Lipids of a Blood Pressure-Lowering Diet: The Dietary Approaches to Stop

Hypertension (DASH) Trial." *The American Journal of Clinical Nutrition* 74 (1): 80–89. https://doi.org/10.1093/ajcn/74.1.80.

64. Estruch, R., E. Ros, J. Salas-Salvadó, M.I. Covas, D. Corella, F. Arós, E. Gómez-Gracia, V. Ruiz-Gutiérrez, et al. 2018. "Primary Prevention of Cardiovascular Disease with a Mediterranean Diet Supplemented with Extra-virgin Olive Oil or Nuts." *New England Journal of Medicine* 378(25): e34.

65. Peters, U., M. F. Leitzmann, N. Chatterjee, Y. Wang, D. Albanes, E. P. Gelmann, M. D. Friesen, E. Riboli, et al. 2007. "Serum Lycopene, Other Carotenoids, and Prostate Cancer Risk: A Nested Case-Control Study in the Prostate, Lung, Colorectal, and Ovarian Cancer Screening Trial." *Cancer Epidemiology Biomarkers & Prevention* 16 (5): 962–68. https://doi.org/10.1158/1055-9965.EPI-06-0861.

66. Chowdhury, R., S. Warnakula, S. Kunutsor, F. Crowe, H.A. Ward, L. Johnson, O.H. Franco, A.S. Butterworth, et al. 2014. "Association of Dietary, Circulating, and Supplement Fatty Acids With Coronary Risk." *Annals of Internal Medicine* 160 (6): 398. https://doi.org/10.7326/M13-1788.

67. Barnard, N.D., W.C. Willett, and E.L. Ding. 2017. "The Misuse of Meta-Analysis in Nutrition Research." *JAMA* 318 (15): 1435. https://doi.org/10.1001/jama.2017.12083.

68. Willett, W. 1999. *Nutritional Epidemiology.* 2nd ed. New York: Oxford University Press.

69. Willett, W. C., L. Sampson, M. J. Stampfer, B. Rosner, C. Bain, J. Witschi, C. H. Hennekens, and F. E. Speizer. 1985. "Reproducibility and Validity of a Semiquantitative Food Frequency Questionnaire." *American Journal of Epidemiology* 122 (1): 51–65. http://www.ncbi.nlm.nih.gov/pubmed/4014201.

70. Powles, J., S. Fahimi, R. Micha, S. Khatibzadeh, P. Shi, M. Ezzati, R.E. Engell, S.S. Lim, et al., and Global Burden of Diseases Nutrition and Chronic Diseases Expert Group. 2013. "Global, Regional and National Sodium Intakes in 1990 and 2010: A Systematic Analysis of 24 h Urinary Sodium Excretion and Dietary Surveys Worldwide." *BMJ Open* 3 (12): e003733. https://doi.org/10.1136/bmjopen-2013-003733.

71. Mozaffarian, D., S. Fahimi, G.M. Singh, R. Micha, S. Khatibzadeh, R.E. Engell, S. Lim, G. Danaei, et al. 2014. "Global Sodium Consumption and Death from Cardiovascular Causes." *New England Journal of Medicine* 371 (7): 624–34. https://doi.org/10.1056/NEJMoa1304127.

72. Morgenstern, H., and E. S. Bursic. 1982. "A Method for Using Epidemiologic Data to Estimate the Potential Impact of an Intervention on the Health Status of a Target Population." *Journal of Community Health* 7 (4): 292–309. http://www.ncbi.nlm.nih.gov/pubmed/7130448.

73. World Bank. 1993. *World Development Report 1993 : Investing in Health.* New York: Oxford University Press. https://doi.org/10.1596/0-1952-0890-0.

74. Salomon, J. A., J. A. Haagsma, A. Davis, C. M. de Noordhout, S. Polinder, A. H. Havelaar, A. Cassini, et al. 2015. "Disability Weights for the Global Burden of Disease 2013 Study." *The Lancet Global Health* 3 (11): e712-23. https://doi.org/10.1016/s2214-109x(15)00069-8.

75. Mozaffarian, D., A. Afshin, N. L. Benowitz, V. Bittner, S. R. Daniels, H. A. Franch, D. R. Jacobs, et al. 2012. "Population Approaches to Improve Diet, Physical

Activity, and Smoking Habits: A Scientific Statement From the American Heart Association." *Circulation* 126 (12): 1514-63. https://doi.org/10.1161/CIR .0b013e318260a20b.

76. Afshin, A., J. Penalvo, L. Del Gobbo, M. Kashaf, R. Micha, K. Morrish, J. Pearson-Stuttard, C. Rehm, et al. 2015. "CVD Prevention Through Policy: A Review of Mass Media, Food/Menu Labeling, Taxation/Subsidies, Built Environment, School Procurement, Worksite Wellness, and Marketing Standards to Improve Diet." *Current Cardiology Reports* 17 (11): 98. https://doi.org/10.1007/s11886 -015-0658-9.

77. Penalvo, J. L., F. Cudhea, R. Micha, C. D. Rehm, A. Afshin, L. Whitsel, P. Wilde, et al. 2017. "The Potential Impact of Food Taxes and Subsidies on Cardiovascular Disease and Diabetes Burden and Disparities in the United States." *BMC Medicine* 15 (1): 208. https://doi.org/10.1186/s12916-017-0971-9.

78. Pearson-Stuttard, J., P. Bandosz, C.D. Rehm, A. Afshin, J.L. Penalvo, L. Whitsel, G. Danaei, R. Micha, et al. 2017. "Comparing Effectiveness of Mass Media Campaigns with Price Reductions Targeting Fruit and Vegetable Intake on US Cardiovascular Disease Mortality and Race Disparities." *The American Journal of Clinical Nutrition* 106 (1): 199-206. https://doi.org/10.3945/ajcn.116.143925.

79. Pearson-Stuttard, J., P. Bandosz, C.D. Rehm, J. Penalvo, L. Whitsel, T. Gaziano, Z. Conrad, P. Wilde, et al. 2017. "Reducing US Cardiovascular Disease Burden and Disparities through National and Targeted Dietary Policies: A Modelling Study." *PLOS Medicine* 14 (6): e1002311. https://doi.org/10.1371/journal .pmed.1002311.

80. Moreira, P.V., L. Hyseni, J.C. Moubarac, A.P.B. Martins, L.G. Baraldi, S. Capewell, M. O'Flaherty, and M. Guzman-Castillo. 2018. "Effects of Reducing Processed Culinary Ingredients and Ultra-Processed Foods in the Brazilian Diet: A Cardiovascular Modelling Study." *Public Health Nutrition* 21 (1): 181-88. https://doi .org/10.1017/S1368980017002063.

81. Moreira, P.V., L.G. Baraldi, J.C. Moubarac, C.A. Monteiro, A. Newton, S. Capewell, and M. O'Flaherty. 2015. "Comparing Different Policy Scenarios to Reduce the Consumption of Ultra-Processed Foods in UK: Impact on Cardiovascular Disease Mortality Using a Modelling Approach." *PLOS One* 10 (2): e0118353. https://doi.org/10.1371/journal.pone.0118353.

82. Huffman, M.D., D.M. Lloyd-Jones, H. Ning, D.R. Labarthe, M. Guzman Castillo, M. O'Flaherty, E.S. Ford, and S. Capewell. 2013. "Quantifying Options for Reducing Coronary Heart Disease Mortality by 2020." *Circulation* 127 (25): 2477-84. https://doi.org/10.1161/CIRCULATIONAHA.112.000769.

83. Powles, J.W., W. Zatonski, S. Vander Hoorn, and M. Ezzati. 2005. "The Contribution of Leading Diseases and Risk Factors to Excess Losses of Healthy Life in Eastern Europe: Burden of Disease Study." *BMC Public Health* 5 (1): 116.

84. He, F.J., S. Pombo-Rodrigues, and G.A. MacGregor, 2014. "Salt Reduction in England from 2003 to 2011: Its Relationship to Blood Pressure, Stroke and Ischaemic Heart Disease Mortality." *BMJ Open* 4 (4): e004549.

85. Rehm, C.D., J.L. Peñalvo, A. Afshin, and D. Mozaffarian. 2016. "Dietary Intake among US Adults, 1999-2012." *JAMA* 315(23): 2542-53.

86. Dandona, L., R. Dandona, G.A. Kumar, D.K. Shukla, V.K. Paul, K. Balakrishnan, D. Prabhakaran, N. Tandon, et al. 2017. "Nations within a Nation: Variations in Epidemiological Transition across the states of India, 1990-2016 in the Global Burden of Disease Study." *The Lancet* 390(10111): 2437-60.

87. Mokdad, A.H., K. Ballestros, M. Echko, S. Glenn, H.E. Olsen, E. Mullany, A. Lee, A.R. Khan, et al. 2018. "The State of US Health, 1990-2016: Burden of Diseases, Injuries, and Risk Factors among US States." *JAMA* 319 (14), 1444-72.

8

A Deeper Look: Obesity

Sara N. Bleich, Johannah M. Frelier, and Kelsey A. Vercammen

LEARNING OBJECTIVES

- Describe current trends in obesity and understand disparities in obesity risk
- Discuss macro-level causes of the obesity epidemic
- Explain the physical, psychosocial, and economic consequences of obesity
- Compare and contrast approaches to combat the obesity epidemic

Case Study: Shape Up Somerville

Somerville is a densely populated, working-class city located in Massachusetts, United States.[1] Somerville has a poverty prevalence of 14.7% and over half of the young children in the community (grades 1-3) participate in a federally subsidized school lunch program that provides meals at low cost or no cost depending on a family's income.[1,2] In 2003, 20% of children in grades 1-3 had overweight and 24% had obesity.[2] This high prevalence of overweight and obesity is understandable considering the **obesogenic environment** that many children in Somerville and other communities in the United States grow up in. Increased access to energy-dense and nutrient-poor meals, rising meal portion sizes, and reduced physical activity may have all contributed to the high levels of childhood obesity observed in the United States in recent years. In an effort to address the high prevalence of overweight and obesity in the city of Somerville, a community-based intervention called "Shape Up Somerville" was developed and implemented in 2003 by researchers from Tufts University, in cooperation with Somerville community partners.[2] The intervention was a multipronged strategy that targeted elementary schools, home life, and the community environment in order to create opportunities for physical activity and increase the availability of healthy food choices for children, with the goal of preventing obesity. Within the school setting, the physical activity and nutrition curriculum were expanded, cafeterias provided more healthy offerings, and school wellness policies were developed. Within the home setting, parents were invited to participate in family events, received bimonthly newsletters that promoted healthy living, and were given free and discounted coupons for healthy foods. Within the community setting, sidewalks were improved and bike lanes were implemented, restaurants enhanced menus, and farmers markets offered promotions on fruits and vegetables.[2] Two years following the implementation of the "Shape Up Somerville" intervention, researchers examined the change in body mass index (BMI) z-scores of children living in Somerville compared to two comparison communities, finding that the BMI z-scores of children in Somerville significantly decreased by 0.06 units compared to controls.[3] Similarly, compared to children in the comparison communities, the odds of overweight and obesity were significantly lower in boys and girls in Somerville (odds ratio = 0.61 for boys, 0.78 for girls).[3] These results are promising and provide evidence that multipronged interventions can be effective in slowing the obesity epidemic.

Over the past few decades, the prevalence of obesity increased drastically in American adults and children. As it would turn out, this obesity epidemic was not isolated to the United States, but rather it was occurring in countries all over the globe. Obesity is one of the most important public health issues of our day. It is extremely prevalent, difficult to prevent and treat, and it increases the risk for many other diseases such as diabetes, hypertension, cardiovascular disease, osteoarthritis, sleep apnea, and multiple cancers.[4] In addition to health consequences, obesity also has economic consequences, including placing a substantial cost burden on health systems. Finally, individuals with obesity often also experience psychosocial consequences due to prevalent bullying, bias, and discrimination against people with obesity. In this chapter, we will take a detailed look at the prevalence of obesity, including disparities in obesity prevalence by socioeconomic status and race/ethnicity. We will examine key underlying causes of obesity and the obesity epidemic and then look briefly at potential approaches that show promise for preventing obesity.

Defining Overweight and Obesity

The human body is composed of two major components: adipose (fat) tissue and lean body mass (which is made up of muscle, bone, and extracellular water).[5] In its simplest definition, overweight and **obesity** can be defined as an excessive amount of adipose tissue. Ideally, then, we would have a way to directly measure adipose tissue and to know what level of adipose tissue is "excessive." However, directly measuring adipose tissue is expensive and requires specialized equipment. It is therefore not frequently measured in large population samples that also function to track the incidence of disease. As a result, few studies have actually been able to relate direct measurements of adipose to disease incidence or prevalence. Instead, many studies have instead used a popular proxy for excessive adipose tissue, body mass index (BMI), and determined what level of BMI is excessive based on the BMI at which disease risk begins to increase substantially. While many anthropometric metrics exist to measure body composition, BMI is the most widely used population-level

Box 8.1. Strengths and Limitations of BMI as a Measure of Adiposity

While body mass index (BMI) is one of the most widely accepted and easily obtained metrics for classifying overweight and obesity, there are some notable limitations. First, BMI does not distinguish between lean body mass and adipose (fat) tissue.[6] Among middle-aged adults, this is not problematic since most of the variation in weight not accounted for by height can be explained by differences in adipose tissue.[6] In some instances, very muscular individuals (e.g., professional athletes or body builders) may be misclassified as overweight or obese using BMI, but this extremely muscular body type does not apply to the majority of the population. However, among older adults, whose lean body mass declines as they age, the variation in weight not accounted for by height is increasingly attributable to differences in lean body mass, not adipose tissue.[7] Therefore, the validity of BMI as a measure of excess adipose tissue is reduced significantly in aging populations.

Another limitation of BMI is that it does not capture the regional distribution of adipose tissue.[5] This is problematic because the distribution of adipose tissue plays an important role in determining the level of risk for diseases associated with obesity. For example, individuals with visceral obesity (excess intra-abdominal adipose tissue) are at the highest risk for cardiovascular disease.[8] Third, variations in body composition across ethnic groups can complicate the use of BMI cutoff values for overweight and obesity.[5] For example, for the same BMI, blacks generally have a lower percentage of body fat than whites, while Asian Americans generally have a higher percentage body fat than whites.[9,10] As a result, different BMI cutoffs for overweight and obesity have been suggested for different race/ethnicities.[11]

Despite these limitations, BMI remains an invaluable tool in classifying overweight and obesity in populations where it is impractical or expensive to utilize gold standard methods such as computed tomography (CT), magnetic resonance imaging (MRI), or dual-energy x-ray absorptiometry (DXA) techniques. Height and weight can easily be obtained through portable scales and stadiometers (to measure height), minimizing the need for expensive equipment and measurement tools. For web- or telephone-based surveys, height and weight can be self-reported.

In addition to BMI, many anthropometric metrics exist to measure body composition including densitometry (underwater weighing), bioelectrical impedance (body fat), imaging methods (e.g., CT, MRI, DXA), skinfold thickness, and circumference measures.[5] While an in-depth discussion of each of these metrics is beyond the scope of this chapter, it is important to point out that each has relative advantages and disadvantages with respect to ease of measurement, cost, accuracy, and ability to assess body composition and fat distribution.[5] Generally, BMI performs well against these measures. For example, the relatively high validity of BMI as a measure of fat mass has been reported in a number of epidemiological studies.[12,13] Also, BMI and circumference measures (waist and waist-to-hip ratio) are similarly strong predictors of type 2 diabetes.[14,15]

measure.[5] BMI requires just a measurement (or self-report) of weight and height, and is therefore low cost, easy to calculate, and involves minimal user error (see box 8.1 for additional information about BMI).

BMI is calculated as the ratio of weight (in kilograms) and the square of height (in meters) using the following equation:

$$BMI = \text{weight in kg} / (\text{height in m})^2$$

Among adult populations, the World Health Organization (WHO) defines overweight as a BMI $\geq 25 \text{kg/m}^2$ and obesity as a BMI $\geq 30 \text{kg/m}^2$, with obesity further classified as class 1 obesity (BMI 30.0–34.9kg/m²), class 2 obesity (BMI 35.0–39.9kg/m²), and class 3 obesity (BMI $\geq 40.0 \text{kg/m}^2$) (table 8.1).[16] Classifi-

Table 8.1. Weight Status Classifications for Adults and Children

	BMI (kg/m²)[a]	BMI percentile[b]
Underweight	<18.5	<5th percentile
Healthy Weight	18.5 to 24.9	5th to <85th percentile
Overweight	≥25.0	85 to <95th percentile
Pre-obese	25.0 to 29.0	—
Obesity	≥30.0	≥95th percentile
Class I Obesity	30.0 to 34.9	—
Class II Obesity	35.0 to 39.9	—
Class III Obesity	≥40.0	—

Source: Adapted from WHO Nutritional Status by Body Mass Index Classification. http://www.euro.who.int/en/health-topics/disease-prevention/nutrition/a-healthy-lifestyle/body-mass-index-bmi.
[a]BMI cutoffs used for adults are consistent with WHO and CDC classifications.
[b]BMI percentile for children is consistent with CDC definition.

cation of overweight and obesity among children and adolescents is more complicated than among adults because both height and body composition are continually changing throughout childhood.[17] Therefore, instead of using BMI cutoff values, children are compared to peers using age- and sex-specific growth standards.[18] Based on these growth standards, for children aged 5-18, the WHO defines overweight as a BMI z-score for age and sex between 1 and 2 standard deviations above the WHO growth standard median and obesity as a BMI z-score for age and sex >2 standard deviations above the median.[19] Among children aged 0-5, WHO thresholds are more lenient, defining overweight as BMI z-score for age and sex >2 standard deviations above the median and obesity as BMI z-score for age and sex >3 standard deviations above the median.[19] Similarly, the US Centers for Disease Control and Prevention (CDC) defines overweight among children as a BMI for age and sex between the 85th and 94th percentiles and obesity as a BMI for age and sex greater than or equal to the 95th percentile.[20]

Obesity Prevalence and Trends
Global Trends and Trends in Developing Countries

Between 1980 and 2013, the global prevalence of overweight and obesity increased by 27.5% for adults and 47.1% for children, resulting in a total of 2.1 billion individuals with overweight or obesity across the world in 2013.[21] Currently, the WHO estimates that 39% of all adults in the world have overweight and 13% have obesity.[22]

There are important geographic trends within the obesity epidemic, with overweight and obesity "hotspots" in North America, Australia and New Zealand, the Pacific Islands, the Eastern Mediterranean, and the Persian Gulf. These are areas where the prevalence of obesity is higher than other parts of the world. Furthermore, greater than half of the world's population with obesity live in just 10 countries: the United States, China, India, Russia, Brazil, Mexico, Egypt, Pakistan, Indonesia, and Germany, although this statistic is influenced by the large population sizes of several of the included countries.

While overweight and obesity was once viewed as a problem of high-income countries, the obesity epidemic is rapidly spreading to low- and middle-income countries.[21] For example, from 1980 to 2013, the prevalence of childhood overweight and obesity in low- and middle-income countries rose from 8.1% to 12.9% among boys and from 8.4% to 13.4% among girls.[21] Moreover, 64% of all individuals with obesity currently live in low- and middle-income countries.[21] This has resulted in the "double burden" of disease, wherein developing countries must face the growing tide of obesity while concurrently addressing existing challenges of malnutrition and infectious diseases.[23] Chapter 10, on the nutrition transition, covers these trends and their causes in more detail.

Trends in High-Income Countries

Since the 1980s, the prevalence of obesity in high-income countries has risen dramatically (figure 8.1). From 1980 to 2008, the age-standardized prevalence of obesity increased from 11.3% to 31.1% in North America, from 11.1% to 20.0% in Western Europe, from 8.3% to 25.3% in Australasia, and from 2.2% to 5.4% in the Asia Pacific region.[24] The current prevalence of overweight and obesity among adults in high-income countries ranges from less than 6% in Japan and Korea to greater than 30% in the United States, Mexico, New Zealand, and Hungary, with 19.5% of the population making up the Organisation for Economic Co-operation and Development (OECD) countries classified as obese.[25] Although the absolute level of obesity varies considerably across the countries, the rate of increase has been quite similar. In general, the prevalence of obesity in high-income countries is higher among women, although the rate of increase in having overweight and obesity is higher among men.[21] With respect to age, prevalence overweight and obesity seems to peak among males in high-income countries around age 55 (of which 33% have overweight and 25% have obesity) and among females in high-income countries around age 60 (of which 31.3% have obesity and 64.5% have overweight or obesity).[21]

Among children and adolescents in high-income countries, the prevalence of overweight and obesity has also increased substantially over the past three decades. From 1980 to 2013, the prevalence of childhood overweight and obesity in high-income countries rose from 16.9% to 23.8% among boys and from 16.2% to 22.6% of girls.[21] The current prevalence of overweight and obesity among children at age 15 ranges from less than 12% in Switzerland, Denmark, Turkey, and France to greater than 20% in Greece, Canada, and the United States, with 15.5% of 15-year-olds in OECD countries classified having obesity.[25]

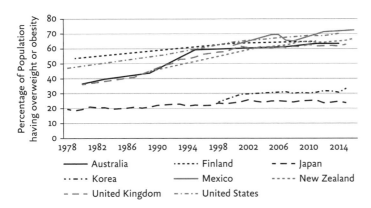

Figure 8.1. Percentage of total population having overweight or obesity in selected OECD countries. *Source:* Data from OECD Health Statistics Database. *Note:* Only countries with frequent and measured BMI data were included in this summary figure.

Following the steep rise in the prevalence of overweight and obesity observed in the 1980s and 1990s, there is a more recent indication that rates of overweight and obesity in high-income countries have begun to level off among the general population. The most consistent evidence for the stabilization of overweight and obesity has been reported for children and adolescents in high-income countries.[26-29] A recent review found that the mean BMI of children has plateaued for both sexes in northwestern Europe, high-income English-speaking countries (e.g., Australia, Canada) and Asia-Pacific regions, for boys in southwestern Europe, and for girls in Central and Andean Latin America.[29] Additionally, important declines in the prevalence of childhood overweight and obesity have been reported in some countries and subgroups. For example, since the early 2000s, childhood obesity in Japan has declined among all age groups except older adolescents (aged 17).[30] Evidence for the leveling off of overweight and obesity rates among adults is less consistent.[31] Increases in overweight and obesity prevalence appear to be slowing among adults in England,[32] but they remain high among adults in European countries, including Austria[33] and Sweden.[34]

Trends in the United States

In line with trends from other high-income countries, the prevalence of obesity has increased among children and adults in the United States.[35] Between 1988 and 2016, the prevalence of obesity among adults in the United States rose from 23% to 39.8%.[35,36] Between 1988 and 2016, the prevalence of childhood obesity in the United States increased from 7.2% to 13.9% among children ages 2 to 5, from 11.3% to 18.4% for children ages 6 to 11, and from 10.5% to 20.6% among adolescents ages 12 to 19.[35]

Disparities in Risk
Socioeconomic Status

The relationship between socioeconomic status (SES) and risk of obesity is complex and differs across high-income and low- and middle-income countries. In low- and many middle-income countries, a higher SES is generally associated with a higher risk of obesity.[37] This is likely in part due to the fact that low-income individuals in low- and middle-income countries are more likely to face food scarcity and be engaged in manual work that requires higher energy expenditure.[37] These characteristics place them at lower risk of obesity.

In high-income countries, however, lower SES is generally associated with a higher risk of obesity, although this association varies somewhat by country, gender, and age.[38] For example, a review of childhood overweight prevalence in 34 countries in Europe reported that children from less affluent families experienced higher levels of overweight than children from more affluent families in 21 of 24 western European countries and 5 of 10 central European countries.[39] Four countries (Poland, Lithuania, Macedonia, and Finland) reported this association only for girls in their population, with boys from more affluent families having higher levels of overweight than boys from less affluent families.[39] In the United States, the inverse relationship between income and risk of overweight and obesity is most consistent for females and children.

There are a number of ways in which SES can influence overweight and obesity risk in high-income countries.[40] First, income is a primary determinant of food insecurity and access to healthy foods. Families in low-income households are often forced to rely on cheap, energy-dense nutrient-poor foods.[41] These types of foods, combined with their high palatability, cause overconsumption of calories and lead to weight gain. Additionally, some research suggests low-income neighborhoods may have fewer full-service supermarkets, further limiting low-income households' access to healthy foods.[42] This can result in a higher consumption of foods from convenience and fast-food stores, which are often higher in calories and of lower nutritional quality than foods purchased from supermarkets. Moreover, low-income neighborhoods generally have limited opportunities for physical activity (e.g., public parks, green space) or residents may not feel safe engaging in physical activity (e.g., higher rates of crime, lack of sidewalks).[43] These reduced opportunities for physical activity may contribute to the higher prevalence of obesity among individuals who live in these neighborhoods. Finally, sleep quantity and quality, stress, and adverse childhood events have all been associated with obesity risk and are more prevalent among populations with lower incomes.

Race/Ethnicity

Racial/ethnic minorities in high-income countries often have a higher burden of overweight and obesity compared to their white and Asian counter-

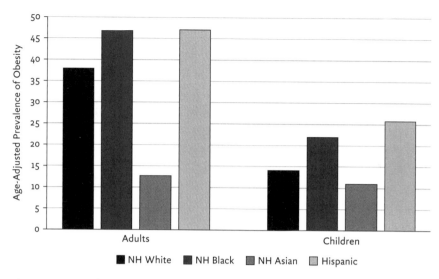

Figure 8.2. Age-adjusted prevalence of obesity for NH white, NH black, NH Asian, and Hispanic adults and children in the United States using NHANES 2015-2016. NH = Non-Hispanic. *Source:* Based on data from Hales, C. M., M. D. Carroll, C. D. Fryar, and C. L. Ogden. 2017. *Prevalence of Obesity Among Adults and Youth: United States, 2015-2016*. NCHS data brief, no 288. Hyattsville, MD: National Center for Health Statistics. https://www.cdc.gov/nchs/data/databriefs/db288.pdf.

parts. For example, in the United States the prevalence of obesity among non-Hispanic (NH) white adults is 37.9%, compared with 46.8% among NH black adults and 47.0% among Hispanic adults (figure 8.2).[36] Similarly, the prevalence of obesity among children is 14.1% for NH white children, compared with 22.0% for NH black children and 25.8% among Hispanic children.

The explanations for disparities in risk across race/ethnicity in the United States are complex and likely involve interactions between socioeconomic status, environments, structural and interpersonal racism, and cultural factors.[44] One explanation is that racial/ethnic minorities in the United States often experience a disproportionately higher poverty rate than their White counterparts (race is closely associated with socioeconomic status). For example, 23.2% of Hispanics and 25.8% of blacks have a household income below the US federal poverty line, compared to 11.6% of whites.[45] In line with the relationship between SES and obesity, racial/ethnic minorities in low-income households may experience higher food insecurity and are forced to rely on cheaper, energy-dense foods of lower nutritional quality. For example, evidence suggests that neighborhoods with higher proportions of blacks have fewer healthy options available outside of the home,[46,47] fast-food restaurants are more prevalent in poorer areas,[47] and consumption of fast food is higher among blacks. Additionally, structural racism may also contribute to these disparities since neighborhoods primarily occupied by racial/ethnic minorities often have limited places to be physically active, with fewer public parks, public pools, and green space available.[48] Related to a stress mechanism, the experience of interpersonal racism may be an added source of stress among racial/ethnic minorities and thereby an additional pathway through which race/ethnicity may augment the risk of obesity. Finally, racial/ethnic minorities are often targeted by the food industry through aggressive marketing of nutritionally poor foods.[49] For example, billboards and other forms of outdoor advertisement for high-calorie/low-nutrient products are reported to be 9 times denser in low-income Hispanic communities compared to white neighborhoods.[50] Another example is that exposure to food and beverage television advertisements is significantly higher in media markets with a higher percentage of blacks.

Indigenous Populations

Indigenous people often experience disproportionately high levels of overweight and obesity. For example, 25.7% of Indigenous people in Canada have obesity compared with 16.9% of non-Indigenous people.[51] In New Zealand, the disparities in risk are even more extreme: while the population average for obesity is 32%, 47% of Māori adults and 67% of Pacific Islands adults have obesity, respectively. In general, there is a lack of high quality, comprehensive health surveillance data among Indigenous populations. For example, the last comprehensive evaluation of obesity prevalence among the American Indian and Alaska Native populations in the United States took place in 1990 and 1991.[52]

As with other racial/ethnic minorities, the reasons for higher rates of obesity among Indigenous populations are multifaceted and may include factors such as disproportionate poverty, discrimination, structural and interpersonal racism, food insecurity, adverse childhood events, and historical trauma. One additional reason is that Indigenous populations often reside in rural and remote areas. Consequently, fresh and healthy foods must be transported long distances to reach the indigenous communities, resulting in limited availability and increased costs. For example, the cost of food products available to a remote indigenous community in Australia was found to be 63% higher than food products from supermarkets in large cities.[53] As a result of this reduced access to healthy foods, the diet of Indigenous people is often high in refined carbohydrates and saturated fats, heightening the risk of overweight and obesity.[54]

Causes of Obesity
Energy Imbalance

On an individual level, we gain or lose weight due to an imbalance between **energy intake** and **energy expenditure**. The long-term, cumulative effect of a positive **energy imbalance** (i.e., energy intake is greater than energy expenditure) is weight gain.[6,55] Increases in energy intake and decreases in energy expenditure have resulted in dramatic population-wide weight gain over the past three decades, which is driving the obesity epidemic. While the change in energy balance has been identified as the primary cause of the obesity, there is debate over the relative contributions of increased energy intake versus decreased energy expenditure in producing the obesity epidemic. One study estimated that increased energy intake accounted for 93% of the change in obesity prevalence observed between 1990 and 2002, with almost all of the countries included in the analysis attributing 60% or more of their population weight gain to excess energy intake.[55] In the United States, the daily number of excess daily calories contributing to the obesity epidemic in adults is 220 calories per day,[56] and in children it is 165 calories per day,[57] with higher levels among adolescents and racial/ethnic minority youth.[58]

Energy Intake

In parallel with obesity trends, the amount of food available for consumption in high-income countries has increased considerably (figure 8.3).[55] Between the 1980s and 2000s, the total amount of calories available for consumption increased by 300 calories/day in the United States, 530 calories/day in Canada, and 190 calories/day in the United Kingdom. This vast increase in the availability of calories has likely contributed to the overall increase in calories consumed by individuals over this same period. Key factors that have likely contributed to increased energy intake over the past 30 years include declines in food prices, increases in the efficiency of food production, greater availability of fast-food and calorie-dense foods, increases in portion size, and aggressive food and beverage marketing.[55]

First, food prices in high-income countries have declined considerably in recent decades, with this decline in price significantly associated with an increase in the number of available calories.[55,59] For example, the United States experienced an 8% decline in food prices between 1980 and 2002, which corresponded to an increase of 25 available calories/day per person.[55] Second, increases in the efficiency of food production through mass processing and distribution have lowered the time costs associated with food preparation.[59] For example, the time required to prepare a meal declined by about 50% from 1965 to 1995.[59] This lower preparation time has likely accelerated overconsumption of calories. Third, fast-food restaurants have proliferated to the point that 33% of children, 41% of adolescents, and 36% of adults are estimated to eat at fast-food restaurants on a typical day in the United States, with a mean caloric intake among consumers of 576 calories, 988 calories, and 877 calories, respectively.[60] Because fast-food meals are known to be high in calories and energy density, the increased presence of fast-food restaurants has likely resulted in higher caloric intake. Fourth, portion sizes for foods consumed outside of the home have increased substantially since the 1970s.[61] These expanding portion sizes mean that consumers are inadvertently

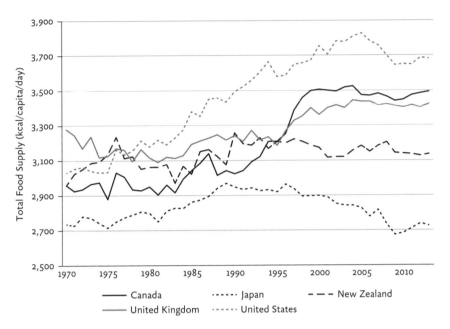

Figure 8.3. Trends in food supply (kcal/capita/day) in high-income countries. *Source:* Data from Food and Agriculture Organization of the United Nations, available until 2013. Adapted from Bleich, S. N., D. Cutler, C. Murray, and A. Adams. 2008. "Why Is the Developed World Obese?" *Annual Review of Public Health* 29 (1): 273–295. doi:10.1146 /annurev.publhealth.29.020907.090954.

consuming many more calories than their counterparts did in previous generations. Experimental evidence indicates that when we are presented with a larger portion size, we eat more total calories.[62] Finally, evidence suggests that the obesity epidemic may be attributable, in part, to the impact of marketing on what we eat and drink.[63,64] Marketing increases awareness of product brands, preferences for those brands, and consumption of those brands.[64,65] For example, an Institute of Medicine committee concluded that "food and beverage marketing influences the preferences and purchase requests of children, influences consumption at least in the short term, likely contributes to less-healthful diets, and may contribute to negative diet-related health outcomes and risk among children and youth."

Energy Expenditure

With respect to energy expenditure, there are a number of indications that populations of high-income countries have reduced energy expenditure in parallel with rising obesity prevalence. The largest declines in energy expenditure have occurred within occupational activity, and in particular, within the highly active work domain, wherein increasingly automated work environments have resulted in decreased energy expenditures for working adults.[55] Additionally, a shift toward sedentary activity (e.g., increased TV watching) has been observed, with consistent evidence demonstrating that a sedentary lifestyle is associated with higher rates of obesity.[66] A rise in passive transportation (e.g., increased car ownership and decreased use of walking or biking) has also likely contributed to the reduction in energy expenditure. For example, one study demonstrated that each additional hour spent in a car per day was associated with a 6% increase in the likelihood of obesity.[67] While energy expenditure has declined over the past 30 years, the magnitude of that change is likely too small to fully explain the obesity epidemic. However, regular physical activity remains an important part of weight maintenance and good health on an individual level.[68,69]

Consequences of Obesity
Physical Health Consequences

There is an abundance of evidence linking overweight and obesity to cardiovascular risk factors (e.g., hypertension), chronic diseases (e.g., cancer), endocrine and metabolic conditions (e.g., insulin resistance), musculoskeletal disorders (e.g., osteoarthritis), and numerous other health problems (e.g., respiratory). Table 8.2 summarizes the physical health consequences associated with overweight and obesity.

Cardiovascular Risk Factors and Cardiovascular Disease

Obesity is strongly associated with many cardiovascular risk factors, including hypertension, increased cholesterol and triglyceride levels, and impaired fasting glucose.[70,71] While these cardiovascular risk factors were primarily seen only among adults with obesity in the past, more recent evidence has consistently documented that children with obesity are increasingly diagnosed with abnormal levels of these cardiometabolic risk factors.[72,73] Partially as a result of the relationship between obesity and cardiovascular risk factors, obesity is also associated with cardiovascular diseases (CVD), including coronary heart disease, stroke, and congestive failure. For example, a meta-analysis of 33 cohort studies pooling data from 310,000 participants in the Asia-Pacific region found positive associations between BMI and risk of ischemic stroke, hemorrhagic stroke, and ischemic heart disease.[74] Similarly, researchers from another study reported that women with obesity had a 2.4 fold greater risk of coronary heart disease compared to women of normal weight.[75] More recently, researchers have come to view obesity as an independent risk factor for CVD, with evidence suggesting that the association between obesity and CVD may not be completely explained by traditional cardiovascular risk factors (e.g., hypertension, high cholesterol).[66] For instance, a 2007 meta-analysis reported that increased BMI remained associated with coronary heart disease events even after adjustment for blood pressure and cholesterol levels, suggesting that obesity may have an independent effect on the occurrence of CVD.[76] Hypothesized

Table 8.2. Physical Health Consequences of Overweight and Obesity

Physical health consequence category	Specific outcomes associated with obesity (selective not exhaustive)
Cardiovascular risk factors	▪ Hypertension[70,71] ▪ Increased cholesterol levels[70,71,67,68] ▪ Increased triglyceride levels[70,67] ▪ Impaired fasting glucose
Chronic diseases	Cardiovascular disease[76] ▪ CHD ▪ Stroke ▪ Peripheral vascular disease Cancer[78] ▪ Endometrial cancer ▪ Colorectal cancer ▪ Adenocarcinoma of the esophagus ▪ Postmenopausal breast cancer Others ▪ Gallbladder disease
Endocrine and metabolic conditions	Endocrine disturbances[6] ▪ Insulin resistance ▪ Reproductive function metabolic disturbances[6] ▪ Metabolic syndrome
Reproductive	▪ Infertility (ovulation disorders) ▪ Miscarriage, stillbirth ▪ Gestational diabetes mellitus
Musculoskeletal	▪ Osteoarthritis[17] ▪ Gout[17]
Other health problems	▪ Pulmonary disease[17]
Mortality	▪ Increased risk of mortality[79,80]

mechanisms through which obesity may independently exert its effect on CVD risk include inflammation, endothelial dysfunction, and thromobogenic factors.[66]

Cancer

There is consistent evidence linking overweight and obesity with certain types of cancer (i.e., hormone-dependent and gastrointestinal cancers), with one study estimating that overweight and obesity account for 14% of deaths from cancer in men and 20% of deaths from cancer in women.[77] Cancers that have the strongest association with overweight and obesity include endometrial cancer, colorectal cancer, adenocarcinoma of the esophagus, and postmenopausal breast cancer.[66] Compared to CVD, there have been considerably fewer studies examining the association between obesity and cancer.[66]

Metabolic and Endocrine Health

Consistent evidence has demonstrated an association between obesity and metabolic and endocrine health. Because adipose tissue produces and is the target of many hormones, individuals with excess adipose tissue often experience endocrine disturbances, particularly in the form of insulin resistance.[66] Consequently, overweight and obesity are considered to be among the most important predictors of type 2 diabetes. For example, in a 16-year cohort study, the risk of type 2 diabetes was 20.1 fold higher for women with obesity compared to women with a BMI less than 23.0.[78] Additional endocrine-related issues associated with obesity include dysfunction in hormones affecting reproductive health (e.g., polycystic ovary syndrome) and adrenocortical function.[17] Abdominal obesity is a component of the "metabolic syndrome," the name for the interconnected collection of symptoms related to metabolic disturbances (e.g., hypertension, high cholesterol, dyslipidemia).

Mortality

Compared to those of healthy weight, individuals with overweight and obesity have increased all-cause mortality risk.[79,80] In a review of over 10 million participants in Asia, Australia, New Zealand, Europe, and North America, researchers reported that those with grade 1 obesity (BMI 30.0–35.0 kg/m^2) had a 45% higher rate of death during the study period (95% CI: 1.41–1.48) compared to healthy weight (BMI 18.5–25.0 kg/m^2) participants.[80] See box 8.2 for an explanation of the phenomenon related to obesity and mortality called the "obesity paradox."

This discussion of physical health consequences is not meant to be exhaustive; obesity affects almost every organ in the body and so is associated with a large number of negative health outcomes.

Economic Consequences

In addition to negative health outcomes, overweight and obesity place a substantial economic burden on health care systems and to broader society. The cost of overweight and obesity can be broken down into *direct costs*, which refer to resources used in the provision of health care services to individuals with overweight or obesity, and *indirect costs*, which include productivity costs (e.g., losses in economic production attributable to overweight and obesity) and transportation costs (e.g., more fuel and larger vehicles are needed to transport heavier travelers).[87] Costs associated with obesity among children and adolescents are particularly concerning because childhood obesity is known to persist in adulthood, resulting in an accumulation of both direct and indirect costs over the life span.[88]

Box 8.2. The Obesity Paradox

The "obesity paradox" refers to the phenomenon in which individuals with overweight or obesity appear to be healthier than individuals with a healthy weight. This has been observed for all-cause mortality, with one highly publicized systematic review and meta-analysis reporting a U-shaped relationship between weight status and all-cause mortality, with the lowest all-cause mortality risk (i.e., the bottom of the U) among overweight individuals.[81] It is now understood that the obesity paradox can be explained by the presence of confounders (e.g., smoking) and reverse causation (e.g., weight loss due to chronic disease).[82] Since the publication of the original systematic review and meta-analysis, a number of reviews have been published with more detailed attention to confounder control and reducing reverse causality.[79,80] The results of these studies have been consistent in finding that overweight and obesity are associated with increased all-cause mortality risk.

A second dimension of the obesity paradox is that individuals with overweight and obesity are associated with a decreased risk of mortality among clinical subpopulations—for example, those with chronic diseases such as cardiovascular disease, cancer, and respiratory disease.[83,84] One study reported that among patients with stable heart failure, those who had overweight and obesity actually lived longer than those who were normal weight.[85] However, it is now well documented that these associations are spurious and occur because of a bias that epidemiologists have called "collider stratification," which occurs when we restrict to or control for a variable that (1) is associated with the exposure (in this case, obesity) and (2) shares common causes with the outcome (mortality in the example above).[84,86] For example, (1) heart failure is associated with obesity (i.e., variable is associated with exposure), and (2) risk factors including genetic factors and lifestyle behaviors contribute to both heart failure and mortality (i.e., variable shares common cause with the outcome), satisfying the conditions of the collider stratification bias.[84] While a complete discussion of how these conditions contribute to bias is beyond the scope of this section, it should be acknowledged that failure to consider collider stratification bias results in a spurious association between obesity and mortality within clinical subpopulations.[84,86]

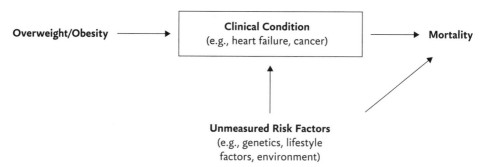

Directed acyclic graph to illustrate collider stratification bias in obesity paradox among clinical subpopulations. *Source:* Figure adapted from Banack, H. R., and A. Stokes. 2017. "The 'Obesity Paradox' May Not Be a Paradox at All." *International Journal of Obesity* 41 (8): 1162–1163. doi:10.1038/ijo.2017.99.

Direct Costs

As discussed in the "Physical Health Consequences" section, obesity is associated with a number of health conditions that may require additional medical care and services. The indirect costs associated with obesity are estimated to account for between 54% and 59% of total costs.[89] Individuals with obesity are estimated to have medical costs approximately 30% greater than their normal-weight counterparts.[90] In a pooled analysis of studies published between 1968 and 2009, the annual per-person direct medical cost of obesity in the United States was estimated at $266 for individuals with overweight and $1,723 for individuals with obesity, resulting in an annual aggregate national cost of overweight and obesity of $113.9 billion.[91] Estimates of direct costs related to overweight and obesity in other countries include CA$6 billion for Canada and €4.85 billion for Germany.[85] Medical expenditures increase with BMI, meaning people with severe obesity incur the largest share of costs associated with overweight and obesity despite making up a smaller proportion of the total population with excess weight.[87]

Indirect Costs

The indirect productivity-related costs associated with obesity include presenteeism, absenteeism, disability, and premature mortality. **Presenteeism** is defined as the costs accrued when an employee is present at work but not able to function at full capacity or productivity due to a health condition. While the evidence linking obesity to presenteeism is limited, there is some indication that higher BMI is associated with presenteeism among working populations.[92] **Absenteeism** refers to time absent from work because of a condition or illness, with costs accrued in the form of lost productivity or increased payouts for sick leave.[87] There is strong evidence that employees with overweight and obesity experience higher levels of absenteeism, with annual obesity-related absenteeism costs in the United States estimated at $6.38 billion.[87] **Disability** in this context refers to both short- and long-term absence from the workplace because a condition or illness precludes one's ability to meet occupational demands.[87] There is a well-established relationship between overweight and obesity and disability in the literature, with the strongest associations found for individuals with obesity. Costs due to **premature mortality** are defined as the lost productivity costs incurred from obesity-related early deaths.[87] Most estimates report that premature mortality makes up the largest proportion of indirect costs, with annual obesity-related premature mortality costs estimated at $30.15 billion.[87]

Obesity may also impact transportation costs because individuals with overweight or obesity require more fuel and larger vehicles to be transported. One study estimated that the weight gained by Americans in the 1990s required the consumption of an additional 350 million gallons of jet fuel in the year 2000.[93] This translated to an added cost of $275 billion to transport this excess adiposity.[93]

Social and Psychosocial Consequences
Weight Stigma

In high-income countries, individuals with overweight or obesity are often highly stigmatized. One study reported that individuals with obesity are 40% to 50% more likely to report any type of stigma, including work-related (e.g., wage penalties), health-related (e.g., inferior medical assistance), lifetime (e.g., professional or academic achievement), or day-to-day stigma.[94]

Within the workplace, evidence points to systematic **weight stigma** against employees with obesity through hiring prejudice and inequity in wages, promotions, and employment termination.[95] One review summarized common stereotypes employers report holding about applicants or employees with obesity, with characteristics including "lacking self-discipline or self-control," "lazy, doesn't try as hard," and "less competent, less ability, less skill."[96] **Wage penalties** (or being paid less for the same work, which have been documented particularly among women with obesity compared to healthy weight counterparts) have serious implications against individuals with overweight or obesity; for example, women with overweight in the United States have lower household incomes and higher rates of household poverty compared to normal-weight women, even after controlling for differences in other characteristics.[97]

Within the health care system, it is well documented that many medical professionals hold negative attitudes toward patients with obesity.[95,98,99] This type of health-related weight stigma is particularly problematic if these negative attitudes have a detrimental impact on clinical judgement, diagnosis and care for patients with obesity. Furthermore, if individuals with obesity perceive the negative attitude of their health professional, they may delay seeking medical care in the future.[100]

Individuals with obesity may also experience weight stigma within the education setting, a domain that is particularly relevant for childhood and adolescent obesity.[99] In particular, children with obesity are more likely to be bullied with teasing, jokes, and derogatory name-calling while at school.[99,101]

Psychological Effects

There is increasing evidence that individuals with overweight or obesity experience heightened mental health disorders. One study conducted among adults in 13 countries reported associations between obesity and both depressive and anxiety disorders, with the strongest associations amongst females and those with severe obesity.[102] A systematic review among children and adolescents found strong evidence that obesity impacts quality of life and self-esteem of children with obesity.[103]

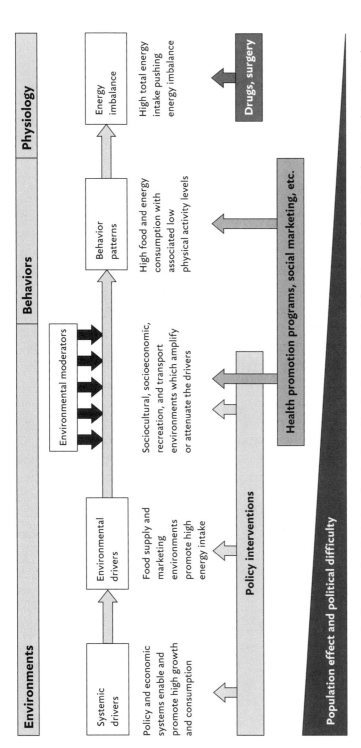

Figure 8.4. Framework of causes of and solutions for obesity epidemic. *Source:* Reprinted from *Lancet*, vol. 378, Swinburn, Boyd A., Gary Sacks, Kevin D. Hall, Klim McPherson, Diane T. Finegood, Marjory L. Moodie, and Steven L. Gortmaker, "The Global Obesity Pandemic: Shaped by Global Drivers and Local Environments," pp. 804–814. Copyright (2011), with permission from Elsevier.

Obesity Interventions

Frameworks for obesity solutions generally consider three main targets for intervention: the environment, behavior, and physiology (figure 8.4).[104] Policy, systems, and/or environmental interventions are needed to affect change in the environmental domain by reducing obesogenic drivers (e.g., food supply and marketing). Interventions in schools, the community, and home can alter the environmental domain but are primarily intended to target the behavior of individuals. Weight-loss medications and surgery are used to change the physiological domain and are beyond the scope of this chapter.

Policy Approaches

High-income and upper-middle-income countries are leading the effort on initiating policies to target systemic and environmental drivers of the obesity epidemic. Policies to reduce obesity include school-based policies (e.g., regulation of vending machines and food served in school meal programs), community-based policies (e.g., restriction of fast-food restaurants through zoning), food industry–based policies (e.g., calorie labeling), and society-wide policies (e.g., regulation of food marketing to children).[104,105] In general, policy interventions may have the potential for greatest population effect because they are more sustainable, are intended to reach the entire population, and often target the root causes of obesity.[104] While policy approaches have the greatest potential to reverse the obesity epidemic, they are often the most difficult to implement.[106] In particular, they are often met with significant opposition from food industry lobbyists, who tend to have significant financial resources.[106] Two examples are provided to illustrate how policy interventions can be used to target environmental risk factors for obesity.

Example 1: Sugar-Sweetened Beverage Tax in Mexico and Berkeley, CA

Sugar-sweetened beverages (SSBs) are drinks with added caloric sweetener (e.g., soda, sports drinks, fruit drinks). There is considerable interest in beverage taxes as a way to reduce SSB intake, as these beverages are strongly linked with obesity, are a risk factor for cancer and type 2 diabetes, and have no nutritional value.[107-112] SSBs are also the largest source of added sugar intake in the US diet[113] with significantly higher consumption in low-income and racial/ethnic minority communities.[114-117] Numerous studies have modeled the effects of taxes on sugar-sweetened beverage consumption and obesity; most of the studies find reduced sugar-sweetened beverage consumption effects with taxes and price increases.[118-120] The most informative real-world evidence to date on the influence of sugar-sweetened beverage taxes on SSB purchases comes from Mexico, and Berkeley, California. Data from Mexico showed that a one peso per fluid ounce SSB tax was associated with a 12% decline in sugar-sweetened beverage purchases (and a 17% decline among low-income consumers) as well as a 4% increase in purchases of non-taxed beverages, mainly bottled plain water.[121] The study of beverage sales in Berkeley found significant declines in sugar-sweetened beverage sales over time compared to control sites (sales, measured in ounces of taxed SSBs, fell by 9.6%).[122] Another study in Berkeley reported that sugar-sweetened beverage intake declined by 25% in low-income neighborhoods compared to control cities six months after tax implementation.[123] To date, no empirical evaluations of beverage taxes have evaluated their impact on obesity risk or other related outcomes.

Example 2: Menu Labeling in the United States

In 2014, the Food and Drug Administration (FDA) issued a final ruling for the implementation of the Affordable Care Act provision that mandated calorie labeling on menus in chain restaurants or similar retail food establishments with more than 20 outlets.[124] After multiple delays, the rule was enforced on May 7, 2018. Policy makers hoped that the menu labeling would catalyze consumers to purchase menu items with fewer calories and that restaurants in turn would reformulate to offer lower-calorie menu items. A recent review evaluating menu labeling prior to the mandate found moderate evidence that menu labeling can indeed reduce calories purchased in restaurants and cafeterias, although more research is needed to tease out how alternative strategies for presenting calorie information (e.g., traffic light labels) may be more effective in altering consumer behavior.[125] Emerging literature suggests that the largest impact of menu labeling may come from restaurants reformulating their menus to offer lower-calorie items.[124,126]

A further discussion of nutrition-related policy approaches is included in chapter 14. Briefly, that chapter looks at examples of nutrition programs and policies across high-income countries and takes a deeper dive into the large suite of nutrition assistance programs in the United States.

School-Based Approaches

Schools have been a focal point for childhood obesity interventions for the past few decades because students spend half of their waking hours and consume at least one-third of their daily calories at school.[127] See, for example, the panel on "Shape Up Somerville," which is based in the school setting, among other locations. Schools are uniquely positioned to implement population-based interventions because they can reach a majority of children using existing infrastructure and without significant adjustments to the children's schedule or lifestyle. Interventions in schools often include a diet-only component (e.g., classes to improve nutrition knowledge), a physical activity-only component (e.g., additional time dedicated each week to physical education classes), or a combined approach using both diet and physical activity. Several recent systematic reviews have identified school-based interventions as having the strongest evidence for success compared to interventions conducted in preschools, the community, or home.[128,129] More specifically, interventions that included a combined diet and physical activity approach and an element of home outreach were often the most effective in controlling weight gain.

Community-Based Approaches

Given the importance of the environmental drivers in the obesity epidemic, researchers are increasingly turning to the community as a point of intervention.[127] Modifiable aspects of the community include the walkability of sidewalks, availability of parks and playgrounds, opportunities to purchase healthy foods, and community-wide social events.[127] Compared to school-based approaches, the evidence for community-based interventions is considerably more limited with additional heterogeneity in intervention characteristics and implementation.[130] One systematic review reported moderate evidence supporting combined diet and physical activity interventions conducted in the community,[130] while another found much weaker evidence (although both were limited by a small number of studies).[129]

Home-Based Approaches

There is strong recognition for the role of the family and home environment in impacting the nutrition and diet-related behaviors of children.[131] Examples of home-based obesity prevention approaches include meal and snack planning,[132] reducing screen time,[132] nutrition education, and family goal setting.[132,133] However, the evidence for exclusively home-based approaches is relatively weak, with most studies finding minimal evidence of success.[128,134] As discussed in the school-based approach section, there is stronger evidence for interventions that are grounded in schools but additionally include home elements.

Conclusion

Across high-income countries, obesity is prevalent, costly, and of consequence. Despite some promising signs that obesity may be leveling and even declining among certain groups, current levels remain unacceptably high. Effective efforts to combat obesity will need to primarily consider the major drivers of excess calorie intake and include multilevel populations approaches that aim to reduce obesity risk in the community, school, and at home.

Review Questions

1. Describe overall trends and patterns in obesity in high-income countries.
2. Give examples of population groups in high-income countries that are at an increased risk for obesity. Discuss some of the proposed reasons for these disparities.

3. List four physical health consequences of obesity.

4. Identify the difference between direct and indirect costs of obesity and provide examples of each.

5. Describe ways in which an individual with obesity may experience weight-related stigma.

6. Discuss how changes in energy balance have contributed to the obesity epidemic.

7. Provide the major advantages of policy approaches to preventing obesity.

8. List an example component of a school-based approach, community-based approach, and home-based approach.

References

1. US Census Bureau. 2016. "Community Facts: Somerville City, Massachusetts." American Fact Finder. https://factfinder.census.gov/faces/nav/jsf/pages/community_facts.xhtml?src=bkmk.

2. Economos, Christina D., Raymond R. Hyatt, Jeanne P. Goldberg, Aviva Must, Elena N. Naumova, Jessica J. Collins, and Miriam E. Nelson. 2007. "A Community Intervention Reduces BMI Z-Score in Children: Shape Up Somerville First Year Results." *Obesity* 15 (5): 1325–36. https://doi.org/10.1038/oby.2007.155.

3. Economos, Christina D., Raymond R. Hyatt, Aviva Must, Jeanne P. Goldberg, Julia Kuder, Elena N. Naumova, Jessica J. Collins, and Miriam E. Nelson. 2013. "Shape Up Somerville Two-Year Results: A Community-Based Environmental Change Intervention Sustains Weight Reduction in Children." *Preventive Medicine* 57 (4): 322–27. https://doi.org/10.1016/j.ypmed.2013.06.001.

4. Guh, Daphne P., Wei Zhang, Nick Bansback, Zubin Amarsi, C. Laird Birmingham, and Aslam H. Anis. 2009. "The Incidence of Co-Morbidities Related to Obesity and Overweight: A Systematic Review and Meta-Analysis." *BMC Public Health* 9 (1): 88. https://doi.org/10.1186/1471-2458-9-88.

5. Willett, Walter. 1998. *Nutritional Epidemiology.* New York: Oxford University Press.

6. Hu, Frank. 2008. *Obesity Epidemiology.* New York: Oxford University Press.

7. Janssen, Ian, Steven B. Heymsfield, ZiMian Wang, and Robert Ross. 2000. "Skeletal Muscle Mass and Distribution in 468 Men and Women Aged 18–88 Yr." *Journal of Applied Physiology* 89 (1): 81–88. https://doi.org/10.1152/jappl.2000.89.1.81.

8. Despres, Jean-Pierre, Sital Moorjani, Paul J. Lupien, Angelo Tremblay, Andre Nadeau, and Claude Bouchard. 1990. "Regional Distribution of Body Fat, Plasma Lipoproteins, and Cardiovascular Disease." *Arteriosclerosis, Thrombosis, and Vascular Biology* 10 (4): 497–511.

9. Deurenberg, P., M. Yap, and W. A. Van Staveren. 1998. "Body Mass Index and Percent Body Fat: A Meta Analysis among Different Ethnic Groups." *International Journal of Obesity* 22 (12): 1164–71.

10. Wagner, Dale R., and Vivian H. Heyward. 2000. "Measures of Body Composition in Blacks and Whites: A Comparative Review." *The American Journal of Clinical Nutrition* 71 (6): 1392–402.

11. WHO Expert Consultation. 2004. "Appropriate Body-Mass Index for Asian Populations and Its Implications for Policy and Intervention Strategies." *The Lancet* 363 (9403): 157-63. https://doi.org/10.1016/S0140-6736(03)15268-3.

12. Sun, Qi, Rob M. Van Dam, Donna Spiegelman, Steven B. Heymsfield, Walter C. Willett, and Frank B. Hu. 2010. "Comparison of Dual-Energy X-Ray Absorptiometric and Anthropometric Measures of Adiposity in Relation to Adiposity-Related Biologic Factors." *American Journal of Epidemiology* 172 (12): 1442-54.

13. Spiegelman, Donna, Richard G. Israel, Claude Bouchard, and Walter C. Willett. 1992. "Absolute Fat Mass, Percent Body Fat, and Body-Fat Distribution: Which Is the Real Determinant of Blood Pressure and Serum Glucose?" *The American Journal of Clinical Nutrition* 55 (6): 1033-44. https://doi.org/10.1093/ajcn/55.6.1033.

14. Qiao, Q., and R. Nyamdorj. 2010. "Is the Association of Type II Diabetes with Waist Circumference or Waist-to-Hip Ratio Stronger than That with Body Mass Index?" *European Journal of Clinical Nutrition* 64 (1): 30-34. https://doi.org/10.1038/ejcn.2009.93.

15. Vazquez, Gabriela, Sue Duval, David R. Jacobs Jr., and Karri Silventoinen. 2007. "Comparison of Body Mass Index, Waist Circumference, and Waist/Hip Ratio in Predicting Incident Diabetes: A Meta-Analysis." *Epidemiologic Reviews* 29 (1): 115-28.

16. "Obesity and Overweight." 2017. World Health Organization. http://www.who.int/mediacentre/factsheets/fs311/en/.

17. *Obesity: Preventing and Managing the Global Epidemic*. 2000. World Health Organization.

18. Onis, Mercedes de. 2007. "WHO Child Growth Standards Based on Length/Height, Weight and Age." *Acta Paediatrica* 95 (S450): 76-85. https://doi.org/10.1111/j.1651-2227.2006.tb02378.x.

19. Onis, M. de, and T. Lobstein. 2010. "Defining Obesity Risk Status in the General Childhood Population: Which Cut-Offs Should We Use?" *International Journal of Pediatric Obesity* 5 (6): 458-60. https://doi.org/10.3109/17477161003615583.

20. Barlow, Sarah E. 2007. "Expert Committee Recommendations Regarding the Prevention, Assessment, and Treatment of Child and Adolescent Overweight and Obesity: Summary Report." *Pediatrics* 120 (Supplement 4): S164-92. https://doi.org/10.1542/peds.2007-2329C.

21. Ng, Marie, Tom Fleming, Margaret Robinson, Blake Thomson, Nicholas Graetz, Christopher Margono, Erin C. Mullany, et al. 2014. "Global, Regional, and National Prevalence of Overweight and Obesity in Children and Adults during 1980-2013: A Systematic Analysis for the Global Burden of Disease Study 2013." *The Lancet* 384 (9945): 766-81. https://doi.org/10.1016/S0140-6736(14)60460-8.

22. "Obesity and Overweight: Factsheet No 311." 2014. World Health Organization. http://www.wpro.who.int/mediacentre/factsheets/obesity/en/.

23. Prentice, Andrew M. 2006. "The Emerging Epidemic of Obesity in Developing Countries." *International Journal of Epidemiology* 35 (1): 93-99. https://doi.org/10.1093/ije/dyi272.

24. Stevens, Gretchen A., Gitanjali M. Singh, Yuan Lu, Goodarz Danaei, John K. Lin, Mariel M. Finucane, Adil N. Bahalim, et al. 2012. "National, Regional, and

Global Trends in Adult Overweight and Obesity Prevalences." *Population Health Metrics* 10 (1): 22. https://doi.org/10.1186/1478-7954-10-22.

25. *Obesity Update 2017*. 2017. OECD. https://www.oecd.org/els/health-systems/Obesity-Update-2017.pdf.

26. Rokholm, Benjamin, Jennifer Lyn Baker, and Thorkild Ingvor A. Sørensen. 2010. "The Levelling Off of the Obesity Epidemic since the Year 1999: A Review of Evidence and Perspectives." *Obesity Reviews* 11 (12): 835–46. https://doi.org/10.1111/j.1467-789X.2010.00810.x.

27. Olds, Tim, Carol Maher, Shi Zumin, Sandrine Péneau, Sandrine Lioret, Katia Castetbon, Jeroen Wilde, et al. 2011. "Evidence That the Prevalence of Childhood Overweight Is Plateauing: Data from Nine Countries." *Pediatric Obesity* 6 (5-6): 342–60.

28. Wabitsch, Martin, Anja Moss, and Katrin Kromeyer-Hauschild. 2014. "Unexpected Plateauing of Childhood Obesity Rates in Developed Countries." *BMC Medicine* 12 (1): 17. https://doi.org/10.1186/1741-7015-12-17.

29. Abarca-Gómez, Leandra, Ziad A. Abdeen, Zargar Abdul Hamid, Niveen M. Abu-Rmeileh, Benjamin Acosta-Cazares, Cecilia Acuin, Robert J. Adams, et al. 2017. "Worldwide Trends in Body-Mass Index, Underweight, Overweight, and Obesity from 1975 to 2016: A Pooled Analysis of 2416 Population-Based Measurement Studies in 128.9 Million Children, Adolescents, and Adults." *The Lancet* 390 (10113): P2627–42. https://doi.org/10.1016/S0140-6736(17)32129-3.

30. Yoshinaga, Masao, Tomoko Ichiki, Yuji Tanaka, Daisuke Hazeki, Hitoshi Horigome, Hideto Takahashi, and Katsuro Kashima. 2010. "Prevalence of Childhood Obesity from 1978 to 2007 in Japan." *Pediatrics International* 52 (2): 213–17.

31. Flegal, Katherine M., M. D. Carroll, C. L. Ogden, and L. R. Curtin. 2010. "Prevalence and Trends in Obesity Among US Adults, 1999-2008." *JAMA* 303 (3): 235. https://doi.org/10.1001/jama.2009.2014.

32. Howel, Denise. 2011. "Trends in the Prevalence of Obesity and Overweight in English Adults by Age and Birth Cohort, 1991-2006." *Public Health Nutrition* 14 (1): 27-33. https://doi.org/10.1017/S136898001000056X.

33. Schober, Edith, Birgit Rami, Sylvia Kirchengast, Thomas Waldhör, and Reinhart Sefranek. 2007. "Recent Trend in Overweight and Obesity in Male Adolescents in Austria: A Population-Based Study." *European Journal of Pediatrics* 166 (7): 709–14. https://doi.org/10.1007/s00431-006-0312-z.

34. Neovius, M., A. Teixeira-Pinto, and .F Rasmussen. 2008. "Shift in the Composition of Obesity in Young Adult Men in Sweden over a Third of a Century." *International Journal of Obesity* 32 (5): 832–36. https://doi.org/10.1038/sj.ijo.0803784.

35. Fryar, Cheryl D., Margaret D. Carroll, and Cynthia L. Ogden. 2012. "Prevalence of Overweight, Obesity, and Extreme Obesity among Adults: United States, Trends 1960-1962 through 2009-2010." Hyattsville, MD: National Center for Health Statistics.

36. Hales, C. M., M. D. Carroll, C. D. Fryar, and C. L. Ogden. 2017. "Prevalence of Obesity Among Adults and Youth: United States, 2015-2016." NCHS data brief, no 288. Hyattsville, MD: National Center for Health Statistics. https://www.cdc.gov/nchs/data/databriefs/db288.pdf.

37. Dinsa, G. Deye, Yevgeniy Goryakin, Elena Fumagalli, and Mark Suhrcke. 2012. "Obesity and Socioeconomic Status in Developing Countries: A Systematic Review." *Obesity Reviews* 13 (11): 1067-79. https://doi.org/10.1111/j.1467-789X.2012 .01017.x.

38. Wang, Youfa, and Hyunjung Lim. 2012. "The Global Childhood Obesity Epidemic and the Association between Socio-Economic Status and Childhood Obesity." *International Review of Psychiatry* 24 (3): 176-88. https://doi.org/10.3109 /09540261.2012.688195.

39. Due, Pernille, Mogens Trab Damsgaard, Mette Rasmussen, Bjørn Evald Holstein, J. Wardle, Juan Merlo, C. Currie, et al. 2009. "Socioeconomic Position, Macroeconomic Environment and Overweight among Adolescents in 35 Coun- tries." *International Journal of Obesity* 33 (10): 1084-93. https://doi.org/10.1038/ijo .2009.128.

40. Drewnowski, Adam. 2009. "Obesity, Diets, and Social Inequalities." *Nutrition Reviews* 67 (Suppl1): S36-39. https://doi.org/10.1111/j.1753-4887.2009.00157.x.

41. Andrieu, Elise, Nicole Darmon, and Adam Drewnowski. 2006. "Low-Cost Diets: More Energy, Fewer Nutrients." *European Journal of Clinical Nutrition* 60 (3): 434.

42. Larson, Nicole I., Mary T. Story, and Melissa C. Nelson. 2009. "Neighbor- hood Environments." *American Journal of Preventive Medicine* 36 (1): 74-81.e10. https://doi.org/10.1016/j.amepre.2008.09.025.

43. Powell, Lisa M., Sandy Slater, Frank J. Chaloupka, and Deborah Harper. 2006. "Availability of Physical Activity-Related Facilities and Neighborhood Demographic and Socioeconomic Characteristics: A National Study." *American Journal of Public Health* 96 (9): 1676-80. https://doi.org/10.2105/AJPH.2005.065573.

44. Caprio, Sonia, Stephen R. Daniels, Adam Drewnowski, Francine R. Kaufman, Lawrence A. Palinkas, Arlan L. Rosenbloom, Jeffrey B. Schwimmer, and M. Sue Kirkman. 2008. "Influence of Race, Ethnicity, and Culture on Childhood Obesity: Implications for Prevention and Treatment." *Obesity* 16 (12): 2566-77.

45. Macartney, Suzanne, Alemayehu Bishaw, and Kayla Fontenot. 2013. *Poverty Rates for Selected Detailed Race and Hispanic Groups by State and Place: 2007-2011*. US Department of Commerce, Economics and Statistics Administration, US Census Bureau. https://www.census.gov/prod/2013pubs/acsbr11-17.pdf.

46. Lewis, LaVonna Blair, David C. Sloane, Lori Miller Nascimento, Allison L. Diamant, Joyce Jones Guinyard, Antronette K. Yancey, and Gwendolyn Flynn. 2005. "African Americans' Access to Healthy Food Options in South Los Angeles Restaurants." *American Journal of Public Health* 95 (4): 668-73. https://doi.org/10.2105 /AJPH.2004.050260.

47. Fleischhacker, S. E., K. R. Evenson, D. A. Rodriquez, and A. S. Ammerman. 2011. "A Systematic Review of Fast Food Access Studies." *Obesity Reviews* 12 (5): e460-71.

48. "Special Report: Racial and Ethnic Disparities in Obesity—Blacks." 2014. The State of Obesity. 2014. https://stateofobesity.org/disparities/blacks/.

49. "Special Report: Racial and Ethnic Disparities in Obesity—Latinos." 2017. The State of Obesity. 2017. https://stateofobesity.org/disparities/latinos/#footnote-19.

50. Yancey, Antronette K., Brian L. Cole, Rochelle Brown, Jerome D. Williams, A. M. Y. Hillier, Randolph S. Kline, Marice Ashe, Sonya A. Grier, Desiree Backman, and William J. McCarthy. 2009. "A Cross-sectional Prevalence Study of Ethnically Targeted and General Audience Outdoor Obesity-related Advertising." *The Milbank Quarterly* 87 (1): 155–84.

51. "Obesity in Canada: Prevalence among Aboriginal Populations." 2011. Government of Canada. https://www.canada.ca/en/public-health/services/health-promotion/healthy-living/obesity-canada/prevalence-among-aboriginal-populations.html.

52. Leadership for Healthy Communities. 2010. "Overweight and Obesity Among American Indian and Alaska Native Youths." Robert Wood Johnson Foundation. http://www.aztribaltransportation.org/htp/pdf/101012_Overweight_Obesity.pdf.

53. Ferguson, Megan, Kerin O'Dea, Mark Chatfield, Marjory Moodie, Jon Altman, and Julie Brimblecombe. 2016. "The Comparative Cost of Food and Beverages at Remote Indigenous Communities, Northern Territory, Australia." *Australian and New Zealand Journal of Public Health* 40 (S1): S21–26. https://doi.org/10.1111/1753-6405.12370.

54. Burns, Jane, and Neil Thomson. 2006. "Summary of Overweight and Obesity among Indigenous Peoples." *Australian Indigenous HealthInfoNet*. https://healthinfonet.ecu.edu.au/key-resources/publications/?id=17506&title=Summary+of+overweight+and+obesity+among+Indigenous+peoples.

55. Bleich, Sara N., David Cutler, Christopher Murray, and Alyce Adams. 2008. "Why Is the Developed World Obese?" *Annual Review of Public Health* 29 (1): 273–95. https://doi.org/10.1146/annurev.publhealth.29.020907.090954.

56. Hall, Kevin D., Gary Sacks, Dhruva Chandramohan, Carson C. Chow, Y. Claire Wang, Steven L. Gortmaker, and Boyd A. Swinburn. 2011. "Quantification of the Effect of Energy Imbalance on Bodyweight." *The Lancet* 378 (9793): 826–37. https://doi.org/10.1016/S0140-6736(11)60812-X.

57. Wang, Y. Claire, Steven L. Gortmaker, Arthur M. Sobol, and Karen M. Kuntz. 2006. "Estimating the Energy Gap Among US Children: A Counterfactual Approach." *Pediatrics* 118 (6): e1721–33. https://doi.org/10.1542/peds.2006-0682.

58. Wang, Y. Claire, C. Tracy Orleans, and Steven L. Gortmaker. 2012. "Reaching the Healthy People Goals for Reducing Childhood Obesity: Closing the Energy Gap." *American Journal of Preventive Medicine* 42 (5): 437–44. https://doi.org/10.1016/j.amepre.2012.01.018.

59. Cutler, David M., Edward L. Glaeser, and Jesse M. Shapiro. 2003. "Why Have Americans Become More Obese?" *The Journal of Economic Perspectives* 17 (3): 93–118.

60. Powell, Lisa M., Binh T. Nguyen, and Euna Han. 2012. "Energy Intake from Restaurants." *American Journal of Preventive Medicine* 43 (5): 498–504. https://doi.org/10.1016/j.amepre.2012.07.041.

61. Young, Lisa R., and Marion Nestle. 2002. "The Contribution of Expanding Portion Sizes to the US Obesity Epidemic." *American Journal of Public Health* 92 (2): 246–49. http://www.ncbi.nlm.nih.gov/pubmed/11818300.

62. Ello-Martin, Julia A., Jenny H. Ledikwe, and Barbara J. Rolls. 2005. "The Influence of Food Portion Size and Energy Density on Energy Intake: Implications

for Weight Management." *The American Journal of Clinical Nutrition* 82 (1): 236S–241S. https://doi.org/10.1093/ajcn/82.1.236S.

63. Zimmerman, Frederick J. 2011. "Using Marketing Muscle to Sell Fat: The Rise of Obesity in the Modern Economy." *Annual Review of Public Health* 32 (April): 285–306. https://doi.org/10.1146/annurev-publhealth-090810-182502.

64. Harris, Jennifer L., Jennifer L. Pomeranz, Tim Lobstein, and Kelly D. Brownell. 2009. "A Crisis in the Marketplace: How Food Marketing Contributes to Childhood Obesity and What Can Be Done." *Annual Review of Public Health* 30 (1): 211–25. https://doi.org/10.1146/annurev.publhealth.031308.100304.

65. Harris, Jennifer L., John A. Bargh, and Kelly D. Brownell. 2009. "Priming Effects of Television Food Advertising on Eating Behavior." *Health Psychology* 28 (4): 404–13. https://doi.org/10.1037/a0014399.

66. Boeing, H. 2013. "Obesity and Cancer—The Update 2013." *Best Practice & Research. Clinical Endocrinology & Metabolism* 27 (2): 219–27.

67. Frank, Lawrence D., Martin A. Andresen, and Thomas L. Schmid. 2004. "Obesity Relationships with Community Design, Physical Activity, and Time Spent in Cars." *American Journal of Preventive Medicine* 27 (2): 87–96. https://doi.org/10.1016/j.amepre.2004.04.011.

68. Vainio, Harri, and Franca Bianchini, eds. 2002. *Weight Control and Physical Activity. IARC Handbooks of Cancer Prevention: Volume 6.* Lyon, France: International Agency for Research on Cancer.

69. Warburton, Darren E. R., Crystal Whitney Nicol, and Shannon S. D. Bredin. 2006. "Health Benefits of Physical Activity: The Evidence." *Canadian Medical Association Journal* 174 (6): 801–9.

70. Freedman, David S., William H. Dietz, Sathanur R. Srinivasan, and Gerald S. Berenson. 1999. "The Relation of Overweight to Cardiovascular Risk Factors among Children and Adolescents: The Bogalusa Heart Study." *Pediatrics* 103 (6 Pt 1): 1175–82. http://www.ncbi.nlm.nih.gov/pubmed/10353925.

71. Wilson, Peter W. F., Ralph B. D'Agostino, Lisa Sullivan, Helen Parise, and William B. Kannel. 2002. "Overweight and Obesity as Determinants of Cardiovascular Risk: The Framingham Experience." *Archives of Internal Medicine* 162 (16): 1867–72. http://www.ncbi.nlm.nih.gov/pubmed/12196085.

72. Freedman, David S., Zuguo Mei, Sathanur R. Srinivasan, Gerald S. Berenson, and William H. Dietz. 2007. "Cardiovascular Risk Factors and Excess Adiposity Among Overweight Children and Adolescents: The Bogalusa Heart Study." *The Journal of Pediatrics* 150 (1): 12–17.e2. https://doi.org/10.1016/j.jpeds.2006.08.042.

73. Goran, Michael I., Geoff D. C. Ball, and Martha L. Cruz. 2003. "Obesity and Risk of Type 2 Diabetes and Cardiovascular Disease in Children and Adolescents." *The Journal of Clinical Endocrinology & Metabolism* 88 (4): 1417–27. https://doi.org/10.1210/jc.2002-021442.

74. Ni Mhurchu, C., A Rodgers, W. H. Pan, D. F. Gu, and M. Woodward. 2004. "Body Mass Index and Cardiovascular Disease in the Asia-Pacific Region: An Overview of 33 Cohorts Involving 310,000 Participants." *International Journal of Epidemiology* 33 (4): 751–58. https://doi.org/10.1093/ije/dyh163.

75. Li, Tricia Y. 2006. "Obesity as Compared With Physical Activity in Predicting Risk of Coronary Heart Disease in Women." *Circulation* 113 (4): 499–506. https://doi.org/10.1161/CIRCULATIONAHA.105.574087.

76. Hubert, Helen B., Manning Feinleib, Patricia M. McNamara, and William P. Castelli. 1983. "Obesity as an Independent Risk Factor for Cardiovascular Disease: A 26-Year Follow-up of Participants in the Framingham Heart Study." *Circulation* 67 (5): 968–77. http://www.ncbi.nlm.nih.gov/pubmed/6219830.

77. Calle, Eugenia E., Carmen Rodriguez, Kimberly Walker-Thurmond, and Michael J. Thun. 2003. "Overweight, Obesity, and Mortality from Cancer in a Prospectively Studied Cohort of US Adults." *New England Journal of Medicine* 348 (17): 1625–38. https://doi.org/10.1056/NEJMoa021423.

78. Hu, Frank B., JoAnn E. Manson, Meir J. Stampfer, Graham Colditz, Simin Liu, Caren G. Solomon, and Walter C. Willett. 2001. "Diet, Lifestyle, and the Risk of Type 2 Diabetes Mellitus in Women." *New England Journal of Medicine* 345 (11): 790–97. https://doi.org/10.1056/NEJMoa010492.

79. Aune, Dagfinn, Abhijit Sen, Manya Prasad, Teresa Norat, Imre Janszky, Serena Tonstad, Pål Romundstad, and Lars J. Vatten. 2016. "BMI and All Cause Mortality: Systematic Review and Non-Linear Dose-Response Meta-Analysis of 230 Cohort Studies with 3.74 Million Deaths among 30.3 Million Participants." *BMJ* 353: i2156.

80. Angelantonio, Emanuele Di, Shilpa N. Bhupathiraju, David Wormser, Pei Gao, Stephen Kaptoge, Amy Berrington de Gonzalez, Benjamin J. Cairns, et al. 2016. "Body-Mass Index and All-Cause Mortality: Individual-Participant-Data Meta-Analysis of 239 Prospective Studies in Four Continents." *The Lancet* 388 (10046): 776–86. https://doi.org/10.1016/S0140-6736(16)30175-1.

81. Flegal, Katherine M., Brian K. Kit, Heather Orpana, and Barry I. Graubard. 2013. "Association of All-Cause Mortality With Overweight and Obesity Using Standard Body Mass Index Categories." *JAMA* 309 (1): 71. https://doi.org/10.1001/jama.2012.113905.

82. Stokes, Andrew, and Samuel H. Preston. 2015. "Smoking and Reverse Causation Create an Obesity Paradox in Cardiovascular Disease." *Obesity* 23 (12): 2485–90.

83. Banack, H. R., and A. Stokes. 2017. "The 'Obesity Paradox' May Not Be a Paradox at All." *International Journal of Obesity* 41 (8): 1162–63. https://doi.org/10.1038/ijo.2017.99.

84. Barnack, Hailey R., and Jay S. Kaufman. 2013. "The 'Obesity Paradox' Explained." *Epidemiology* 24 (3): 461–62.

85. Curtis, Jeptha P., Jared G. Selter, Yongfei Wang, Saif S. Rathore, Ion S. Jovin, Farid Jadbabaie, Mikhail Kosiborod, et al. 2005. "The Obesity Paradox." *Archives of Internal Medicine* 165 (1): 55. https://doi.org/10.1001/archinte.165.1.55.

86. Hernán, Miguel A., Sonia Hernández-Díaz, and James M. Robins. 2004. "A Structural Approach to Selection Bias." *Epidemiology* 15 (5): 615–25.

87. Lehnert, Thomas, Diana Sonntag, Alexander Konnopka, Steffi Riedel-Heller, and Hans-Helmut König. 2013. "Economic Costs of Overweight and Obesity." *Best Practice & Research Clinical Endocrinology & Metabolism* 27 (2): 105–15. https://doi.org/10.1016/j.beem.2013.01.002.

88. Sonntag, Diana, Shehzad Ali, and Freia De Bock. 2016. "Lifetime Indirect Cost of Childhood Overweight and Obesity: A Decision Analytic Model." *Obesity* 24 (1): 200-206.

89. Dee, Anne, Karen Kearns, Ciaran O'Neill, Linda Sharp, Anthony Staines, Victoria O'Dwyer, Sarah Fitzgerald, et al. 2014. "The Direct and Indirect Costs of Both Overweight and Obesity: A Systematic Review." *BMC Research Notes* 7 (1): 242. https://doi.org/10.1186/1756-0500-7-242.

90. Withrow, David, and D. A. Alter. 2011. "The Economic Burden of Obesity Worldwide: A Systematic Review of the Direct Costs of Obesity." *Obesity Reviews* 12 (2): 131-41.

91. Tsai, Adam Gilden, David F. Williamson, and Henry A. Glick. 2011. "Direct Medical Cost of Overweight and Obesity in the USA: A Quantitative Systematic Review." *Obesity Reviews* 12 (1): 50-61.

92. Janssens, Heidi, Els Clays, France Kittel, Dirk De Bacquer, Annalisa Casini, and Lutgart Braeckman. 2012. "The Association Between Body Mass Index Class, Sickness Absence, and Presenteeism." *Journal of Occupational and Environmental Medicine* 54 (5): 604-9. https://doi.org/10.1097/JOM.0b013e31824b2133.

93. Dannenberg, Andrew L., Deron C. Burton, and Richard J. Jackson. 2004. "Economic and Environmental Costs of Obesity." *American Journal of Preventive Medicine* 27 (3): 264. https://doi.org/10.1016/j.amepre.2004.06.004.

94. Carr, Deborah, and Michael A. Friedman. 2005. "Is Obesity Stigmatizing? Body Weight, Perceived Discrimination, and Psychological Well-Being in the United States." *Journal of Health and Social Behavior* 46 (3): 244-59. https://doi.org/10.1177/002214650504600303.

95. Puhl, Rebecca, and Kelly D. Brownell. 2001. "Bias, Discrimination, and Obesity." *Obesity Research* 9 (12): 788-805. https://doi.org/10.1038/oby.2001.108.

96. Roehling, Mark V. 1999. "Weight-based Discrimination in Employment: Psychological and Legal Aspects." *Personnel Psychology* 52 (4): 969-1016.

97. Gortmaker, Steven L., Aviva Must, James M. Perrin, Arthur M. Sobol, and William H. Dietz. 1993. "Social and Economic Consequences of Overweight in Adolescence and Young Adulthood." *New England Journal of Medicine* 329 (14): 1008-12. https://doi.org/10.1056/NEJM199309303291406.

98. Blumberg, Phyllis, and Linda P. Mellis. 1985. "Medical Students' Attitudes toward the Obese and the Morbidly Obese." *International Journal of Eating Disorders* 4 (2): 169-75. https://doi.org/10.1002/1098-108X(198505)4:2<169::AID-EAT2260040204>3.0.CO;2-F.

99. Budd, Geraldine M., Megan Mariotti, Diane Graff, and Kathleen Falkenstein. 2011. "Health Care Professionals' Attitudes about Obesity: An Integrative Review." *Applied Nursing Research* 24 (3): 127-37.

100. Olson, Cheri L., Howard D. Schumaker, and Barbara P. Yawn. 1994. "Overweight Women Delay Medical Care." *Archives of Family Medicine* 3 (10): 888.

101. Geel, M. Van, P. Vedder, and J. Tanilon. 2014. "Are Overweight and Obese Youths More Often Bullied by Their Peers? A Meta-Analysis on the Relation between Weight Status and Bullying." *International Journal of Obesity* 38 (10): 1263.

102. Scott, Kate M., Ronny Bruffaerts, Gregory E. Simon, Jordi Alonso, Matthias Angermeyer, Giovanni de Girolamo, Koen Demyttenaere, et al. 2008. "Obesity and Mental Disorders in the General Population: Results from the World Mental Health Surveys." *International Journal of Obesity* 32 (1): 192-200. https://doi.org/10.1038/sj.ijo.0803701.

103. Griffiths, Lucy J., Tessa J. Parsons, and Andrew J. Hill. 2010. "Self-esteem and Quality of Life in Obese Children and Adolescents: A Systematic Review." *Pediatric Obesity* 5 (4): 282-304.

104. Swinburn, Boyd A., Gary Sacks, Kevin D. Hall, Klim McPherson, Diane Finegood, Marjory L. Moodie, and Steven L. Gortmaker. 2011. "The Global Obesity Pandemic: Shaped by Global Drivers and Local Environments." *The Lancet* 378 (9793): 804-14. https://doi.org/10.1016/S0140-6736.

105. Zhang, Qi, Shiyong Liu, Ruicui Liu, Hong Xue, and Youfa Wang. 2014. "Food Policy Approaches to Obesity Prevention: An International Perspective." *Current Obesity Reports* 3 (2): 171-82.

106. Gortmaker, Steven L., Boyd A. Swinburn, David Levy, Rob Carter, Patricia L. Mabry, Diane T. Finegood, Terry Huang, et al. 2011. "Changing the Future of Obesity: Science, Policy, and Action." *The Lancet* 378 (9793): 838-47. https://doi.org/10.1016/S0140-6736(11)60815-5.

107. Dong, Di, Marcel Bilger, Rob M. van Dam, and Eric A. Finkelstein. 2015. "Consumption of Specific Foods and Beverages and Excess Weight Gain among Children and Adolescents." *Health Affairs* 34 (11): 1940-48.

108. Ebbeling, Cara B., Henry A. Feldman, Virginia R. Chomitz, Tracy A. Antonelli, Steven L. Gortmaker, Stavroula K. Osganian, and David S. Ludwig. 2012. "A Randomized Trial of Sugar-Sweetened Beverages and Adolescent Body Weight." *New England Journal of Medicine* 367 (15): 1407-16. https://doi.org/10.1056/NEJMoa1203388.

109. Hu, Frank B. 2013. "Resolved: There Is Sufficient Scientific Evidence That Decreasing Sugar-Sweetened Beverage Consumption Will Reduce the Prevalence of Obesity and Obesity-Related Diseases." *Obesity Reviews* 14 (8): 606-19. https://doi.org/10.1111/obr.12040.

110. Ludwig, David S., Karen E. Peterson, and Steven L. Gortmaker. 2001. "Relation between Consumption of Sugar-Sweetened Drinks and Childhood Obesity: A Prospective, Observational Analysis." *The Lancet* 357 (9255): 505-8. https://doi.org/10.1016/S0140-6736(00)04041-1.

111. Malik, Vasanti S., Walter C. Willett, and Frank B. Hu. 2009. "Sugar-Sweetened Beverages and BMI in Children and Adolescents: Reanalyses of a Meta-Analysis." *The American Journal of Clinical Nutrition* 89 (1): 438-39. https://doi.org/10.3945/ajcn.2008.26980.

112. Malik, Vasanti S., Matthias B. Schulze, and Frank B. Hu. 2006. "Intake of Sugar-Sweetened Beverages and Weight Gain: A Systematic Review1-3." *The American Journal of Clinical Nutrition* 84 (2): 274-88. https://doi.org/10.1093/ajcn/84.1.274.

113. "Sources of Calories from Added Sugars among the US Population, 2005-06." 2018. Epidemiology and Genomics Research Program. National Cancer Institute. 2018. http://epi.grants.cancer.gov/diet/foodsources/added_sugars/.

114. Beck, Amy L., Anisha Patel, and Kristine Madsen. 2013. "Trends in Sugar-Sweetened Beverage and 100% Fruit Juice Consumption among California Children." *Academic Pediatrics* 13 (4): 364-70.

115. Bleich, Sara N., Y. Claire Wang, Youfa Wang, and Steven L. Gortmaker. 2009. "Increasing Consumption of Sugar-Sweetened Beverages among US Adults: 1988-1994 to 1999-2004." *The American Journal of Clinical Nutrition* 89 (1): 372-81. https://doi.org/10.3945/ajcn.2008.26883.

116. Han, Euna, and Lisa M. Powell. 2013. "Consumption Patterns of Sugar-Sweetened Beverages in the United States." *Journal of the Academy of Nutrition and Dietetics* 113 (1): 43-53. https://doi.org/10.1016/j.jand.2012.09.016.

117. Wang, Y. Claire, Sara N. Bleich, and Steven L. Gortmaker. 2008. "Increasing Caloric Contribution From Sugar-Sweetened Beverages and 100% Fruit Juices Among US Children and Adolescents, 1988-2004." *Pediatrics* 121 (6): e1604-14. https://doi.org/10.1542/peds.2007-2834.

118. Andreyeva, Tatiana, Frank J. Chaloupka, and Kelly D. Brownell. 2011. "Estimating the Potential of Taxes on Sugar-Sweetened Beverages to Reduce Consumption and Generate Revenue." *Preventive Medicine* 52 (6): 413-16.

119. Backholer, Kathryn, Danja Sarink, Alison Beauchamp, Catherine Keating, Venurs Loh, Kylie Ball, Jane Martin, et al. 2016. "The Impact of a Tax on Sugar-Sweetened Beverages According to Socio-Economic Position: A Systematic Review of the Evidence." *Public Health Nutrition* 19 (17): 3070-84.

120. Brownell, Kelly D., Thomas Farley, Walter C. Willett, Barry M. Popkin, Frank J. Chaloupka, Joseph W. Thompson, and David S. Ludwig. 2009. "The Public Health and Economic Benefits of Taxing Sugar-Sweetened Beverages." *New England Journal of Medicine* 361 (16): 1599-1605. https://doi.org/10.1056/NEJMhpr0905723.

121. Colchero, M. Arantxa, Barry M. Popkin, Juan A. Rivera, and Shu Wen Ng. 2016. "Beverage Purchases from Stores in Mexico under the Excise Tax on Sugar Sweetened Beverages: Observational Study." *BMJ* 352 (January): h6704. https://doi.org/10.1136/bmj.h6704.

122. Silver, Lynn D., Shu Wen Ng, Suzanne Ryan-Ibarra, Lindsey Smith Taillie, Marta Induni, Donna R. Miles, Jennifer M. Poti, and Barry M. Popkin. 2017. "Changes in Prices, Sales, Consumer Spending, and Beverage Consumption One Year after a Tax on Sugar-Sweetened Beverages in Berkeley, California, US: A Before-and-After Study." Edited by Claudia Langenberg. *PLOS Medicine* 14 (4): e1002283. https://doi.org/10.1371/journal.pmed.1002283.

123. Falbe, Jennifer, Hannah R. Thompson, Christina M. Becker, Nadia Rojas, Charles E. McCulloch, and Kristine A. Madsen. 2016. "Impact of the Berkeley Excise Tax on Sugar-Sweetened Beverage Consumption." *American Journal of Public Health* 106 (10): 1865-71. https://doi.org/10.2105/AJPH.2016.303362.

124. Bleich, Sara N., Julia A. Wolfson, Marian P. Jarlenski, and Jason P. Block. 2015. "Restaurants With Calories Displayed On Menus Had Lower Calorie Counts Compared To Restaurants Without Such Labels." *Health Affairs* 34 (11): 1877-84. https://doi.org/10.1377/hlthaff.2015.0512.

125. Bleich, Sara N., Christina D. Economos, Marie L. Spiker, Kelsey A. Vercammen, Eric M. VanEpps, Jason P. Block, Brian Elbel, et al. 2017. "A

Systematic Review of Calorie Labeling and Modified Calorie Labeling Interventions: Impact on Consumer and Restaurant Behavior." *Obesity* 25 (12): 2018-44. https://doi.org/10.1002/oby.21940.

126. Bleich, Sara N., Julia A. Wolfson, and Marian P. Jarlenski. 2016. "Calorie Changes in Large Chain Restaurants." *American Journal of Preventive Medicine* 50 (1): e1-8. https://doi.org/10.1016/j.amepre.2015.05.007.

127. Committee on Accelerating Progress in Obesity Prevention, Food and Nutrition Board, and Institute of Medicine. 2012. *Accelerating Progress in Obesity Prevention: Solving the Weight of the Nation*. Edited by D. Glickman, L. Parker, L. J. Sim, H. Del Valle Cook, and E. A. Miller. Washington, DC: National Academies Press.

128. Wang, Y., L. Cai, Y. Wu, R. F. Wilson, Christine Weston, O. Fawole, Sara N. Bleich, et al. 2015. "What Childhood Obesity Prevention Programmes Work? A Systematic Review and Meta-Analysis." *Obesity Reviews* 16 (7): 547-65. https://doi.org/10.1111/obr.12277.

129. Bleich, Sara N., Kelsey A. Vercammen, Laura Y. Zatz, Johannah M. Frelier, Cara B. Ebbeling, and Anna Peeters. 2018. "Interventions to Prevent Global Childhood Overweight and Obesity: A Systematic Review." *The Lancet Diabetes & Endocrinology* 6 (4): 332-46. https://doi.org/10.1016/S2213-8587(17)30358-3.

130. Bleich, Sara N., Jodi Segal, Yang Wu, Renee Wilson, and Youfa Wang. 2013. "Systematic Review of Community-Based Childhood Obesity Prevention Studies." *Pediatrics* 132 (1): e201-10. https://doi.org/10.1542/peds.2013-0886.

131. Novilla, M. Lelinneth B., Michael D. Barnes, G. Natalie, Patrick N. Williams, and Janice Rogers. 2006. "Public Health Perspectives on the Family: An Ecological Approach to Promoting Health in the Family and Community." *Family & Community Health* 29 (1): 28-42.

132. Hull, P. C., M. Buchowski, J. R. Canedo, B. M. Beech, L. Du, T. Koyama, and R. Zoorob. 2016. "Childhood Obesity Prevention Cluster Randomized Trial for Hispanic Families: Outcomes of the Healthy Families Study." *Pediatric Obesity*. https://doi.org/10.1111/ijpo.12197.

133. Fulkerson, Jayne A., Sarah Friend, Colleen Flattum, Melissa Horning, Michelle Draxten, Dianne Neumark-Sztainer, Olga Gurvich, et al. 2015. "Promoting Healthful Family Meals to Prevent Obesity: HOME Plus, a Randomized Controlled Trial." *International Journal of Behavioral Nutrition and Physical Activity* 12 (1): 154. https://doi.org/10.1186/s12966-015-0320-3.

134. Showell, Nakiya N., Oluwakemi Fawole, Jodi Segal, Renee F. Wilson, Lawrence J. Cheskin, Sara N. Bleich, Yang Wu, et al. 2013. "A Systematic Review of Home-Based Childhood Obesity Prevention Studies." *Pediatrics* 132 (1): e193-200. https://doi.org/10.1542/peds.2013-0786.

9

Nutrition-Related Diseases in Low- and Middle-Income Countries

Valerie M. Friesen, Mduduzi N. N. Mbuya, Alison Tumilowicz, and Lynnette M. Neufeld

LEARNING OBJECTIVES

- List the leading causes death and disability in low- and middle-income countries
- Identify the key nutrition-related risk factors contributing to the leading causes of death and disability
- Describe the mechanistic relationships that underlie the contribution of the key nutrition-related risk factors to death and disability
- Compare how these nutrition-related risk factors for death and disability differ over time and by region and population group

Case Study: A Story from Zimbabwe

As dawn breaks on what promised to be a sunny February morning, NakaNomsa is awakened by her squirming, colicky, youngest child. Struggling to recall where she had placed the remedy her mother had helped her prepare to help relieve the little one's discomfort, she offers her breast instead. As the child suckles, NakaNomsa's mind runs through the many tasks that face her that day, visualizing her maize field and the grain filling crop as the priority for the day.

A different person would relish the scenic view of the green field at the root of a mountain. Her mind's eye instead knows that a herd of baboons lurk, eagerly awaiting the harvest and anticipating their share. She dreads the thought of spending most of the day keeping watch and protecting her crop. More so than she does the other chores that await around the homestead. She sighs, "You cannot tell a hungry child that you gave him food yesterday" [Zimbabwean proverb].

Her wandering mind quickly remembers that the herbal mixture is within arm's reach. Determined to protect her newborn from any ailment, including whatever it was that took her first-born child, Nomsa, at the early age of 4, she smears the concoction on the roof of the baby's mouth and rises to start her new day.

Many deaths are attributable to preventable causes globally, and most of these occur in low- to middle-income countries. Public health officials need to understand the risk factors that underlie the major causes of death and disability for two reasons: first, to find ways to prevent disease and injury, and second, to inform health policy and prioritize interventions to improve global health. The term **risk factor** is defined in this chapter as "a factor that raises the probability of adverse health outcomes" as per the definition used by the World Health Organization (WHO).[1] A risk factor may therefore be an attribute or characteristic of an individual, or an exposure that increases the likelihood of developing a disease or injury and may be a causative agent (such as a food contaminant) or a condition (such as micronutrient deficiency) that makes one likely to develop a disease or suffer more severely from its effects.

The leading causes of death and disability in low- and middle-income countries (LMIC) are a combination of predominantly childhood **communicable diseases** (e.g., respiratory infections) and **noncommunicable**, which previously were only common in high-income countries. Specifically, the leading causes of death across the total population in low-income countries are lower respiratory infections, diarrheal disease, and stroke (accounting for 84.9, 57.2, and 49.6 deaths per 100,000 population, respectively, in 2015). In lower-middle-income countries, the leading causes of death include ischemic heart disease, followed by stroke and lower respiratory infections (accounting for 111.9, 68.8, and 51.5 deaths per 100,000 population, respectively, in 2015). In middle-income countries, the leading causes of death are ischemic heart disease, stroke, and chronic obstructive pulmonary disease (133.4, 120.9, and 50.4 deaths per 100,000 population, respectively, in 2015).[2]

In this chapter, we will identify the key nutrition-related risk factors for the aforementioned leading causes of death and disability in low- and middle-income countries and discuss the mechanisms by which each of these risk factors contribute to death and disability. We will focus more attention on the communicable diseases, which still contribute to a sizable burden of illness and deaths in low-income, lower-middle-income, and among some populations in middle-income countries. Finally, we will conclude by discussing how these risk factors differ over time, by region, and by population group.

Nutrition-Related Risk Factors for Death and Disability in Low- and Middle-Income Countries

Nearly all the leading causes of death and disability in LMIC described above have nutrition- and/or dietary-related risk factors. Estimates of the burden of maternal and child mortality that can be attributed to **undernutrition** have been critical in highlighting the need for optimal nutrition to improve survival.[3-5] In this section, we cover the key nutrition-related risk factors related to the three leading causes of death mentioned above: lower respiratory infections, diarrheal disease, and stroke. We also discuss the mechanistic relationships that underlie their contribution to death and disability.

Lower Respiratory Infections

Lower respiratory infections are the number one cause of death in low-income countries and the third leading cause of death in lower-middle-income countries.[2] Acute lower respiratory infections are defined as acute infections that disturb the airways underneath the epiglottis and include laryngitis, tracheitis, bronchitis, bronchiolitis, lung infections, or any combination of them according to the International Classification of Diseases. The WHO considers pneumonia and bronchiolitis to be the major components of acute lower respiratory infections, and most disease reduction programs focus on identifying children with these conditions.[6] The highest burden of **morbidity** and **mortality** from acute lower respiratory infections, such as pneumonia and bronchiolitis, is among children under 5 years of age, with 95% of all deaths from acute lower respiratory infections occurring in LMIC.[7] The key nutrition-related risk factors that contribute to the development of acute lower respiratory infections among children under 5 years of age are suboptimal breastfeeding, undernutrition, and low birth weight.[8]

Suboptimal Breastfeeding as a Risk Factor

Children who are not optimally breastfed (commonly defined as exclusively breastfed during the first six months of life, followed by continued breastfeeding with appropriate complementary foods up to 24 months of age and beyond) are at an increased risk of morbidity and mortality from pneumonia and other forms of acute lower respiratory infections. Specifically, compared to infants who are optimally breastfed, infants in LMIC who are suboptimally breastfed have a higher risk of severe acute lower respiratory infections (odds ratio [OR]: 2.34; 95% CI: 1.42-3.88), higher hospitalization for respiratory infection,[9] and higher mortality from acute lower respiratory infections.[7] For pneumonia specifically, evidence from a systematic review and meta-analysis of 10 studies indicates that, among children aged 0-6 months and those aged 6-23 months, those who had suboptimal breastfeeding were at substantially increased risk of death from pneumonia.[10]

The protective benefits of breastfeeding on acute lower respiratory infections are believed to be due to the transfer of antibodies and lymphocytes (such as lactoferrin, lysozyme, secretory IgA, and leukocytes) from mother to infant that strengthen the innate immune response, which provides protection against infections.[11] Additionally, breastmilk promotes maturation of the immune system in infants, which can reduce risk of infection later in life.[12]

Undernutrition as a Risk Factor

Undernutrition and infection (of all kinds) are inextricably linked, and the relationship between them has been widely studied over many decades.[13-15] To begin with, inadequate diet among children results in weight loss or lack of adequate weight gain (even if no loss is evident) and reduced immune function due to low intake of necessary nutrients. Undernourished children do not grow properly and become underweight, weak, and susceptible to infections (figure 9.1).[16] Consequently, the combination of infection and undernourishment causes damage to the epithelial mucosa of the intestines, leading to malabsorption, diarrhea, and loss of appetite. Further exacerbating this is the fact that infection is metabolically expensive: it is characterized by increased catabolism and sequestration of nutrients that are required for tissue synthesis and growth. This impaired absorption and utilization of nutrients with attendant lethargy leads to reduction in dietary intake, which continues the cycle. Too often, this vicious cycle culminates in death.

In epidemiologic studies, being underweight (defined as weight-for-age less than 2 standard deviations) has been associated with substantially increased risk for developing severe acute lower respiratory infection (OR 4.47; 95% CI 2.10-9.49).[17] Additionally, undernutrition, as indicated by anthropometric indicators, is strongly and consistently associated with increased death from acute lower respiratory infection.[7,18] Findings from a systematic review indicate that among children who develop pneumonia, those who are moderately and severely malnourished have substantially higher risk of dying from pneumonia compared to children who are adequately nourished (relative risks [RR] ranged from 1.2 to 36.5 and 2.9 to 121.2, respectively).[19] That said, the number and types of pathogens that cause bacterial pneumonia in severely undernourished children have been shown to differ from those isolated in children without severe malnutrition. This may lead to challenges in diagnosing and treating acute lower respiratory conditions in undernourished children, suggesting that further research into pneumonia etiology is warranted.[19]

Low Birth Weight as a Risk Factor

For many children in LMIC, the process of becoming undernourished begins during the prenatal period when maternal health and nutrition as well as the genetic and constitutional characteristics of the fetus influence fetal growth and development. Although there are many known risk factors for

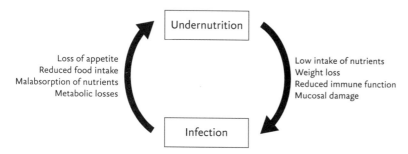

Figure 9.1. Synergistic relationship between undernutrition and infection.

low birth weight, a child is generally born too small because they were either born too soon, grew too slowly in utero, or a combination of the two. Both factors (being born too soon and growing too slowly in utero) are independent predictors of mortality. Compared with their normal birth weight counterparts, low birth weight infants (defined as birth weight less than 2.5 kg regardless of gestational age) were shown in early studies to be up to 40 times more likely to die in the neonatal period and 5 times more likely in the postneonatal period.[20] Low birth weight and, in particular, very low birth weight infants are often frail, experience difficulty in thriving, and are predisposed to a variety of neurodevelopmental disorders and later suboptimal health.[20] These include, but are not limited to, cerebral palsy and lung disorder that are likely related to the increased risk of mortality seen among these infants. Multiple systematic reviews[7,17] have confirmed that low birth weight is a risk factor for acute lower respiratory infections among children under 5 years of age. Concerningly, in a follow-up study of men born during 1911-1930 whose birth weights, weights at 1 year, and childhood illnesses were recorded, lower birth weight was associated with worse adult lung function.[21] This suggests that intrauterine influences that retard fetal weight gain may pose irrecoverable constraints on the growth and development of the airways.

Diarrheal Disease

Diarrheal disease is the second leading cause of death in low-income countries[2] and among children under the age of 5 globally.[22] In LMIC, diarrhea from infection is prevalent in young children. Defined as the passage of three or more loose or liquid stools per day, diarrhea is most often a symptom of an infection in the intestinal tract that is spread through contaminated food or drinking water, or from inadequate hygiene. Diarrheal disease is preventable when the oral transmission of causative pathogens is interrupted through the safe disposal of feces (preferably in acceptable toilet facilities), handwashing with soap after potential contamination events, handwashing before handling food, fly control, separation of children from exposure to animals/animal feces, and providing safe drinking water. These interventions are frequently defined as adequate water, sanitation, and hygiene (WASH). Diarrhea is treatable with oral rehydration solution (a mixture made up of clean water, salt, and sugar to replace water and electrolytes lost in stools) and, in some cases, additional supplementation with zinc.[22] The key nutrition-related risk factors that contribute to the development of diarrheal disease among children under 5 years of age are suboptimal breastfeeding, undernutrition, and micronutrient deficiencies.

Suboptimal Breastfeeding as a Risk Factor

Children who are not optimally breastfeed are at an increased risk of morbidity and mortality from diarrhea due to reduced immunity. Breastfeeding, as previously described, is protective against infections, such as those in the intestinal tract that cause diarrhea, by transferring antibodies and lymphocytes from mother to infant that strengthen the immune response and promote maturation of the immune system.[11,12] In addition to the protective qualities of breastmilk itself, exclusively breastfeeding children means that potentially contaminated food and water are excluded from their diet, making it inherently protective by eliminating these other sources of contamination.

Exclusively breastfed infants have lower risk of diarrhea and other infections compared to those given other foods or liquids.[23,24] Breastfeeding is protective against incidence of diarrhea and hospitalization for diarrhea.[9] A meta-analysis of 18 studies found not breastfeeding to be associated with excess risk of diarrhea mortality in comparison to exclusive breastfeeding among infants 0-5 months of age (RR: 10.52) and to any breastfeeding among children aged 6-23 months (RR: 2.18).[25]

Undernutrition as a Risk Factor

Children who are undernourished or have reduced immunity are at greatest risk of death from diarrhea. As described previously (figure 9.1), malnutrition and infection can cause a vicious cycle where infection can cause children to become malnourished and malnourished children are at a greater risk of contracting infection. In the case of diarrhea, which is most often a symptom of infection in the intestinal tract, each diarrheal episode limits the absorption of nutrients needed for growth, which can lead to malnutrition. Consequently, malnourished children are more likely to get, or experience more severe, diarrhea due to reduced immune function and impaired absorption.[22]

Both underweight and **stunting** are strongly and consistently associated with increased death from diarrhea.[18] Underweight (low weight-for-age) specifically is estimated to account for approximately 60% of the deaths due to diarrhea among children.[26] Preexisting undernutrition is also associated with increased severity of diarrhea.[27]

Micronutrient Deficiencies as a Risk Factor

Micronutrient deficiencies can increase the risk of infections, such as diarrhea. Inadequate zinc reduces immunity and prevents the liver from releasing vitamin A, which can cause malabsorption syndromes. Inadequate vitamin A can cause damage to the epithelial mucosa.[16] Vitamin A is required to sustain the epithelium of the respiratory and gastrointestinal tracts and thus plays an essential role in protecting the body against infection. Supplementation of vitamin A and zinc has been shown to be associated with the prevention and/or treatment of diarrheal diseases by enhancing the integrity of the gut and immune function. High-dose vitamin A supplementation has been shown to reduce severity of diarrhea in most supplementation trials (but not all).[28] High-dose zinc supplementation in children in developing countries is associated with a reduction in diarrheal incidence by nearly 20%,[29] as well as a 24% reduction in duration when provided during diarrhea.[30]

Stroke

A stroke occurs when blood flow to an area of the brain is either interrupted or reduced. Essentially a brain attack (as opposed to a heart attack), this results in the brain not receiving enough oxygen (cerebral hypoxia) or nutrients, causing brain cells to die and therefore leading to outcomes ranging from trouble walking, speaking, and understanding, as well as paralysis or death.[31] Stroke (also referred to as one of the components of cerebrovascular disease) is etiologically related to hypertension, atherosclerosis leading to coronary artery disease, dyslipidemia, heart disease, and hyperlipidemia. All of these conditions are related also to overweight, obesity, and poor diet quality, and, in some cases, undernutrition. The leading nutrition-related risk factors for stroke in high-income countries discussed in chapter 7 are relevant in LMIC (see table 7.1). This section will cover additional nutrition-related risk factors that are specific to all population groups in LMIC, specifically undernutrition, overweight/obesity, and poor diet.

In LMIC, the incidence of stroke has increased by 100% between 1970 and 2008 (from 52 [95% CI 33-71] to 117 [95% CI 79-156] per 100,000 person years) compared to a 40% *decrease* in high-income countries. Furthermore, stroke incidence rates were 20% higher in LMIC compared to high-income countries for the first time in 2000-2008.[32] During this time, economic development, urbanization, and globalization caused significant food and lifestyle changes globally, which likely contributed to the increase in LMIC stroke incidence.[33,34]

Undernutrition as a Risk Factor

A lack of essential nutrients, most often in the form of calories and protein during the in-utero, infancy, and childhood life stages, increases the risk of stroke later in life. For example, poor maternal nutrition can lead to development of a flat pelvis, which impairs fetal growth[35] and may be linked to increased hypertension of the baby in adulthood, which is associated with increased risk of stroke.[36] Similarly, childhood undernutrition postnatally (from birth to 2 years of age) can lead to poor growth, which is also associated with increased risk of hypertension in adulthood, which in turn is associated with increased risk of stroke.[35] The mechanisms that explain the predisposition to stroke of persons who were undernourished in early life are unclear, though it is hypothesized that the development of hypertension as a result of poor growth in childhood may be due to impaired development of cerebral vasculature at this critical stage of brain growth.[35]

Overweight/Obesity as a Risk Factor

Chronic excess intake of calories results in weight gain and eventually excess body fat, or overweight/obesity. As described in chapter 8, excess body fat increases risk for many diseases, including stroke, through inflammation, which triggers the accumulation of plaques and blockages in blood vessels. In addition to impacting risk for stroke directly through the inflammation mechanism, overweight and obesity also increase the risk for a multitude of other conditions that are also risk factors for stroke, including hypertension, hyperlipidemia, and diabetes, that are causal risk factors for stroke in both LMIC and high-income countries.[37]

Poor Diet as a Risk Factor

Independent of the contribution of excess calories and overweight or obesity status, there is convincing evidence that certain dietary patterns and dietary components contribute to the risk of stroke. As shown in chapter 7 (table 7.1), low fruit, vegetable, and whole-grain intake as well as high sodium intake and sugar-sweetened beverage intake have been associated with substantially increased risk for stroke. At the same time, quality of the overall diet, including energy intake and expenditure balance, is considered to be more important than individual nutrients or foods in reducing risk of stroke.[36,38] There is some evidence to support the hypothesis that certain diets can prevent stroke, such as those that are rich in minimally processed fruits, vegetables, legumes, and whole grains, and low in salt, added sugars, and red meat, such as the Mediterranean diet or DASH (Dietary Approaches to Stop Hypertension) diet.[36] Also, the association between alcohol intake and risk of stroke has been widely studied with varied results dependent on quantities consumed and stroke type. Light to moderate drinking has been shown to reduce risk of coronary heart disease, ischemic stroke, and diabetes, while heavy drinking/binge drinking increases risk of hemorrhagic stroke.[38]

Differences in Nutrition-Related Risk Factors for Death and Disability over Time and by Region and Population Group

Health outcomes, such as morbidity and mortality, tend to be both a determinant and consequence of population differences and population change. While this chapter provides an overview of the nutrition-related drivers of death and disability in LMIC, it is important to acknowledge and discuss the heterogeneity of nutrition-related risk factors of death and disability across space and time. This section covers them briefly.

Differences across Geographies

The 2001 Global Burden of Disease study estimated that in LMIC, non-communicable diseases were responsible for more than 50% of deaths in adults 15 to 59 years of age in all regions except South Asia and Sub-Saharan Africa, where communicable diseases remain responsible for one-third and two-thirds of deaths, respectively.[39] It is important to note that these aggregated summary statistics for all LMIC mask the heterogeneity that exists within regions (and subnationally). For instance, as mentioned above, South Asia and Sub-Saharan Africa still have substantial burdens of extreme poverty, undernutrition, and communicable diseases, and living conditions and risk factors that give rise to communicable diseases (indoor smoke from household use of solid fuels; poor water, sanitation, and hygiene; and unsafe sex) are prevalent. Risk factors for noncommunicable diseases (such as, smoking, alcohol, high blood pressure and cholesterol, and overweight and obesity) are widespread globally and increasing over time.

Differences over Time: The Epidemiological Transition

The type and prevalence of nutrition-related risk factors for death and disability have changed over time, and staggering differences continue to exist between regions and population groups in LMIC compared to high-income countries. As a country develops, there is transition in disease risk in the population from mainly infectious diseases, including diarrhea and pneumonia, to mainly noncommunicable diseases, including stroke and cardiovascular diseases.[40] This transition is the result of improved health care (reducing preventable deaths from conditions such as diarrhea among children), an aging population (higher incidence of noncommunicable diseases among adults as they age), and improved public health interventions (reduced infectious diseases due to vaccinations and improved water and sanitation).[1] This epidemiological transition in LMIC resulted in a 20% reduction in the per capita communicable, and 10% increase in noncommunicable, disease burden between 1990 and 2001.[39] However, in certain regions, particularly in sub-Saharan Africa, where a high proportion of LMIC remain, this shift is occurring more slowly and the leading risk factors continue to be those affecting the poor (demographic segment) and children (age group). The disease burden for childhood communicable diseases has fallen substantially, but underweight and suboptimal breastfeeding remain leading causes of disease.[41] Simultaneously, many LMIC are now dealing with a double burden of malnutrition (described further in chapter 10), as there is an increase in noncommunicable diseases due to changes in diet and lifestyle patterns while communicable diseases remain high.

Conclusion

Currently, the leading causes of death and disability in LMIC are lower respiratory infections and diarrheal disease, predominantly affecting children, and stroke in adulthood. Suboptimal breastfeeding and undernutrition are the major risk factors for death and disability from lower respiratory infections and diarrheal disease by contributing to the vicious cycle of malnutrition and infection. Poor diets and various other factors that contribute to under- and overnutrition are the major risk factors for stroke, partially due to their impact on associated conditions, such as obesity, hypertension, hyperlipidemia, and diabetes.

LMIC are in various stages of the demographic, epidemiologic, and nutrition transitions and thus are experiencing rapid changes in the patterns of disease. These transitions have resulted in the emergence of a double burden of preventable communicable childhood diseases alongside chronic, noncommunicable diseases in adults in LMIC.

Poorer subpopulations of LMIC live in conditions of overcrowding, inadequate housing, poor water, sanitation and hygiene, indoor biomass fuel exposure, food chain contaminant exposure, food insecurity, and suboptimal feeding. These living conditions predispose people to poor nutritional status, adverse health outcomes, and the interactions between the two, through the mechanisms presented in this chapter. Further complicating this picture is the fact that people often lack the resources to mitigate this vicious cycle. In other words, *poverty begets poverty* is one way of summarizing the poverty trap—the self-reinforcing mechanism that causes poverty to persist. This explanation can be extended to a health–poverty trap.

Conversely, good nutritional status and health are key to agricultural and economic productivity. In states of disease, people work less, produce less, and earn less. For people like NakaNomsa, their surviving families, and the communities in which they reside, emergence from this health–poverty trap requires coherent policy actions that address the factors underlying the specific conditions that predispose them to death and disability. Governments, policy makers, and program implementers need to first understand, and then simultaneously address, the multiple causes of death and disability. Nutrition is a key part of this equation.

Review Questions

1. List the leading causes of death and disability in low- and middle-income countries, and discuss how and why they differ from those in high-income countries.
2. What factors perpetuate the vicious cycle of malnutrition and infection, and how?
3. How does breastfeeding reduce the risk of morbidity and mortality from infectious diseases, such as pneumonia and diarrhea, among infants and young children?
4. Undernutrition and overnutrition are respectively considered conditions of deprivation and excess. Describe how each condition contributes to the increased risk of developing a stroke.
5. Describe the epidemiological transition that is occurring in low- and middle-income countries.

References

1. World Health Organization. 2008. "The Global Burden of Disease: 2004 Update." Geneva, Switzerland: World Health Organization.

2. "The Top 10 Causes of Death." 2018. http://www.who.int/news-room/fact -sheets/detail/the-top-10-causes-of-death.

3. Black, Robert E., Cesar G. Victora, Susan P. Walker, Zulfiqar A. Bhutta, Parul Christian, Mercedes De Onis, Majid Ezzati, et al. 2013. "Maternal and Child Undernutrition and Overweight in Low-Income and Middle-Income Countries." *The Lancet* 382 (9890): 427–51. https://doi.org/10.1016/S0140-6736(13)60937-X.

4. Fishman, Steven M., Laura E. Caulfield, Mercedes De Onis, Monika Blossner, Adnan A. Hyder, Luke Mullany, and Robert E. Black. 2004. "Childhood and Maternal Underweight." In *Comparative Quantification of Health Risks: Global and Regional Burden of Disease Attributable to Selected Major Risk Factors*, 1:39–161. Geneva, Switzerland: World Health Organization.

5. Pelletier, D. L., E. A. Frongillo, and J. P. Habicht. 1993. "Epidemiologic Evidence for a Potentiating Effect of Malnutrition on Child Mortality." *American Journal of Public Health* 83 (8): 1130–33.

6. Lanata, Claudio F., Igor Rudan, Cynthia Boschi-Pinto, Lana Tomaskovic, Thomas Cherian, Martin Weber, and Harry Campbell. 2004. "Methodological and Quality Issues in Epidemiological Studies of Acute Lower Respiratory Infections in Children in Developing Countries." *International Journal of Epidemiology* 33 (6): 1362–72. https://doi.org/10.1093/ije/dyh229.

7. Sonego, Michela, Maria Chiara Pellegrin, Genevieve Becker, and Marzia Lazzerini. 2015. "Risk Factors for Mortality from Acute Lower Respiratory Infections (ALRI) in Children under Five Years of Age in Low and Middle-Income Countries: A Systematic Review and Meta-Analysis of Observational Studies." *PLoS ONE* 10 (1). https://doi.org/10.1371/journal.pone.0116380.

8. Roth, Daniel, Laura E. Caulfield, Majid Ezzati, and Robert E. Black. 2008. "Acute Lower Respiratory Infections in Childhood: Opportunities for Reducing the Global Burden through Nutritional Interventions." *Bulletin of the World Health Organization* 86 (5): 356–64. https://doi.org/10.2471/BLT.07.049114.

9. Horta, Bernardo L., Cesar G. Victora, and World Health Organization. 2013. "Short-Term Effects of Breastfeeding: A Systematic Review on the Benefits of Breastfeeding on Diarrhoea and Pneumonia Mortality." https://apps.who.int/iris /handle/10665/95585.

10. Lamberti, Laura M., Irena Zakarija-Grković, Christa L. Fischer Walker, Evropi Theodoratou, Harish Nair, Harry Campbell, and Robert E. Black. 2013. "Breastfeeding for Reducing the Risk of Pneumonia Morbidity and Mortality in Children under Two: A Systematic Literature Review and Meta-Analysis." *BMC Public Health* 13 (3): S18. https://doi.org/10.1186/1471-2458-13-S3-S18.

11. Newburg, David S., and W. Allan Walker. 2007. "Protection of the Neonate by the Innate Immune System of Developing Gut and of Human Milk." *Pediatric Research* 61 (1): 2–8. https://doi.org/10.1203/01.pdr.0000250274.68571.18.

12. Moore, Sophie E., Andrew C. Collinson, Pa Tamba N'Gom, and Andrew M. Prentice. 2005. "Maternal Malnutrition and the Risk of Infection in Later Life."

The Impact of Maternal Nutrition on the Offspring, Nestlé Nutrition Workshop Series Pediatric Program, 55: 153-67. https://doi.org/10.1159/000082600.

13. Beisel, William R. 1996. "Nutrition and Immune Function: Overview." *The Journal of Nutrition* 126 (suppl_10): 2611S-2615S. https://doi.org/10.1093/jn/126 .suppl_10.2611S.

14. Keusch, Gerald T. 2003. "The History of Nutrition: Malnutrition, Infection and Immunity." *The Journal of Nutrition* 133 (1): 336S-340S. https://doi.org/10.1093 /jn/133.1.336S.

15. Scrimshaw, Nevin Stewart, Carl Ernest Taylor, and John Everett Gordon. 1968. "Interactions of Nutrition and Infection," 37. WHO Monograph Series no. 57. Geneva, Switzerland: World Health Organization.

16. Katona, Peter, and Judit Katona-Apte. 2008. "The Interaction between Nutrition and Infection." *Clinical Infectious Diseases* 46 (10): 1582-88. https://doi.org /10.1086/587658.

17. Jackson, Stewart, Kyle H. Mathews, Dražen Pulanić, Rachel Falconer, Igor Rudan, Harry Campbell, and Harish Nair. 2013. "Risk Factors for Severe Acute Lower Respiratory Infections in Children-a Systematic Review and Meta-Analysis." *Croatian Medical Journal* 54 (2): 110-21.

18. Rice, A. L., L. Sacco, A. Hyder, and R. E. Black. 2000. "Malnutrition as an Underlying Cause of Childhood Deaths Associated with Infectious Diseases in Developing Countries." *Bulletin of the World Health Organization* 78 (10): 1207-21.

19. Chisti, Mohammod Jobayer, Marc Tebruegge, Sophie La Vincente, Stephen M. Graham, and Trevor Duke. 2009. "Pneumonia in Severely Malnourished Children in Developing Countries—Mortality Risk, Aetiology and Validity of WHO Clinical Signs: A Systematic Review." *Tropical Medicine & International Health* 14 (10): 1173-89. https://doi.org/10.1111/j.1365-3156.2009.02364.x.

20. McCormick, Marie C. 1985. "The Contribution of Low Birth Weight to Infant Mortality and Childhood Morbidity." *New England Journal of Medicine* 312 (2): 82-90.

21. Barker, D. J., K. M. Godfrey, C. Fall, C. Osmond, P. D. Winter, and S. O. Shaheen. 1991. "Relation of Birth Weight and Childhood Respiratory Infection to Adult Lung Function and Death from Chronic Obstructive Airways Disease." *British Medical Journal* 303 (6804): 671-75. https://doi.org/10.1136/bmj.303.6804.671.

22. World Health Organization. 2017. "Diarrhoeal Disease." https://www.who .int/news-room/fact-sheets/detail/diarrhoeal-disease.

23. Brown, Kenneth H., Robert E. Black, Guillermo Lopez de Romaña, and Hilary Creed de Kanashiro. 1989. "Infant-Feeding Practices and Their Relationship with Diarrheal and Other Diseases in Huascar (Lima), Peru." *Pediatrics* 83 (1): 31-40.

24. Popkin, Barry M., Linda Adair, John S. Akin, Robert Black, John Briscoe, and Wilhelm Flieger. 1990. "Breast-Feeding and Diarrheal Morbidity." *Pediatrics* 86 (6): 874-82.

25. Lamberti, Laura M., Christa L. Fischer Walker, Adi Noiman, Cesar Victora, and Robert E. Black. 2011. "Breastfeeding and the Risk for Diarrhea Morbidity and Mortality." *BMC Public Health* 11 (3): S15. https://doi.org/10.1186/1471-2458-11-S3-S15.

26. Caulfield, Laura E., Mercedes de Onis, Monika Blössner, and Robert E. Black. 2004. "Undernutrition as an Underlying Cause of Child Deaths Associated

with Diarrhea, Pneumonia, Malaria, and Measles." *The American Journal of Clinical Nutrition* 80 (1): 193-98. https://doi.org/10.1093/ajcn/80.1.193.

27. Brown, Kenneth H. 2003. "Diarrhea and Malnutrition." *Journal of Nutrition* 133 (1): 328S-332S. https://doi.org/10.1093/jn/133.1.328S.

28. Villamor, Eduardo, and Wafaie W. Fawzi. 2000. "Vitamin A Supplementation: Implications for Morbidity and Mortality in Children." *The Journal of Infectious Diseases* 182 (Supplement_1): S122-33. https://doi.org/10.1086/315921.

29. Bhutta, Z. A., R. E. Black, K. H. Brown, J. M. Gardner, S. Gore, A. Hidayat, F. Khatun, et al. 1999. "Prevention of Diarrhea and Pneumonia by Zinc Supplementation in Children in Developing Countries: Pooled Analysis of Randomized Controlled Trials. Zinc Investigators' Collaborative Group." *The Journal of Pediatrics* 135 (6): 689-97.

30. Bhutta, Z. A., S. M. Bird, R. E. Black, K. H. Brown, J. M. Gardner, A. Hidayat, F. Khatun, et al. 2000. "Therapeutic Effects of Oral Zinc in Acute and Persistent Diarrhea in Children in Developing Countries: Pooled Analysis of Randomized Controlled Trials." *The American Journal of Clinical Nutrition* 72 (6): 1516-22. https://doi.org/10.1093/ajcn/72.6.1516.

31. World Health Organization. 2018. "Stroke, Cerebrovascular Accident." http://www.emro.who.int/health-topics/stroke-cerebrovascular-accident/index.html.

32. Feigin, Valery L, Carlene MM Lawes, Derrick A Bennett, Suzanne L Barker-Collo, and Varsha Parag. 2009. "Worldwide Stroke Incidence and Early Case Fatality Reported in 56 Population-Based Studies: A Systematic Review." *The Lancet Neurology* 8 (4): 355-69. https://doi.org/10.1016/S1474-4422(09)70025-0.

33. Dans, Antonio, Nawi Ng, Cherian Varghese, E Shyong Tai, Rebecca Firestone, and Ruth Bonita. 2011. "The Rise of Chronic Non-Communicable Diseases in Southeast Asia: Time for Action." *The Lancet* 377 (9766): 680-89. https://doi.org/10.1016/S0140-6736(10)61506-1.

34. Lock, Karen, Richard D. Smith, Alan D. Dangour, Marcus Keogh-Brown, Gessuir Pigatto, Corinna Hawkes, Regina Mara Fisberg, and Zaid Chalabi. 2010. "Health, Agricultural, and Economic Effects of Adoption of Healthy Diet Recommendations." *The Lancet* 376 (9753): 1699-1709. https://doi.org/10.1016/S0140-6736(10)61352-9.

35. Osmond, Clive, Eero Kajantie, Tom J. Forsén, Johan G. Eriksson, and David J. P. Barker. 2007. "Infant Growth and Stroke in Adult Life: The Helsinki Birth Cohort Study." *Stroke* 38 (2): 264-70. https://doi.org/10.1161/01.STR.0000254471.72186.03.

36. Hankey, Graeme J. 2012. "Nutrition and the Risk of Stroke." *The Lancet Neurology* 11 (1): 66-81. https://doi.org/10.1016/S1474-4422(11)70265-4.

37. O'Donnell, Martin J., Denis Xavier, Lisheng Liu, Hongye Zhang, Siu Lim Chin, Purnima Rao-Melacini, Sumathy Rangarajan, et al. 2010. "Risk Factors for Ischaemic and Intracerebral Haemorrhagic Stroke in 22 Countries (the INTER-STROKE Study): A Case-Control Study." *The Lancet* 376 (9735): 112-23. https://doi.org/10.1016/S0140-6736(10)60834-3.

38. Kuklina, Elena V., Xin Tong, Mary G. George, and Pooja Bansil. 2012. "Epidemiology and Prevention of Stroke: A Worldwide Perspective." *Expert Review of Neurotherapeutics* 12 (2): 199-208. https://doi.org/10.1586/ern.11.99.

39. Lopez, Alan D., Colin D. Mathers, Majid Ezzati, Dean T. Jamison, and Christopher J. L. Murray, eds. 2006. *Global Burden of Disease and Risk Factors*. Washington, DC: World Bank.

40. Omran, Abdel R. 2005. "The Epidemiologic Transition: A Theory of the Epidemiology of Population Change." *Milbank Quarterly* 83 (4): 731-57. https://doi.org/10.1111/j.1468-0009.2005.00398.x.

41. Lim, Stephen S., Theo Vos, Abraham D. Flaxman, Goodarz Danaei, Kenji Shibuya, Heather Adair-Rohani, Markus Amann, et al. 2012. "A Comparative Risk Assessment of Burden of Disease and Injury Attributable to 67 Risk Factors and Risk Factor Clusters in 21 Regions, 1990-2010: A Systematic Analysis for the Global Burden of Disease Study 2010." *The Lancet* 380 (9859): 2224-60. https://doi.org/10.1016/S0140-6736(12)61766-8.

10

The Nutrition Transition

Lindsay M. Jaacks and Alexandra L. Bellows

LEARNING OBJECTIVES

- Define the stages of the nutrition transition and key indicators of this phenomenon
- Describe historical, economic, political, social, and cultural factors that have shaped the nutrition transition globally
- Understand the consequences of the nutrition transition in terms of the epidemiological transition, and which subpopulations are most impacted by the nutrition transition as it advances
- Give examples of approaches to addressing the nutrition transition to promote health and prevent disease

As a result of economic development, industrialization, urbanization, and globalization, societies around the world have witnessed dramatic changes in dietary intake and physical activity patterns, known as the nutrition transition. As a consequence, the primary form of malnutrition has shifted from **underweight** to **overweight** and **obesity** (box 10.1).[1] Herein we describe in detail two case studies, the first of Brazil, which is in the later stages of the nutrition transition, and the second of India, which is in the earlier stages of the transition. We then discuss the history and development of the theory of the nutrition transition, the key components of the theory, underlying drivers, and major consequences. The chapter concludes with a discussion of the main challenges and gaps that remain in our understanding of the nutrition transition, and future directions for research and policy.

Case Study: Nutrition Transitions in Brazil and India

Brazil

Brazil is the fifth most populous country, home to an estimated 207 million people,[2] and has the ninth-largest gross domestic product (GDP) in the world.[3] It is the most populous country and largest economy in South America, and it was named "one of the fastest rising emerging powers" in 2012.[4] Brazil has also witnessed significant urbanization. Today, the vast majority of Brazilians—86%—live in urban areas compared to just 56% in 1970.[5]

Scholars have posited that the unprecedented growth of Brazil is a result of a foreign policy that emphasizes development in terms of South-South cooperation, leadership in preventing and treating AIDS and tropical dis-

Box 10.1. Malnutrition in All Its Forms

The nutrition transition is monitored using the anthropometric measures of weight and height, which in turn are used to calculate *body mass index (BMI)*: weight in kilograms divided by height in meters-squared.

The malnutrition spectrum ranges from undernutrition to over-nutrition. *Underweight* is defined as BMI <18.5 kg/m² in adults and <−1 SD in children. Over-nutrition includes:

- *Overweight*,[1] defined as BMI ≥25 to <30 kg/m² in adults and >1 to 2 SD in children aged >5 to 18 years and >2 to 3 SD in children from birth to five years.

- *Obesity*,[1] defined as BMI ≥30 kg/m² in adults and >2 SD in children aged >5 to 18 years and >3 SD in children from birth to five years.

Often times in low- and middle-income countries, overweight and obesity are combined into a single category representing over-nutrition.

A second commonly used indicator of under-nutrition is *stunting*, defined as height-for-age <-2 SD in children.

Other terms used in this chapter include:

Gini index: A measure of the extent to which the distribution of income within an economy deviates from a perfectly equal distribution. A Gini index of 0 represents perfect equality, while an index of 100 implies perfect inequality.

Gross domestic product (GDP): The monetary value of all goods and services produced within a country over a specified period of time.

Gross national product (GNP): The market value of all goods and services produced by citizens of a country (either within the country itself or abroad) over a specified period of time.

---

eases, and advocacy on renewable energy rather than military power.[4] With these progressive policies in place, Brazil saw its economy flourish at the turn of the twenty-first century. Indeed, economic growth in Brazil outpaced many developed countries before the 2008-2009 recession.[4] However, the economic gains were not distributed equally, and as a result, Brazil has one of the highest levels of income inequality in the world, as measured by the **Gini index**.[6] This inequality may partially explain the persistent double burden of under- and over-nutrition discussed in greater detail later on in this chapter.

As a result of these historical, economic, and political factors, dietary intake has changed dramatically in Brazil over the past 50 years. In 2003, Brazil surpassed Australia as the world's largest exporter of beef and is neck and neck with the United States as the world's largest exporter of soya—Brazil's most abundant food crop.[7] This intensification of the beef and soya industries has led to deforestation in the Brazilian Amazon[8]—one of the many pathways by which the nutrition transition is related to climate change.

While Brazil lacks robust longitudinal individual-level dietary data, data from household food expenditure surveys conducted from 1974 to 2008 indicate a decrease in household purchases of foods typically seen as "traditional" staples in the Brazilian diet, such as rice, beans, and cassava.[9,10] At the same time, purchases of processed foods such as cookies, sugar-sweetened beverages, and processed meats increased.[9-11]

Ultra-processed foods, including sugar-sweetened beverages, industrialized breads, pizzas, hamburgers, cakes, and cookies, now account for approximately 30% of total calories in the Brazilian diet.[12] Sugar-sweetened beverages alone account for approximately 17% of total calories, with the most commonly consumed sugar-sweetened beverages being caloric coffee beverages.[13] Higher income and education are associated with a greater proportion of total calories from ultra-processed foods.[12] For example, Brazilian adolescents and adults with higher income and education are more likely to consume high-caloric beverages, including caloric soft drinks, fruit/vegetable juices, and caloric milk/soymilk beverages.[13]

With these shifts toward unhealthy eating patterns, it is not surprising that Brazil has seen rates of overweight and obesity increase significantly. From 1974 to 2008, the prevalence of overweight in men increased from 15% to 37% and in women from 20% to 31%; and the prevalence of obesity increased from 3% to 13% in men and 7% to 17% in women.[14] If trends continue, an estimated 95% of men and 52% of women will be overweight or obese by 2050.[15] Coinciding with this increase in overweight and obesity, the burden of noncommunicable diseases such as hypertension and diabetes has increased.[9] In 2007, 72% of all deaths in Brazil were attributed to noncommunicable diseases, with the greatest burden in the North and Northeast regions, the poorest areas of the country.[9]

Importantly, the rate of increase of overweight and obesity is greater among adults in lower socioeconomic strata.[14] In fact, among wealthy women, obesity rates are actually decreasing.[16] These observations suggest that Brazil is progressing to later stages of the nutrition transition, where the highest burden of over-nutrition and noncommunicable diseases shifts from individuals with higher socioeconomic status to those with lower socioeconomic status. These stages will be described in greater detail later in this chapter.

The recognition of overweight and obesity as important nutrition challenges in Brazil can be traced to the publication of the National Food and Nutrition Policy in 1999.[17] Twelve years later, in 2011, this policy was updated and the Strategic Action Plan to Tackle NCDs (noncommunicable diseases) 2011–2022 was launched.[17] Essential components of that action plan are the promotion of physical activity and healthy eating.[18] Main actions include, for physical activity:

- Health Academy: building spaces for health promotion activities, including physical activity and educational programs nested in the primary health care system;
- Health in School: development of nutritional assessment and promotion of physical activity and healthy eating in schools;
- National Program for Healthy Sidewalks and building bike lanes, parks, squares, and jogging trails; and

- public health messaging campaigns to promote physical activity integrated into major events such as the FIFA 2014 Soccer World Cup and the 2016 Olympic Games.

And, for healthy eating:

- improving the healthfulness of food provided through the National Program of School Meals;
- supporting intersectoral partnerships and agreements in order to increase the production and supply of minimally processed foods;
- supporting agreements with the private sector aimed at reducing salt and sugar in food;
- recommending the adoption of fiscal measures to reduce the price of fruits and vegetables; and
- establishing regulations for the advertising of food to children. Unfortunately, a governmental proposal in 2006 to regulate the advertising of foods high in sugar, salt, and saturated and *trans* fat was challenged in court by food industry representatives.[17]

Building off of this action plan, in 2014, Brazil's Ministry of Health updated the National Dietary Guidelines to promote the consumption of minimally processed foods and the avoidance of processed and ultra-processed foods, oils, fats, salt, and sugar. In addition, these guidelines promote family household meals and the avoidance of fast-food chains and exposure to food advertising.[19] Together, these policies represent one of the most comprehensive government responses to the nutrition transition of any country to date, and thus Brazil is an important case study that may be applied to other countries at earlier stages of this transition.

India

India is the second-largest country in the world, with an estimated population of 1.3 billion people,[2] and the seventh-largest economy.[3] Following the implementation of economic liberalization policies in 1991, the country has experienced continuous growth of per capita GDP[20] and a decrease in poverty rates, though the rate remains high, with an estimated 37% of the population living on less than a $1.25 a day.[21] India's per capita GDP (US$1,709.60) is substantially smaller than Brazil's (US$8,649.90)[20,22] (figure 10.1), and so India is a case study of a rapidly developing country in the earlier stages of the nutrition transition. This observation is further supported by trends in urbanization in India: just 33% of the country lives in urban areas, a small increase from 23% in 1980,[23] though this number is expected to rise to 50% by 2050.[24] (Recall that 56% of Brazilians lived in urban areas in 1970.[5])

Similar to Brazil, these historical, economic, and political factors in India have contributed to changes in dietary intake. The percentage of calories

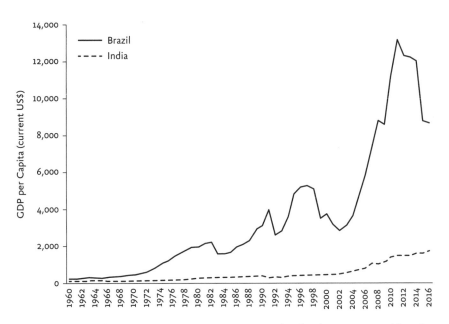

Figure 10.1. Growth in GDP per capita over time in Brazil and India. *Source:* World Bank.

from cereals is declining while the percentage from fat is increasing.[25] India is now the second-largest producer and largest consumer of sugar,[26] and while sales of sugar-sweetened beverages are significantly lower than in Latin America, they have increased 13% year on year since 1998.[27] Much of this increase has been attributed to the increasing presence of roadside restaurants selling sugar-sweetened beverages.[26] Because India is still in the early stages of the nutrition transition, the poorest dietary habits (related to noncommunicable disease risk factors) are seen in the wealthiest third of the population.[27]

Concurrent with these shifts in dietary intake, the burden of over-nutrition in India has increased. From 1980 to 2013, the prevalence of overweight and obesity in Indian men increased from 15% to 20% and 15% to 21% in women.[28] Today, in all 29 states of India, noncommunicable diseases pose a higher burden on the population than communicable diseases, even in the poorest states where undernutrition is still a major public health concern.[29] The country is now facing the daunting task of addressing a substantial double burden of under- and over-nutrition.

Around the same time that Brazil adopted its Strategic Action Plan to Tackle NCDs, the Indian government launched its National Programme for Prevention and Control of Cancer, Diabetes, Cardiovascular Diseases, and Stroke. However, in stark contrast to Brazil's action plan, India's program does not include a clear set of actions to address unhealthy diets and physical inactivity. The program is almost entirely focused on screening, early diagnosis, and treatment rather than primary prevention. This reflects a common phenomenon in low-income countries that continue to carry significant undernutrition burdens: nutrition and food policies largely focus on preventing/reducing hunger by providing adequate calories from staple grains,[30] whereas policies aimed at improving diets for noncommunicable disease prevention are lacking.

Recent evidence from a policy space analysis in India suggests that stakeholders acknowledge opportunities for integrated food-based approaches to addressing the double burden, particularly as it relates to dietary diversity and the following foods: fruits, vegetables, pulses, coarse cereals, nuts, milk, eggs, fish, and healthy oils.[31] These opportunities are highlighted in the 2011 Dietary Guidelines for Indians, which clearly recognize the nutrition transition as a "shift from traditional to 'modern' foods . . . increased intake of processed and ready-to-eat foods, intensive marketing of junk foods and 'health' beverages."[32] Most of the 15 specific recommendations in the guidelines focus on improving unhealthy diets that have resulted from the nutrition transition, including eating plenty of vegetables and fruits, moderate use of edible oils and animal-based foods, restricting ghee/butter/Vanaspati (margarine) and salt, avoiding overeating, minimizing processed foods, and exercising regularly.[32]

Importantly, these guidelines were distributed and discussed with multiple sectors in India, including agriculture, health, education, rural development, and state-level departments of women and children.[33] However, to date, they have not been translated into policies or regulations that could improve nutrition and health such as taxes on sugar-sweetened beverages[27] or the reformulation of partially hydrogenated vegetable oils to eliminate dietary *trans* fat.[34]

Defining the Nutrition Transition

The term **nutrition transition** encompasses changing patterns in diet and physical activity. After World War II, dietary patterns shifted from diets high in complex carbohydrates (e.g., whole grains) and fiber to diets high in simple carbohydrates (e.g., refined grains), animal-based foods, saturated fat, and added sugars.[35-39] In recent decades, increased consumption of processed foods including sugar-sweetened beverages and fast food are also considered key indicators of the nutrition transition.[39] Changes in diet coincide with changes in physical activity, particularly declines in occupation- and transport-related physical activity.[35,36] This transition first occurred in high-income countries such as the United States and countries in Western Europe and is now occurring at an unprecedented rate in low- and middle-income countries.[36]

Barry Popkin, who first proposed the nutrition transition in 1993,[40] has described five key stages:[37]

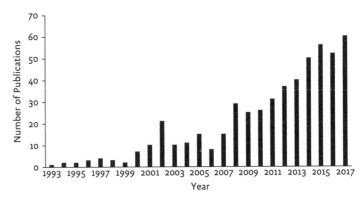

Figure 10.2. Publications in PubMed with the search term "Nutrition Transition" by year.

1. *Collecting food*: hunter-gathering stage with a healthy diet and low life expectancy
2. *Famine*: staple grains predominant and nutritional deficiencies are high
3. *Receding famine*: increased fruits and vegetables and animal-based foods, diets improve, but nutritional deficiencies persist
4. *Degenerative disease*: increased fat, sugar, and processed foods with an increase in obesity
5. *Behavioral change*: higher-quality fat, increased consumption of whole grains and obesity decreases

The first two stages of the transition have already occurred in the majority of countries, and an increasing number of countries are transitioning from stage 3 to stage 4, including Brazil and India. A few high-income countries have begun the transition from stage 4 to stage 5. For example, in the United States, from 1977 to 1996, total calories, away-from-home food, snacks, and sugar-sweetened beverages all increased,[41] but more recently, from 2004-2010, total calories decreased for the first time in decades.[42] Moreover, whole-grain consumption has increased,[43] while consumption of sugar-sweetened beverages has decreased,[44] thus supporting a shift to stage 5 of the nutrition transition.

Since 1993, the number of publications on the nutrition transition has increased dramatically (figure 10.2). We describe in greater detail specific changes in diet and physical activity that characterize the nutrition transition in the sections that follow.

Diet

Populations in many low- and middle-income countries are increasingly adopting a "Western diet," a phrase used to describe a diet high in fat, simple carbohydrates, added sugar, and animal-based foods. In particular, due to decreases in the cost of production resulting from technological advances, there have been large increases in the consumption of vegetable oils such as rapeseed/canola oil, palm oil, and soya oil.[38] Added sugars are entering diets primarily through increased consumption of sugar-sweetened beverages, but also processed foods such as cakes and cookies.[38] A review by Popkin and Corinna Hawkes found that from 2009 to 2014 sales of sugar-sweetened beverages decreased in many high-income countries but increased in many low- and middle-income countries.[45] Similarly, the increases in production of animal-based foods such as beef, poultry, and fish have primarily occurred in these rapidly developing countries.[46]

In addition to these overall changes in dietary patterns, the nutrition transition is marked by changes in (1) food processing, (2) food packaging, and (3) eating patterns (e.g., frequency and location of eating); each of these is discussed in detail in the sections that follow.

Food Processing

Carlos Monteiro has pioneered research on the distinct role of food processing in the nutrition transition and obesity.[47] He classifies foods according to their level of processing: (1) minimally processed foods (e.g., frozen vegetables, canned legumes, and pasteurized dairy products), (2) ingredients extracted from whole foods such as flour and oil, and (3) ultra-processed foods, which are foods made up entirely of extracted ingredients plus added sugar and salt (e.g., burgers, chips, cookies, and sugar-sweetened beverages).[47] Ultra-processed foods are typically high in calories and low in essential nutrients, are the primary source of *trans* fat in the diet, and have come to dominate the global food system due to their hyper-palatability, low cost, and pervasive marketing. They are favored by large transnational corporations because of their long shelf life and high profit margins: Monteiro estimates that production of ultra-processed foods costs just 5% to 10% of the selling value of these products.[47]

In the United States, an estimated 60% of calories are from ultra-processed foods, which have significantly higher levels of saturated fat, sugar, and salt than other less-processed foods.[48,49] In Canada, ultra-processed foods accounted for just 24% of calories in 1938, more than doubling to 55% in 2001.[50] In Sweden, the consumption of ultra-processed foods increased by 142% from 1960 to 2010, from 125 to 302 kg/capita per annum, with especially large increases in sugar-sweetened beverages, chips, and candies.[51] An ecological study of 19 European countries found a positive association between household availability of ultra-processed foods and obesity.[52]

While trends have remained relatively consistent in high-income countries, sales of ultra-processed foods have increased significantly over the past 20 years in low- and middle-income countries.[53] In Mexico, for example, ultra-processed foods contribute 50% of calories, and the proportion continues to increase.[54] In Brazil, the proportion is lower at 26% in 2008–2009,[55] but it is similarly increasing over time.[56] In Asia, processed foods have entered the market more slowly than in Latin America. Approximately 28% of calories are from processed foods in China.[57] In East and Southern Africa (Ethiopia, Uganda, Tanzania, Mozambique, Malawi, and Zambia), the proportion is estimated to be 36% of all food purchases.[58] In most of these developing country settings, the proportion of calories from ultra-processed foods is significantly higher among those living in urban areas and those with higher incomes, though the rate of increase is higher in some countries among poorer households—suggesting a future shift in the over-nutrition burden.

Food Packaging

Not only are ultra-processed foods high in energy, added sugar, and salt, and low in essential nutrients, they are also more likely to be packaged in materials containing synthetic chemicals associated with metabolic disorders including obesity and diabetes. Bisphenol A (BPA) is one such example. BPA is used in the production of polycarbonate plastics found in some food and beverage packaging as well as epoxy resins used to coat metal products such as food cans and bottle tops. While production of BPA is increasing worldwide, trends in its use vary across regions: it is decreasing in the United States and Western Europe,[59] increasing in emerging markets, particularly in Asia,[60] and banned in France.[61] A recent meta-analysis found that BPA exposure was significantly associated with general obesity, abdominal obesity, diabetes, and hypertension.[62] This BPA-obesity exposure-response relation is associated with significant economic costs in the United States and Europe.[63,64]

Similar to BPA, phthalates are a chemical added to plastics to make them more flexible, transparent, and/or durable. A recent analysis of the US National Health and Nutrition Examination Survey (NHANES) found that certain phthalates were associated with increased risk of diabetes in adults,[65] and a previous study reported an association between phthalates and insulin resistance in adolescents.[66] To date, most studies, particularly on phthalates, have been cross-sectional, conducted in the United States, and do not adjust for confounding by ultra-processed food intake. More research is needed to explore the role of changes in food packaging in the nutrition transition—especially considering that food labeling, which requires packaging, is one of the proposed strategies to address the adverse consequences of the nutrition transition.

Eating Patterns

As countries progress through the nutrition transition and household income increases, frequency and location of eating have shifted from traditional meals at home to increased consumption of "Westernized" foods outside of the home. Foods consumed outside of the home, whether they be a snack from a vending machine, a meal from a fast-food restaurant, or a meal from a full-service restaurant, are typically higher in calories, saturated fat, and added sugar than foods consumed inside the home.[67] Prospective studies from the United States, Australia, and Spain have found that eating outside of the home is associated with weight gain.[68]

The way in which food is cooked inside the home is also undergoing a transition. In China, for example, steaming and boiling are used less frequently as households shift toward frying,[69] a transition related to the increased availability and consumption of vegetable oils discussed earlier in the chapter. In the United States, approximately 68% of women and 42% of men reported preparing food (includes cleaning up after food preparation) in 2007-2008 compared to 92% of women and 29% of men in 1965-1966.[70] Time spent cooking at home decreased from 1965 to the mid-1990s among women who cook but has since leveled off at approximately 65 minutes per day. Among men, it has steadily increased and was, on average, 45 minutes per day in 2007-2008 for those who cook.[70]

Snacking, defined as the consumption of food outside of the "traditional" three meals—breakfast, lunch, and dinner—is on the rise. This trend is well documented in high-income countries such as the United States,[71,72] and evidence is accumulating that a similar pattern is emerging in middle-income countries such as China, Mexico, and Brazil.[73-76] In the United States, where 97% of children and adults reported snacking in 2006, an average of two or three snacks per day are consumed and the energy density of snacks has increased over time.[71,72] Similarly, data from Brazil and Mexico suggest that two-thirds of individuals report consuming at least one snack during the day and on average people are consuming one or two snacks per day.[73,74] In China, the overall snacking prevalence (60% in children and 35% in adults) is lower, although it is increasing over time.[76]

Physical Activity

Low physical activity is another major aspect of the nutrition transition contributing to energy imbalance and obesity. Global data from 2004 indicated 3.2 million deaths could be attributed to physical inactivity, with the majority (50%) of deaths occurring in middle-income countries.[77]

The World Health Organization recommends that adults aged 18-64 should do 150 minutes of moderate-intensity physical activity every week.[78] Adequate physical activity can mitigate the risk of heart disease, diabetes, and some cancers,[77] all of which are also considered diet-related noncommunicable diseases. In 2012, a cross-sectional analysis of 122 countries found that at least 30% of adults and 80% of adolescents are not meeting physical activity recommendations.[79]

Unfortunately, data on long-term trends in physical activity are limited because a standardized physical activity measurement instrument was not adopted until the late 1990s.[79] What data are available (in China, the United States, the United Kingdom, Brazil, and India) indicate that the decrease in total physical activity is largely due to significant declines in occupation and domestic physical activity rather than transportation or leisure physical activity.[80] In fact, China, the United States, the United Kingdom, and Brazil are experiencing slight increases in leisure physical activity, but this increase is not enough to offset large declines in the other physical activity domains.[80]

Related to this, in all of these countries, sedentary time is increasing.[80] This is particularly worrisome because sedentary time, independent of physical activity, is associated with weight gain and obesity.[81]

Drivers of the Nutrition Transition
Economic Development

Global per capita income is projected to rise 2% a year worldwide, with even greater increases seen in low- and middle-income countries.[39] Economic development, both personal and countrywide, allows for greater interaction with technology that can reduce physical activity and increase caloric intake. At the country level, increased economic development allows for citizens to have increased access to marketing and processed food through technology.[37] Results from an analysis that included 100 countries found that body mass index (BMI) was positively associated with rising national income particularly in low- and middle-income countries, but for higher income countries the association is not as strong.[82]

Gross national product (GNP) has been identified as a modifier of the effect of household income on overweight and obesity. For countries with a per capita GNP greater than US$2,500, people with lower socioeconomic status are more likely to be overweight or obese.[83] For countries with a per capita GNP less than US$2,500 (all country GNP values deflated to 2001), overweight and obesity are associated with higher socioeconomic status.[83] These results indicate that early in economic growth, countries may still be struggling with food insecurity and undernutrition, therefore overweight is associated with the ability to purchase food. As a country becomes wealthier, food insecurity decreases but healthy food options remain prohibitively expensive for people of lower socioeconomic status. Thus, these individuals are at increased risk of over-nutrition in these contexts.

Economic development is closely linked with both rising household income and industrialization. Typically, as countries industrialize, occupations shift from agriculture to manufacturing or service sectors.[36] This has important implications in terms of increasing household income and purchasing power. Rising household income increases access to transnational food products such as sugar-sweetened beverages, fast food, and processed foods. For example, a recent analysis found that in 79 of 82 countries analyzed from

1990 to 2016 there was an increase in affordability of sugar-sweetened beverages due to rapid increases in household income.[84]

This increase in purchasing power also enables the purchase of technology to reduce time spent on household chores such as clothes washing and food preparation. Increased wealth is further associated with increased use of technology such as TV and video games during leisure time in lieu of more active leisure activities such as outdoor recreation, active play for children, and domestic activities.[36,37,39]

Urbanization

According to the United Nation's 2014 World Urbanization Prospects Report, 54% of the world's population now lives in an urban setting. In 2050, it is predicted that two-thirds of the population will live in an urban setting.[24] Urbanization can promote obesity through changes in the built environment, which facilitate a more sedentary lifestyle, less laborious employment opportunities, availability of food options—particularly ready-made foods—and increased interaction with marketing for transnational food products.[38,39]

Increased urbanization in a country can also result in changes in a country's food system, with less land and labor devoted to the agricultural sector. This can limit the types of foods available locally, particularly if government policies promote cash crop production (e.g., sugar cane, maize, palm oil, and animal-based foods) in order to promote economic development.[39] These policies result in the increased accessibility in terms of price and abundance for cash crops, while other crops such as fruits and vegetables remain costly to produce and consume.[38]

Urbanization increases access to health facilities and education, which are associated with decreased risk of obesity in high-income countries. Unfortunately, many countries moving up the economic ladder are experiencing rapid urbanization, but health care and education infrastructure are not keeping pace. Unsustainable urban development can result in increased economic inequality, pollution, and crime, all of which may further reduce physical activity, particularly leisure activity.[24] Urbanization is also associated with decreased sleep time and increased stress, both of which are positively associated with overweight and obesity.[39] On the other hand, in higher income countries such as the United States, living in an urban area may decrease the risk of obesity because people in urban areas may be more physically active, have greater access to healthy food choices, higher socioeconomic status, and have better access to health care.[85-88]

Globalization

The World Health Organization defines **globalization** as "the increased interconnectedness and interdependence of peoples and countries," which is associated with movement of goods, services, and ideas across international borders.[89] Foreign direct investment facilitated by liberal global trade agreements have facilitated greater access to a variety of foods and have allowed transnational corporations to expand into developing markets.[39,90] Low- and middle-income countries that enter free trade agreements with the United States have a 63% higher level of sugar-sweetened beverage consumption per capita than countries who have not entered such agreements, adjusting for GDP, urbanization, and other macroeconomic factors.[91] For example, in 2007 Vietnam joined the World Trade Organization, which resulted in the allowance of significantly greater foreign direct investment from transnational corporations. Sales of sugar-sweetened beverages rose significantly faster compared to the Philippines, where these restrictions were still in place.[92]

Worldwide, there is an increasing number of supermarkets—typically owned by transnational or regional companies that displace local vendors of fresh food.[39] The expansion of supermarkets into low- and middle-income countries has been driven by foreign direct investment from transnational corporations and increased household income due to economic growth.[93] While supermarkets can increase dietary diversity by increasing access to a wider variety of foods, supermarkets can also increase access to cheap processed foods and sugary sweets and beverages.[94] Since 2000 in China, all villages included in a nationally represented survey had a supermarket,[54] and sales of processed foods via supermarkets increased from 20% in 1999 to over 60% in 2013.[95] Similarly, in Thailand, 85% of participants from a nationally representative survey in 2009 had access to a supermarket, and frequent shopping at supermarkets and convenience stores was associated with consumption of sugar-sweetened beverages, snack foods, processed meats, Western-style bakery items, instant foods, and deep-fried foods.[96] These findings are consistent across the globe; in Latin America, the percentage of food purchased in supermarkets increased from 15% to 60% between 1990 and 2000.[97]

These changes in food purchasing patterns have important implications for health. For example, in Kenya, after controlling for socioeconomic status, purchasing food at a supermarket was positively associated with higher BMI and increased risk of metabolic syndrome.[98,99] These and other consequences of the nutrition transition are explored further in the next section.

Consequences of the Nutrition Transition: Obesity and the Double Burden

The most obvious consequence of the nutrition transition is overweight and obesity. In 2014, nearly 2 billion adults were classified as overweight and over 600 million adults were classified as obese.[100] Overweight and obesity are risk factors for many chronic diseases such as diabetes, cardiovascular diseases, and some cancers, which put significant strain on health systems, decrease quality of life, reduce productivity, and result in significant economic losses—both at the individual and country level.[39]

The increase in these noncommunicable diseases is known as the epidemiologic transition. First described in 1971 by Omran, the epidemiologic transition is a shift away from infectious diseases and nutrient deficiencies, which typically affect younger members of the population, toward chronic diseases such as cardiovascular disease, mental health disorders, and cancers, which typically affect older members of the population.[101] As low- and middle-income countries rapidly progress through the epidemiologic transition, there exists a period during which substantial burdens of both over- and undernutrition coexist. This is known as the double burden of malnutrition and can occur within a community, household, or even within an individual.

At the community level, increasing rates of diet-related noncommunicable diseases may occur while a large percentage of individuals still suffer from diseases related to undernutrition. At the household level, individuals within a household may be experiencing the effects of over- and undernutrition simultaneously. Typically, this presents as a child under 5 years of age who is stunted while the mother is overweight or obese. Finally, at the individual level, an individual can be overweight or obese while suffering from micronutrient deficiencies or in the case of children, a child can be overweight yet stunted.[102]

In many low-income countries, particularly in sub-Saharan Africa and South Asia, the burden of undernutrition is still quite large. While stunting rates have decreased globally, in 2016, over 130 million children were considered to be stunted, with 40% of stunted children living in South Asia.[100] The double burden of malnutrition is also occurring in countries such as Tanzania, where undernutrition is still perceived to be the primary nutrition concern. Unpublished data from a rural district found that in 2017 nearly 35% of women of reproductive age were either overweight or obese. Another study in rural Tanzania found that increased BMI was positively correlated with dietary patterns dominated by the consumption of bread and cakes, a dietary pattern typically seen amongst wealthier individuals.[103] These two studies indicate that the nutrition transition is taking place in rural areas of countries where undernutrition remains a significant public health problem.

The Nutrition Transition and Climate Change

The nutrition transition and climate change share the underlying drivers of economic development, industrialization, and globalization. However, until recently,[104-107] the links between these two global challenges were not explicitly evaluated. The impact of our food system on the environment is indisputable: agriculture alone accounts for nearly one-fifth of all greenhouse gas emissions, and livestock production in particular accounts for nearly

80% of these emissions.[108] As discussed earlier in this chapter, as the nutrition transition progresses, demand for animal-based foods increases, and thus the greenhouse gas emissions from our food system are likely to increase.[104] Given that we live in a globalized world, changes in food consumption in one country may drive environmental impacts of food production in other countries; for example, increased demand for pig meat in China has been linked to increasing soya production in Brazil (for animal feed).[106]

Greenhouse gas emissions are not the only environmental impact of our food system. Intensive water and land use, biodiversity loss, and excessive nutrient (e.g., nitrogen) runoff are also important impacts of the nutrition transition. With respect to water use, changes in supply over the past 10 years of cow meat in Brazil, pig meat in China, and cereals in China and India were associated with the greatest water requirements of all supply changes evaluated for these three countries.[106] The increase in vegetable oil consumption, particularly in India and Brazil, was associated with the greatest increase in land use.[106] Going back to greenhouse gases, the increased supply of cow meat and milk in Brazil and cereals in India were associated with the greatest emissions.[106] Thus, the impacts of dietary changes resulting from the nutrition transition are numerous.

Luckily, there are many win–win interventions that would mitigate climate change while also promoting health.[109] For example, reducing consumption of meat would drastically reduce greenhouse gas emissions, while also preventing many diet-related noncommunicable diseases. Similarly, promoting active transportation, especially in urban environments, would reduce greenhouse gas emissions from vehicles while also increasing physical activity. Thus, emphasizing the environmental co-benefits of diet and physical activity interventions may be one more way to gain government support for policies and regulations addressing the nutrition transition.

Conclusion

The nutrition transition is a theory describing how changes in diet and physical activity are affecting health outcomes worldwide and within countries. Key aspects of the transition include a shift away from traditional foods high in fiber to "Westernized" foods high in fat, sugar, and salt, and low in fiber and essential nutrients. In addition to changes in the types of foods and beverages consumed, the source of food is becoming more global, foods are undergoing more processing and packaging, and they are being consumed outside of the home and outside typical meal times. These phenomena have been described in detail in the Americas, especially the United States, Mexico, and Brazil, and in India, China, and South Africa.

There are major gaps in our understanding of the specific characteristics and effects of this transition, especially in low-income and lower-middle-income countries in Asia and sub-Saharan Africa. Nonetheless, to date, few countries have escaped the ill effects of this transition, namely overweight and obesity.[110] One exception may be South Korea, where fat intake has remained low, and fruit and vegetable intakes have increased greatly.[111] Indeed, South Korea is poised to be the first country to achieve an average female life expectancy greater than 90 years by 2030.[112]

Many challenges remain in studying the nutrition transition and should be kept in mind as policy makers, public health professionals, and researchers move forward. Nationally representative food consumption data are limited, particularly in low- and middle-income countries. Surveillance is a critical component for monitoring the nutrition transition and evaluating policies or regulations. A great example of this is Mexico's tax on nonessential energy-dense foods and sugar-sweetened beverages. The availability of longitudinal national household purchasing data enabled researchers to determine that purchases of both of these food groups significantly declined in the first year after the implementation of the tax.[113,114] While the need for a standardized instrument to monitor the nutrition transition, particularly individual-level intake of ultra-processed foods both inside and outside the home, is recognized,[115] such an instrument does not currently exist.

If we are to address the triple threat of undernutrition, overweight and obesity, and climate change, multisectoral actions to improve the healthfulness of our global food system are urgently needed. Dietary change is complex, especially in settings where over- and undernutrition coexist, and the shift from achieving nutritional adequacy to excessive consumption is occurring rapidly in low- and middle-income countries. Efforts to maintain healthy aspects of traditional diets should be strengthened and policies put in place to encourage and enable widespread diversification of diets with an emphasis on whole grains, vegetables, fruits, beans and legumes, and nuts and seeds.

Review Questions

1. Similar to Brazil and India, the United States adopted food-based dietary guidelines in 2015. In fact, according to the Food and Agriculture Organization, over 100 countries worldwide have adopted context-specific food-based dietary guidelines. However, most of these countries are stuck in stage 4 (Degenerative Disease) of the nutrition transition. How might countries implement these guidelines to have a greater impact on diets and the food system?

2. Most countries in sub-Saharan Africa are in the early stages of the nutrition transition. What are some steps that policy makers and public health professionals can take now to prevent the adverse consequences of the "Westernization" of diets observed in other parts of the world? How might these actions impact persistent undernutrition in these settings?

3. In this chapter, you learned about the impact of the nutrition transition on climate change. Conversely, climate change will influence crop production patterns around the world. How might this scenario lead to a "stage 6" of the nutrition transition? Describe the identifying characteristics of this new stage.

4. The Minimum Dietary Diversity for Women (MDD-W) was developed by the Food and Agriculture Organization as a measure of diet quality and micronutrient adequacy. It includes 10 food groups: (1) grains, white roots and tubers, and plantains; (2) pulses (beans, peas and lentils); (3) nuts and seeds; (4) dairy; (5) meat, poultry, and fish; (6) eggs; (7) dark-green leafy vegetables; (8) other vitamin A-rich fruits and vegetables; (9) other vegetables; and (10) other fruits. Scores are calculated by adding up the number of food groups consumed over a specified time period, with a higher score indicating a higher-quality diet. What are the limitations of adopting this tool for national diet surveillance in low- and middle-income countries? What food groups would you add or remove from this tool, if any, to improve our understanding of the nutrition transition in these settings?

5. There is currently no standardized metric for classifying countries according to their stage in the nutrition transition, thus making it difficult for governments to prioritize this issue over other pressing issues. Imagine that you are tasked with creating such a metric for the World Health Organization. What indicators would you include and why?

References

1. Onis, Mercedes De, and Tim Lobstein. 2010. "Defining Obesity Risk Status in the General Childhood Population: Which Cut-Offs Should We Use?" *International Journal of Pediatric Obesity* 5 (6): 458-60. https://doi.org/10.3109/17477161003615583.

2. "Population 2017." 2018. *World Development Indicators Database*. Washington, DC: World Bank. http://databank.worldbank.org/data/download/POP.pdf.

3. "Gross Domestic Product 2017." 2018. *World Development Indicators Database*. Washington, DC: World Bank. http://databank.worldbank.org/data/download /GDP.pdf.

4. Dauvergne, Peter, and Déborah B. L. Farias. 2012. "The Rise of Brazil as a Global Development Power." *Third World Quarterly* 33 (5): 903-17. https://doi.org/10 .1080/01436597.2012.674704.

5. "Urban Population (% of Total): Brazil." 2017. Washington, DC: World Bank. https://data.worldbank.org/indicator/SP.URB.TOTL.IN.ZS?locations=BR.

6. "GINI Index (World Bank Estimate): Brazil." 2017. Washington, DC: World Bank. https://data.worldbank.org/indicator/SI.POV.GINI.

7. Tollefson, Jeff. 2010. "The Global Farm: With Its Plentiful Sun, Water and Land, Brazil Is Quickly Surpassing Other Countries in Food Production and Exports. But Can It Continue to Make Agricultural Gains without Destroying the Amazon? Jeff Tollefson Reports from Brazil." *Nature* 466 (7306): 554-57.

8. Pfaff, Alexander, and Robert Walker. 2010. "Regional Interdependence and Forest 'Transitions': Substitute Deforestation Limits the Relevance of Local Reversals." *Land Use Policy* 27 (2): 119-29.

9. Schmidt, Maria Inês, Bruce Bartholow Duncan, Gulnar Azevedo e Silva, Ana Maria Menezes, Carlos Augusto Monteiro, Sandhi Maria Barreto, Dora Chor, and Paulo Rossi Menezes. 2011. "Chronic Non-Communicable Diseases in Brazil: Burden and Current Challenges." *The Lancet* 377 (9781): 1949-61. https://doi.org/10 .1016/s0140-6736(11)60135-9.

10. Levy, Renata Bertazzi, Rafael Moreira Claro, and Carlos Augusto Monteiro. 2009. "Sugar and Total Energy Content of Household Food Purchases in Brazil." *Public Health Nutrition* 12 (11): 2084. https://doi.org/10.1017/S1368980009005588.

11. Carvalho, Aline Martins de, Chester Luiz Galvão César, Regina Mara Fisberg, and Dirce Maria Marchioni. 2014. "Meat Consumption in Sao Paulo—Brazil: Trend in the Last Decade." Edited by Suminori Akiba. *PLoS One* 9 (5): e96667. https://doi.org/10.1371/journal.pone.0096667.

12. Louzada, Maria Laura da Costa, Larissa Galastri Baraldi, Euridice Martinez Steele, Ana Paula Bortoletto Martins, Daniela Silva Canella, Jean-Claude Moubarac, Renata Bertazzi Levy, et al. 2015. "Consumption of Ultra-Processed Foods and Obesity in Brazilian Adolescents and Adults." *Preventive Medicine* 81 (December): 9-15. https://doi.org/10.1016/j.ypmed.2015.07.018.

13. Pereira, Rosangela A., Amanda M. Souza, Kiyah J. Duffey, Rosely Sichieri, and Barry M. Popkin. 2015. "Beverage Consumption in Brazil: Results from the First National Dietary Survey." *Public Health Nutrition* 18 (07): 1164-72. https://doi.org/10.1017/S1368980014001657.

14. Conde, Wolney Lisboa, and Carlos Augusto Monteiro. 2014. "Nutrition Transition and Double Burden of Undernutrition and Excess of Weight in Brazil." *The American Journal of Clinical Nutrition* 100 (6): 1617S-22S. https://doi.org/10.3945/ajcn.114.084764.

15. Rtveladze, Ketevan, Tim Marsh, Laura Webber, Fanny Kilpi, David Levy, Wolney Conde, Klim McPherson, et al. 2013. "Health and Economic Burden of Obesity in Brazil." Edited by Bruno Caramelli. *PLoS ONE* 8 (7): e68785. https://doi.org/10.1371/journal.pone.0068785.

16. Monteiro, Carlos A., Wolney L. Conde, and Barry M. Popkin. 2007. "Income-Specific Trends in Obesity in Brazil: 1975-2003." *American Journal of Public Health* 97 (10): 1808-12. https://doi.org/10.2105/ajph.2006.099630.

17. Jaime, P. C., A. C. F. da Silva, P. C. Gentil, Rafael Moreira Claro, and Carlos Augusto Monteiro. 2013. "Brazilian Obesity Prevention and Control Initiatives." *Obesity Reviews* 14 (November): 88-95. https://doi.org/10.1111/obr.12101.

18. "Strategic Action Plan to Tackle Noncommunicable Diseases (NCD) in Brazil 2011-2022." 2011. Brasília: Brazil Ministry of Health, Health Surveillance Secretariat, Health Situation Analysis Department.

19. "Dietary Guidelines for the Brazilian Population." 2015. Brasilia: Brazil Ministry of Health. http://bvsms.saude.gov.br/bvs/publicacoes/dietary_guidelines_brazilian_population.pdf.

20. "GDP per Capita (Current US$): India." 2017. Washington, DC: World Bank. https://data.worldbank.org/indicator/NY.GDP.PCAP.CD?locations=IN.

21. Varadharajan, Kiruba S., Tinku Thomas, and Anura V. Kurpad. 2013. "Poverty and the State of Nutrition in India." *Asia Pacific Journal of Clinical Nutrition* 22 (3): 326-39. https://doi.org/10.6133/apjcn.2013.22.3.19.

22. "GDP per Capita (Current US$): Brazil." 2017. Washington, DC: World Bank. https://data.worldbank.org/indicator/NY.GDP.PCAP.CD?locations=BR.

23. "Urban Population (% of Total): India." 2017. Washington, DC: World Bank. https://data.worldbank.org/indicator/SP.URB.TOTL.IN.ZS?locations=IN&view=chart.

24. "World Urbanization Prospects: The 2014 Revision (Highlights) (ST/ESA/ SER.A/352)." 2014. New York: United Nations Department of Economic and Social Affairs.

25. Misra, Anoop, Neha Singhal, Bhattiprolu Sivakumar, Namita Bhagat, Abhishek Jaiswal, and Lokesh Khurana. 2011. "Nutrition Transition in India: Secular Trends in Dietary Intake and Their Relationship to Diet-Related Non-Communicable Diseases." *Journal of Diabetes* 3 (4): 278-92. https://doi.org/10.1111/j .1753-0407.2011.00139.x.

26. Gulati, Seema, and Anoop Misra. 2014. "Sugar Intake, Obesity, and Diabetes in India." *Nutrients* 6 (12): 5955-74. https://doi.org/10.3390/nu6125955.

27. Basu, Sanjay, Sukumar Vellakkal, Sutapa Agrawal, David Stuckler, Barry Popkin, and Shah Ebrahim. 2014. "Averting Obesity and Type 2 Diabetes in India through Sugar-Sweetened Beverage Taxation: An Economic-Epidemiologic Modeling Study." Edited by Tony Blakely. *PLoS Medicine* 11 (1): e1001582. https:// doi.org/10.1371/journal.pmed.1001582.

28. Ng, Marie, Tom Fleming, Margaret Robinson, Blake Thomson, Nicholas Graetz, Christopher Margono, Erin C. Mullany, et al. 2014. "Global, Regional, and National Prevalence of Overweight and Obesity in Children and Adults during 1980-2013: A Systematic Analysis for the Global Burden of Disease Study 2013." *The Lancet* 384 (9945): 766-81. https://doi.org/10.1016/S0140-6736(14)60460-8.

29. Dandona, Lalit, Rakhi Dandona, G. Anil Kumar, D. K. Shukla, Vinod K. Paul, Kalpana Balakrishnan, Dorairaj Prabhakaran, et al. 2017. "Nations within a Nation: Variations in Epidemiological Transition across the States of India, 1990-2016 in the Global Burden of Disease Study." *The Lancet* 390 (10111): 2437-60. https://doi.org/10.1016/S0140-6736(17)32804-0.

30. Pingali, Prabhu. 2015. "Agricultural Policy and Nutrition Outcomes–Getting beyond the Preoccupation with Staple Grains." *Food Security* 7 (3): 583-91.

31. Thow, Anne Marie, Suneetha Kadiyala, Shweta Khandelwal, Purnima Menon, Shauna Downs, and K Srinath Reddy. 2016. "Toward Food Policy for the Dual Burden of Malnutrition." *Food and Nutrition Bulletin* 37 (3): 261-74. https://doi .org/10.1177/0379572116653863.

32. "Dietary Guidelines for Indians: A Manual." 2011. 2nd ed. Hyderabad, India: Indian Council of Medical Research, National Institute of Nutrition.

33. Krishnaswamy, K. 2008. "Developing and Implementing Dietary Guidelines in India." *Asia Pacific Journal of Clinical Nutrition* 17 Suppl 1: 66-69.

34. Downs, Shauna M., Vidhu Gupta, Suparna Ghosh-Jerath, Karen Lock, Anne Marie Thow, and Archna Singh. 2013. "Reformulating Partially Hydrogenated Vegetable Oils to Maximise Health Gains in India: Is It Feasible and Will It Meet Consumer Demand?" *BMC Public Health* 13 (1): 1139. https://doi.org/10.1186/1471 -2458-13-1139.

35. Drewnowski, Adam, and Barry M. Popkin. 1997. "The Nutrition Transition: New Trends in the Global Diet." *Nutrition Reviews* 55 (2): 31-43. https://www.ncbi .nlm.nih.gov/pubmed/9155216.

36. Popkin, Barry M. 2001. "The Nutrition Transition and Obesity in the Developing World." *Journal of Nutrition* 131 (3): 871S-873S. https://www.ncbi.nlm .nih.gov/pubmed/11238777.

37. Popkin, Barry M. 2006. "Global Nutrition Dynamics: The World Is Shifting Rapidly toward a Diet Linked with Noncommunicable Diseases." *American Journal of Clinical Nutrition* 84 (2): 289-98. https://www.ncbi.nlm.nih.gov/pubmed/16895874.

38. Popkin, Barry M. 2015. "Nutrition Transition and the Global Diabetes Epidemic." *Current Diabetes Reports* 15 (9): 64. https://doi.org/10.1007/s11892-015-0631-4.

39. Malik, Vasanti S., Walter C. Willett, and Frank B. Hu. 2013. "Global Obesity: Trends, Risk Factors and Policy Implications." *Nature Reviews Endocrinology* 9 (1): 13-27. https://doi.org/10.1038/nrendo.2012.199.

40. Popkin, Barry M. 1993. "Nutritional Patterns and Transitions." *Population and Development Review* 19 (1): 138-57.

41. Nielsen, Samara Joy, Anna Maria Siega-Riz, and Barry M. Popkin. 2002. "Trends in Energy Intake in US between 1977 and 1996: Similar Shifts Seen across Age Groups." *Obesity Research* 10 (5): 370-78. https://doi.org/10.1038/oby.2002.51.

42. Ford, Earl S., and William H. Dietz. 2013. "Modeling Dietary Patterns to Assess Sodium Recommendations for Nutrient Adequacy." *The American Journal of Clinical Nutrition* 97 (4): 848-53. https://doi.org/10.3945/ajcn.112.052662.

43. Albertson, Ann M., Marla Reicks, Nandan Joshi, and Carolyn K Gugger. 2015. "Whole Grain Consumption Trends and Associations with Body Weight Measures in the United States: Results from the Cross Sectional National Health and Nutrition Examination Survey 2001-2012." *Nutrition Journal* 15 (1): 8. https://doi.org/10.1186/s12937-016-0126-4.

44. Kit, Brian K., Tala H. I. Fakhouri, Sohyun Park, Samara Joy Nielsen, and Cynthia L. Ogden. 2013. "Trends in Sugar-Sweetened Beverage Consumption among Youth and Adults in the United States: 1999-2010." *The American Journal of Clinical Nutrition* 98 (1): 180-88. https://doi.org/10.3945/ajcn.112.057943.

45. Popkin, Barry M., and Corinna Hawkes. 2016. "Sweetening of the Global Diet, Particularly Beverages: Patterns, Trends, and Policy Responses." *The Lancet Diabetes & Endocrinology* 4 (2): 174-86. https://doi.org/10.1016/s2213-8587(15)00419-2.

46. Delgado, Christopher L. 2003. "Rising Consumption of Meat and Milk in Developing Countries Has Created a New Food Revolution." *Journal of Nutrition* 133 (11 Suppl 2): 3907S-3910S. https://www.ncbi.nlm.nih.gov/pubmed/14672289.

47. Monteiro, Carlos A. 2009. "Nutrition and Health. The Issue Is Not Food, nor Nutrients, so Much as Processing." *Public Health Nutrition* 12 (5): 729. https://doi.org/10.1017/S1368980009005291.

48. Poti, Jennifer M., Michelle A. Mendez, Shu Wen Ng, and Barry M. Popkin. 2015. "Is the Degree of Food Processing and Convenience Linked with the Nutritional Quality of Foods Purchased by US Households?" *The American Journal of Clinical Nutrition* 101 (6): 1251-62. https://doi.org/10.3945/ajcn.114.100925.

49. Martínez Steele, Eurídice, Larissa Galastri Baraldi, Maria Laura da Costa Louzada, Jean-Claude Moubarac, Dariush Mozaffarian, and Carlos Augusto Monteiro. 2016. "Ultra-Processed Foods and Added Sugars in the US Diet: Evidence from a Nationally Representative Cross-Sectional Study." *BMJ Open* 6 (3): e009892. https://doi.org/10.1136/bmjopen-2015-009892.

50. Monteiro, Carlos A., J. C. Moubarac, Geoffrey Cannon, Shu Wen Ng, and Barry Popkin. 2013. "Ultra-processed Products Are Becoming Dominant in the Global Food System." *Obesity Reviews* 14 (S2): 21-28.

51. Juul, Filippa, and Erik Hemmingsson. 2015. "Trends in Consumption of Ultra-Processed Foods and Obesity in Sweden between 1960 and 2010." *Public Health Nutrition* 18 (17): 3096-107.

52. Monteiro, Carlos Augusto, Jean-Claude Moubarac, Renata Bertazzi Levy, Daniela Silva Canella, Maria Laura da Costa Louzada, and Geoffrey Cannon. 2018. "Household Availability of Ultra-Processed Foods and Obesity in Nineteen European Countries." *Public Health Nutrition* 21 (1): 18-26. https://doi.org/10.1017/S1368980017001379.

53. Stuckler, David, and Marion Nestle. 2012. "Big Food, Food Systems, and Global Health." *PLoS Medicine* 9 (6): e1001242. https://doi.org/10.1371/journal.pmed.1001242.

54. Popkin, Barry M. 2014. "Nutrition, Agriculture and the Global Food System in Low and Middle Income Countries." *Food Policy* 47 (August): 91-96. https://doi.org/10.1016/j.foodpol.2014.05.001.

55. Canella, Daniela Silva, Renata Bertazzi Levy, A. P. Martins, Rafael Moreira Claro, Jean-Claude Moubarac, Larissa Galastri Baraldi, Geoffrey Cannon, et al. 2014. "Ultra-Processed Food Products and Obesity in Brazilian Households (2008-2009)." *PLoS One* 9 (3): e92752.

56. Martins, Ana Paula Bortoletto, Renata Bertazzi Levy, Rafael Moreira Claro, Jean Claude Moubarac, and Carlos Augusto Monteiro. 2013. "Increased Contribution of Ultra-Processed Food Products in the Brazilian Diet (1987-2009)." *Revista de Saude Publica* 47 (4): 656-65.

57. Zhou, Yijing, Shufa Du, Chang Su, Bing Zhang, Huijun Wang, and Barry M. Popkin. 2015. "The Food Retail Revolution in China and Its Association with Diet and Health." *Food Policy* 55 (August): 92-100. https://doi.org/10.1016/j.foodpol.2015.07.001.

58. Tschirley, David L., Jason Snyder, Michael Dolislager, Thomas Reardon, Steven Haggblade, Joseph Goeb, Lulama Traub, et al. 2015. "Africa's Unfolding Diet Transformation: Implications for Agrifood System Employment." *Journal of Agribusiness in Developing and Emerging Economies* 5 (2): 102-36.

59. Liu, Buyun, Hans-Joachim Lehmler, Yangbo Sun, Guifeng Xu, Yuewei Liu, Geng Zong, Qi Sun, et al. 2017. "Bisphenol A Substitutes and Obesity in US Adults: Analysis of a Population-Based, Cross-Sectional Study." *The Lancet Planetary Health* 1 (3): e114-22. https://doi.org/10.1016/S2542-5196(17)30049-9.

60. Corrales, Jone, Lauren A. Kristofco, W. Baylor Steele, Brian S. Yates, Christopher S. Breed, E. Spencer Williams, and Bryan W. Brooks. 2015. "Global Assessment of Bisphenol A in the Environment." *Dose Response* 13 (3): 155932581559830. https://doi.org/10.1177/1559325815598308.

61. Seltenrich, Nate. 2015. "A Hard Nut to Crack: Reducing Chemical Migration in Food-Contact Materials." *Environmental Health Perspectives* 123 (7): A174-79. https://doi.org/10.1289/ehp.123-A174.

62. Rancière, Fanny, Jasmine G. Lyons, Venurs H. Y. Loh, Jérémie Botton, Tamara Galloway, Tiange Wang, Jonathan E. Shaw, et al. 2015. "Bisphenol A and

the Risk of Cardiometabolic Disorders: A Systematic Review with Meta-Analysis of the Epidemiological Evidence." *Environmental Health* 14 (1): 46. https://doi.org/10.1186/s12940-015-0036-5.

63. Attina, Teresa M., Russ Hauser, Sheela Sathyanarayana, Patricia A. Hunt, Jean-Pierre Bourguignon, John Peterson Myers, Joseph DiGangi, et al. 2016. "Exposure to Endocrine-Disrupting Chemicals in the USA: A Population-Based Disease Burden and Cost Analysis." *The Lancet Diabetes & Endocrinology* 4 (12): 996-1003. https://doi.org/10.1016/S2213-8587(16)30275-3.

64. Trasande, Leonardo. 2014. "Further Limiting Bisphenol A In Food Uses Could Provide Health and Economic Benefits." *Health Affairs* 33 (2): 316-23. https://doi.org/10.1377/hlthaff.2013.0686.

65. James-Todd, Tamarra, Richard Stahlhut, John D. Meeker, Sheena-Gail Powell, Russ Hauser, Tianyi Huang, and Janet Rich-Edwards. 2012. "Urinary Phthalate Metabolite Concentrations and Diabetes among Women in the National Health and Nutrition Examination Survey (NHANES) 2001-2008." *Environmental Health Perspectives* 120 (9): 1307-13. https://doi.org/10.1289/ehp.1104717.

66. Trasande, Leonardo, Adam J. Spanier, Sheela Sathyanarayana, Teresa M. Attina, and Jan Blustein. 2013. "Urinary Phthalates and Increased Insulin Resistance in Adolescents." *Pediatrics* 132 (3): e646-55.

67. Lachat, C., E. Nago, R. Verstraeten, D. Roberfroid, J. Van Camp, and P. Kolsteren. 2012. "Eating Out of Home and Its Association with Dietary Intake: A Systematic Review of the Evidence." *Obesity Reviews* 13 (4): 329-46. https://doi.org/10.1111/j.1467-789X.2011.00953.x.

68. Bezerra, Ilana N., Cintia Curioni, and Rosely Sichieri. 2012. "Association between Eating Out of Home and Body Weight." *Nutrition Reviews* 70 (2): 65-79. https://doi.org/10.1111/j.1753-4887.2011.00459.x.

69. Wang, Zhihong, Fengying Zhai, Shufa Du, and Barry Popkin. 2008. "Dynamic Shifts in Chinese Eating Behaviors." *Asia Pacific Journal of Clinical Nutrition* 17 (1): 123-30. https://www.ncbi.nlm.nih.gov/pubmed/18364337.

70. Smith, Lindsey P., Shu Wen Ng, and Barry M. Popkin. 2013. "Trends in US Home Food Preparation and Consumption: Analysis of National Nutrition Surveys and Time Use Studies from 1965-1966 to 2007-2008." *Nutrition Journal* 12 (1): 45.

71. Piernas, Carmen, and Barry M. Popkin. 2010. "Trends in Snacking Among US Children." *Health Affairs* 29 (3): 398-404. https://doi.org/10.1377/hlthaff.2009.0666.

72. Piernans, Carmen, and Barry M. Popkin. 2010. "Snacking Increased among US Adults between 1977 and 2006." *The Journal of Nutrition* 140 (2): 325-32. https://doi.org/10.3945/jn.109.112763.

73. Duffey, Kiyah J., Rosangela A. Pereira, and Barry M. Popkin. 2013. "Prevalence and Energy Intake from Snacking in Brazil: Analysis of the First Nationwide Individual Survey." *European Journal of Clinical Nutrition* 67 (8): 868-74. https://doi.org/10.1038/ejcn.2013.60.

74. Duffey, Kiyah J., Juan A. Rivera, and Barry M. Popkin. 2014. "Snacking Is Prevalent in Mexico." *The Journal of Nutrition* 144 (11): 1843-49. https://doi.org/10.3945/jn.114.198192.

75. Adair, Linda S., and Barry M. Popkin. 2005. "Are Child Eating Patterns Being Transformed Globally?" *Obesity Research* 13 (7): 1281-99. https://doi.org/10.1038/oby.2005.153.

76. Wang, Zhihong, Fengying Zhai, Bing Zhang, and Barry M. Popkin. 2012. "Trends in Chinese Snacking Behaviors and Patterns and the Social-Demographic Role between 1991 and 2009." *Asia Pacific Journal of Clinical Nutrition* 21 (2): 253-62. https://www.ncbi.nlm.nih.gov/pubmed/22507613.

77. "Global Health Risks: Mortality and Burden of Disease Attributable to Selected Major Risks." 2009. Geneva, Switzerland: World Health Organization.

78. "Global Recommendations on Physical Activity for Health." 2010. Geneva, Switzerland: World Health Organization. http://apps.who.int/iris/bitstream/10665/44399/1/9789241599979_eng.pdf.

79. Hallal, Pedro C., Lars Bo Andersen, Fiona C. Bull, Regina Guthold, William Haskell, and Ulf Ekelund. 2012. "Global Physical Activity Levels: Surveillance Progress, Pitfalls, and Prospects." *The Lancet* 380 (9838): 247-57. https://doi.org/10.1016/s0140-6736(12)60646-1.

80. Ng, S. W., and Barry M. Popkin. 2012. "Time Use and Physical Activity: A Shift Away from Movement across the Globe." *Obesity Reviews* 13 (8): 659-80. https://doi.org/10.1111/j.1467-789X.2011.00982.x.

81. Golubic, R., K. Wijndaele, S. J. Sharp, R. K. Simmons, S. J. Griffin, N. J. Wareham, U. Ekelund, and S. Brage. 2015. "Physical Activity, Sedentary Time and Gain in Overall and Central Body Fat: 7-Year Follow-up of the ProActive Trial Cohort." *International Journal of Obesity* 39 (1): 142-48. https://doi.org/10.1038/ijo.2014.66.

82. Ezzati, Majid, Stephen Vander Hoorn, Carlene M. M. Lawes, Rachel Leach, W. Philip T. James, Alan D. Lopez, Anthony Rodgers, et al. 2005. "Rethinking the 'Diseases of Affluence' Paradigm: Global Patterns of Nutritional Risks in Relation to Economic Development." Edited by Thomas Novotny. *PLoS Medicine* 2 (5): e133. https://doi.org/10.1371/journal.pmed.0020133.

83. Monteiro, Carlos A., Wolney L. Conde, B. Lu, and Barry M. Popkin. 2004. "Obesity and Inequities in Health in the Developing World." *International Journal of Obesity* 28 (9): 1181-86. https://doi.org/10.1038/sj.ijo.0802716.

84. Blecher, Evan, Alex C. Liber, Jeffrey M. Drope, Binh Nguyen, and Michal Stoklosa. 2017. "Global Trends in the Affordability of Sugar-Sweetened Beverages, 1990-2016." *Preventing Chronic Disease* 14 (May): 160406. https://doi.org/10.5888/pcd14.160406.

85. Johnson, James Allen, and Asal Mohamadi Johnson. 2015. "Urban-Rural Differences in Childhood and Adolescent Obesity in the United States: A Systematic Review and Meta-Analysis." *Childhood Obesity* 11 (3): 233-41. https://doi.org/10.1089/chi.2014.0085.

86. Lutfiyya, M. Nawal, Linda F. Chang, and Martin S. Lipsky. 2012. "A Cross-Sectional Study of US Rural Adults' Consumption of Fruits and Vegetables: Do They Consume at Least Five Servings Daily?" *BMC Public Health* 12 (1): 280. https://doi.org/10.1186/1471-2458-12-280.

87. Befort, Christie A., Niaman Nazir, and Michael G. Perri. 2012. "Prevalence of Obesity Among Adults From Rural and Urban Areas of the United States:

Findings From NHANES (2005-2008)." *The Journal of Rural Health* 28 (4): 392-97. https://doi.org/10.1111/j.1748-0361.2012.00411.x.

88. Parks, S. E., R. A. Housemann, and R. C. Brownson. 2003. "Differential Correlates of Physical Activity in Urban and Rural Adults of Various Socioeconomic Backgrounds in the United States." *Journal of Epidemiology and Community Health* 57 (1): 29-35. https://www.ncbi.nlm.nih.gov/pubmed/12490645.

89. "Globalization." n.d. Geneva, Switzerland: World Health Organization. http://www.who.int/topics/globalization/en/.

90. Hawkes, Corinna. 2005. "The Role of Foreign Direct Investment in the Nutrition Transition." *Public Health Nutrition* 8 (4): 357-65. https://www.ncbi.nlm.nih.gov/pubmed/15975180.

91. Stuckler, D., M. McKee, S. Ebrahim, and S. Basu. 2012. "Manufacturing Epidemics: The Role of Global Producers in Increased Consumption of Unhealthy Commodities Including Processed Foods, Alcohol, and Tobacco." *PLoS Med* 9 (6): e1001235. https://doi.org/10.1371/journal.pmed.1001235.

92. Schram, Ashley, Ronald Labonte, Phillip Baker, Sharon Friel, Aaron Reeves, and David Stuckler. 2015. "The Role of Trade and Investment Liberalization in the Sugar-Sweetened Carbonated Beverages Market: A Natural Experiment Contrasting Vietnam and the Philippines." *Globalization and Health* 11 (1): 41. https://doi.org/10.1186/s12992-015-0127-7.

93. Reardon, Thomas, Peter C. Timmer, and Bart Minten. 2012. "Supermarket Revolution in Asia and Emerging Development Strategies to Include Small Farmers." *Proceedings of the National Academy of Sciences* 109 (31): 12332-37. https://doi.org/10.1073/pnas.1003160108.

94. Hawkes, Corinna. 2008. "Dietary Implications of Supermarket Development: A Global Perspective." *Development Policy Review* 26 (6): 35.

95. Baker, Phillip, and Sharon Friel. 2016. "Food Systems Transformations, Ultra-Processed Food Markets and the Nutrition Transition in Asia." *Globalization and Health* 12 (1): 80. https://doi.org/10.1186/s12992-016-0223-3.

96. Kelly, Matthew, Sam-ang Seubsman, Cathy Banwell, Jane Dixon, and Adrian Sleigh. 2014. "Thailand's Food Retail Transition: Supermarket and Fresh Market Effects on Diet Quality and Health." *British Food Journal* 116 (7): 1180-93.

97. Popkin, Barry M., Linda S. Adair, and Shu Wen Ng. 2012. "Global Nutrition Transition and the Pandemic of Obesity in Developing Countries." *Nutrition Reviews* 70 (1): 3-21. https://doi.org/10.1111/j.1753-4887.2011.00456.x.

98. Demmler, Kathrin M., Stephan Klasen, Jonathan M. Nzuma, and Matin Qaim. 2017. "Supermarket Purchase Contributes to Nutrition-Related Non-Communicable Diseases in Urban Kenya." Edited by Bhavani Shankar. *PLoS One* 12 (9): e0185148. https://doi.org/10.1371/journal.pone.0185148.

99. Kimenju, Simon C., Ramona Rischke, Stephan Klasen, and Matin Qaim. 2015. "Do Supermarkets Contribute to the Obesity Pandemic in Developing Countries?" *Public Health Nutrition* 18 (17): 3224-33. https://doi.org/10.1017/S1368980015000919.

100. Hawkes, Corinna, and Jess Fanzo. 2017. "Global Nutrition Report 2017: Nourishing the SDGs." New York: UNICEF.

101. Omran, A. R. 1977. "Epidemiologic Transition in the United States: The Health Factor in Population Change." *Population Bulletin* 32 (2): 1-42. http://www.ncbi.nlm.nih.gov/pubmed/12335110.

102. Tziomis, Emma, and Linda B. Adair. 2014. "Childhood Dual Burden of Under- and Over-Nutrition in Low- and Middle-Income Countries: A Critical Review." *Food Nutrition Bulletin* 35 (2): 13.

103. Keding, Gudrun B., John M. Msuya, Brigitte L. Maass, and Michael B. Krawinkel. 2011. "Dietary Patterns and Nutritional Health of Women: The Nutrition Transition in Rural Tanzania." *Food and Nutrition Bulletin* 32 (3): 218-26. https://doi.org/10.1177/156482651103200306.

104. Aleksandrowicz, Lukasz, Rosemary Green, Edward J. M. Joy, Pete Smith, and Andy Haines. 2016. "The Impacts of Dietary Change on Greenhouse Gas Emissions, Land Use, Water Use, and Health: A Systematic Review." *PLoS One* 11 (11): e0165797.

105. An, R., M. Ji, and S. Zhang. 2018. "Global Warming and Obesity: A Systematic Review." *Obesity Reviews* 19 (2): 150-63. https://doi.org/10.1111/obr.12624.

106. Gill, Margaret, Diana Feliciano, Jennie Macdiarmid, and Pete Smith. 2015. "The Environmental Impact of Nutrition Transition in Three Case Study Countries." *Food Security* 7 (3): 493-504.

107. Tilman, David, and Michael Clark. 2014. "Global Diets Link Environmental Sustainability and Human Health." *Nature* 515 (7528): 518-22. https://doi.org/10.1038/nature13959.

108. McMichael, Anthony J., John W. Powles, Colin D. Butler, and Ricardo Uauy. 2007. "Food, Livestock Production, Energy, Climate Change, and Health." *The Lancet* 370 (9594): 1253-63. https://doi.org/10.1016/s0140-6736(07)61256-2.

109. Bloomberg, Michael R., and Rohit T. Aggarwala. 2008. "Think Locally, Act Globally." *American Journal of Preventive Medicine* 35 (5): 414-23. https://doi.org/10.1016/j.amepre.2008.08.029.

110. Swinburn, Boyd A., Gary Sacks, Kevin D. Hall, Klim McPherson, Diane T. Finegood, Marjory L. Moodie, and Steven L. Gortmaker. 2011. "The Global Obesity Pandemic: Shaped by Global Drivers and Local Environments." *The Lancet* 378 (9793): 804-14. https://doi.org/10.1016/S0140-6736.

111. Lee, Min-June, Barry M. Popkin, and Soowon Kim. 2002. "The Unique Aspects of the Nutrition Transition in South Korea: The Retention of Healthful Elements in Their Traditional Diet." *Public Health Nutrition* 5 (1a): 197-203.

112. Kontis, Vasilis, James E. Bennett, Colin D. Mathers, Guangquan Li, Kyle Foreman, and Majid Ezzati. 2017. "Future Life Expectancy in 35 Industrialised Countries: Projections with a Bayesian Model Ensemble." *The Lancet* 389 (10076): 1323-35.

113. Batis, Carolina, Juan A. Rivera, Barry M. Popkin, and Lindsey Smith Taillie. 2016. "First-Year Evaluation of Mexico's Tax on Nonessential Energy-Dense Foods: An Observational Study." *PLoS Medicine* 13 (7): e1002057.

114. Colchero, M. Arantxa, Barry M. Popkin, Juan A. Rivera, and Shu Wen Ng. 2016. "Beverage Purchases from Stores in Mexico under the Excise Tax on Sugar

Sweetened Beverages: Observational Study." *BMJ* 352 (January): h6704. https://doi
.org/10.1136/bmj.h6704.

115. Walls, Helen L., Deborah Johnston, Jacob Mazalale, and Ephraim W.
Chirwa. 2018. "Why We Are Still Failing to Measure the Nutrition Transition."
BMJ Global Health 3 (1): e000657.

11

A Deeper Look: Stunting

Lora L. Iannotti and Melissa Chapnick

LEARNING OBJECTIVES

- Describe the burden of stunting in terms of prevalence, trends, and disparities across different contexts
- Delineate the determinants of stunting across multiple levels: biological, child, household, and community
- Identify key stakeholders working to improve child growth and development
- Characterize policy, program, and research solutions that have been applied globally for stunting prevention

Case Study: A Vignette from Ecuador

Martha lives with her family in a small, thatched-roof dwelling high in the mountains of Ecuador. Although she is nearly 3 years of age, Martha appears to be only reaching the beginning of toddlerhood; she is stunted in both growth and development. Her family and neighbors in the community of Tingo Pucara come from the indigenous group of Kichwa. Indigenous groups around the world are often marginalized and lack basic services, such as education, health care, and economic inputs, leading to poor health outcomes (figure 11.1). Stunting prevalence among indigenous groups in Ecuador is nearly double the national average.

The Kichwa have strong connections to their land and ecosystems more broadly, as manifest in the entity *Pacha Mama*, Mother Earth in Kichwa. Unfortunately, Tingo Pucara and other Andean communities have experienced the negative effects of drought and encroaching modernization, both contributing to food insecurity and stunting. Martha's diet largely consists of the potatoes grown by her family; sometimes fava beans, quinoa, or rice; and on special occasions eggs or meat. Despite living in this fairly remote part of Ecuador, processed foods and sugary drinks are part of the diet. Martha and many of the children are also chronically affected by respiratory and enteric infections. All of these factors converge to cause stunted growth and development for Martha in an intergenerational cycle, perpetuating the problem in the community for years to come.

The term **stunting** refers to deficits in linear growth, which is often associated with deficits in cognitive and socio-emotional development. Stunting means

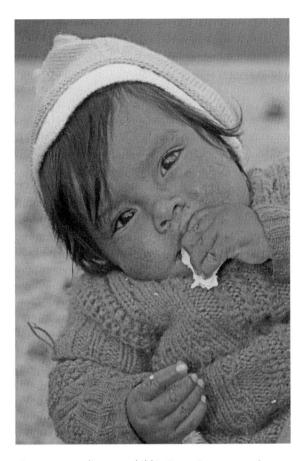

Figure 11.1. Indigenous child in Peru. *Source:* urosr/
Shutterstock.com.

that individuals are not meeting their full growth or developmental potential, which has important implications for health, human development, and economic development. As a result, the first nutrition goal of the World Health Assembly is to reduce stunting by 40% by 2025. However, despite global consensus of the importance of this issue and likely due to the difficulty in moving the needle on the underlying causes of stunting, if current trends continue, this goal will not be met. In this chapter we discuss the prevalence and trends in stunting and its consequences. We then examine the key proximal and distal factors that contribute to stunting, using the UNICEF framework to examine causes at multiple levels. We conclude by examining the policy, programming, and research solutions that have been implemented to date.

Stunting: Definitions and Global Milestones

The World Health Organization (WHO) defines stunting as length/height-for-age z-score (LAZ/HAZ; among infants and children aged 0-24 months, we measure recumbent length, among children older than 24 months, we measure standing height) less than 2 standard deviations below the WHO

Child Growth Standards median. However, stunting can be applied more broadly to refer to children with both stunted linear growth and cognitive development. In this chapter we will refer to these two types of stunting as *growth stunting* and *developmental stunting*, respectively. In the spectrum of malnutrition problems, stunting represents the more chronic form of undernutrition, compared to **underweight** (weight-for-age z-score <-2 standard deviations) and **wasting** (weight-for-height z-score <-2 standard deviations), which are considered acute forms of undernutrition.

Stunting together with underweight, wasting, and other markers such as mid-upper arm circumference (MUAC) or head circumference are classified as anthropometric indicators. **Anthropometry** literally means the measurement of man, and in the field of public health nutrition it has been defined as "measurements of the variations of the physical dimensions and the gross composition of the human body at different age levels and degrees of nutrition."[1] Stunting and other anthropometric markers are often used in low- and middle-income countries (LMIC) to assess nutritional status because collecting height or weight measures in a community setting is low-cost and relatively easy, compared to other methods of assessing nutritional status, such as drawing blood for nutrition biomarkers, bioelectrical impedance for body composition, or imaging for bone growth. Population prevalence of stunting, underweight, and wasting provide important insight into an array of nutrition and public health problems. For example, population prevalence of growth stunting is an indicator of chronically undernourished populations, whereas an increase in the prevalence of wasting often represents an acute cause of malnutrition such as famine.

WHO Child Growth Standards

Introduced in 2006, the WHO Child Growth Standards are the first internationally representative set of growth curves. The standards were based on data collected longitudinally from six different countries in the WHO Multicentre Growth Reference Study from 1997 to 2003. Several observations motivated the global nutrition community to develop the new standards and replace the NCHS 1977/98 charts that had been derived from a population of non-breastfed children in the United States. One key motivation was to test whether children from different ethnicities and regions of the world grow similarly when they experience environments supportive of growth in the absence of key environmental differences such as poverty, sanitation, smoke exposure, or formula exposure. Importantly, growth depends on particular breastfeeding and complementary feeding practices, but it was also important to show that interethnic variability in growth was due to environment and not genetics. Thus, they set out to establish normative standards in which children would be provided optimal growing conditions across all six countries.

The findings from the Multicentre Growth Reference Study affirmed these hypotheses and confirmed that children from different ethnic origins could grow similarly under optimal conditions.[2,3] Findings from this study also demonstrated that exclusive and predominantly breastfed children grew taller and were thinner, in general, compared to non-breastfed children from the NCHS study. The WHO Growth Standards are now widely applied around the world with some exceptions, including the United States and China.

United Nations Decade on Nutrition and World Health Assembly Nutrition Targets

In April 2016, the United Nations General Assembly declared 2016-2025 the UN Decade of Action on Nutrition, with an ambitious goal to end hunger and eradicate malnutrition worldwide.[4] The proclamation affirmed the world's commitment to Sustainable Development Goal #2: *Zero Hunger*. The WHO and the Food and Agriculture Organization (FAO) will lead the effort adhering to the normative Framework for Action established during the Second International Conference on Nutrition (ICN2). The Framework for Action is intended to coordinate and mobilize nutrition champions from around the world to confront the most serious nutrition issues, including stunting. Member States in the World Health Assembly (WHA) have also now established six nutrition targets to be met by 2025 (figure 11.2).[5] First among the goals is the target to reduce stunting by 40% among children less than 5 years of age. These high-level UN policies demonstrate global consensus for the importance and urgency of ending this chronic form of malnutrition. Several other global policies, norms, and standards underlie and guide the overarching decade and targets and will be discussed below.

The Problem
Prevalence, Trends, and Disparities

Growth and developmental stunting exists in most parts of the world, however it is more prevalent in lower- and middle-income countries compared to high-income countries. Recent joint estimates from UNICEF, WHO, and the World Bank indicate that, globally, 154.8 million (22.9%) children under the age of 5 are growth stunted. In absolute numbers, Asia exceeds all regions with 87 million stunted children, followed by Africa (59 million), Latin America and the Caribbean (6 million), and Oceania (0.5 million) (figure 11.3).[6] Trends indicate a decreasing number and percentage of young children stunted globally, down from 198.4 million (32.7%) in 2000. Again, there are important differences across regions such that progress to reduce stunting has been greater in Latin America and the Caribbean (−40%) and Asia (−37%), compared to Africa (−18%) and Oceania (+4%). Africa is the only region where the absolute number of stunted children has increased (figure 11.4).[6]

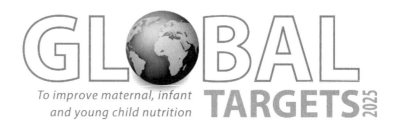

To improve maternal, infant and young child nutrition

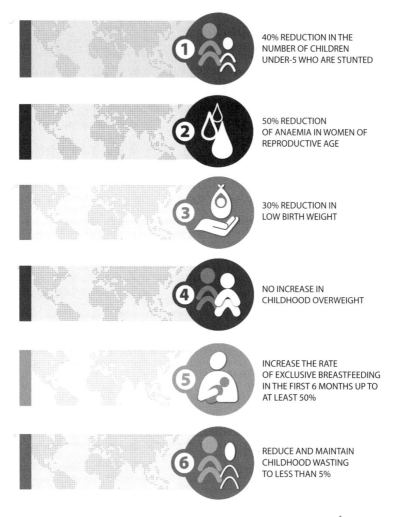

1 40% REDUCTION IN THE NUMBER OF CHILDREN UNDER-5 WHO ARE STUNTED

2 50% REDUCTION OF ANAEMIA IN WOMEN OF REPRODUCTIVE AGE

3 30% REDUCTION IN LOW BIRTH WEIGHT

4 NO INCREASE IN CHILDHOOD OVERWEIGHT

5 INCREASE THE RATE OF EXCLUSIVE BREASTFEEDING IN THE FIRST 6 MONTHS UP TO AT LEAST 50%

6 REDUCE AND MAINTAIN CHILDHOOD WASTING TO LESS THAN 5%

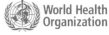

Figure 11.2. Global Nutrition Targets 2025. *Source:* "Global Targets to Improve Maternal, Infant and Young Child Nutrition 2025," Poster A. World Health Organization. http://www.who.int/nutrition/topics/English_Poster_A_Global_Target_2025.pdf?ua=1.

LEVELS AND TRENDS IN CHILD MALNUTRITION

UNICEF / WHO / World Bank Group
Joint Child Malnutrition Estimates

Key findings of the 2017 edition

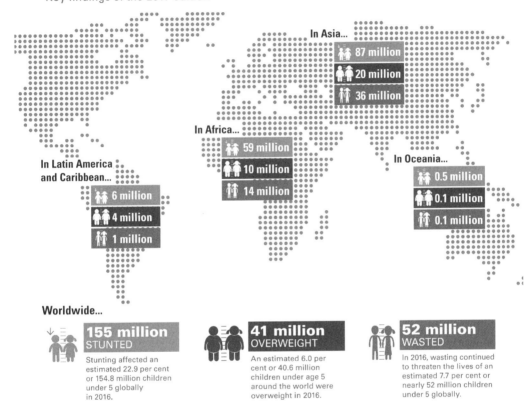

In Asia...
87 million
20 million
36 million

In Africa...
59 million
10 million
14 million

In Latin America and Caribbean...
6 million
4 million
1 million

In Oceania...
0.5 million
0.1 million
0.1 million

Worldwide...

155 million
STUNTED

Stunting affected an estimated 22.9 per cent or 154.8 million children under 5 globally in 2016.

41 million
OVERWEIGHT

An estimated 6.0 per cent or 40.6 million children under age 5 around the world were overweight in 2016.

52 million
WASTED

In 2016, wasting continued to threaten the lives of an estimated 7.7 per cent or nearly 52 million children under 5 globally.

These new estimates supersede former analyses and results published by UNICEF, WHO and the World Bank Group.

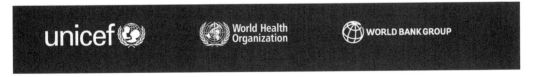

unicef · World Health Organization · WORLD BANK GROUP

Figure 11.3. Joint malnutrition estimates. *Source:* "Joint Child Malnutrition Estimates: Key Findings of the 2017 Edition." UNICEF, WHO, World Bank Group. 2017; p. 1. http://www.who.int/nutgrowthdb/jme_brochoure2017.pdf?ua=1.

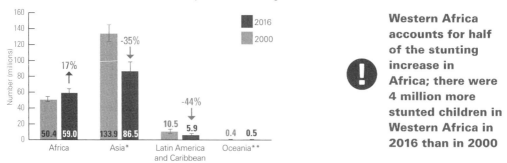

Africa is the only region where the number of stunted children has risen
Number (millions) of stunted children under 5, by United Nations region, 2000 and 2016

Western Africa accounts for half of the stunting increase in Africa; there were 4 million more stunted children in Western Africa in 2016 than in 2000

Figure 11.4. African region stunting. *Source:* "Joint Child Malnutrition Estimates: Key Findings of the 2017 Edition." UNICEF, WHO, World Bank Group. 2017; p. 5. http://www.who.int/nutgrowthdb/jme_brochoure2017.pdf?ua=1.

While global figures tend to focus on regional and national estimates, there are important disparities across different populations within a given country that merit attention. For example, in the indigenous population of Ecuador from the case study above, stunting prevalence is 42.3% compared to the national average of 25.2%.[7] In some Kichwa communities of Cotopaxi Province, stunting prevalence nears 60%.[8] There is well-established evidence that stunting prevalence varies with income and wealth at the global and national levels. The second of the seminal *Lancet* Series on Maternal and Child Nutrition (2013) first highlighted the stark difference in stunting prevalence between LMIC (28%) compared to high-income countries (7.2%).[9] This work additionally documented large disparities based on wealth quintiles within a given country, with stunting prevalence much greater among children in the lower wealth quintiles compared to those in higher wealth quintiles. In some countries there are also differences between boys and girls in terms of stunting prevalence. One meta-analysis of national data from 16 sub-Saharan African countries showed boys were more stunted than girls.[10] Disparities similarly exist by rural and urban residence, maternal education, and other factors that we discuss below. These disparities point to critical stunting determinants to be discussed below and should be considered for appropriate targeting of programming and policy to be most impactful for vulnerable populations.

First 1,000 Days and Beyond

The period from conception to approximately 2 years of life was labeled the **"first 1,000 days,"** in part to leverage the catchy phrase in messaging but as well because it represents a highly vulnerable stage of the life cycle when nutrition insults may have irreparable consequences. Combined data from nationally representative studies in LMIC indicates that linear growth, in-

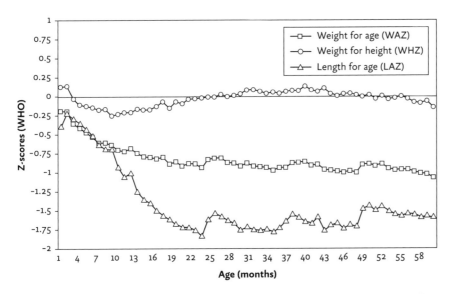

Figure 11.5. Mean anthropometric z-scores according to age. *Source:* Reproduced with permission from *Pediatrics,* 125 (3), e473–480. Copyright © 2010 by the AAP.

dicated by length-for-age z-score (LAZ), precipitously falters during infancy and is not regained during the first five years of life (figure 11.5).[11] Within the nutrition programming and policy arena, the initial response to this finding was to focus on the periods of exclusive breastfeeding (0–6 months) and complementary feeding (6–24 months). However, more recent analyses have highlighted the importance of maternal nutrition prior to birth, showing that in utero growth faltering, indicated by **small for gestational age (SGA)**, contributes more substantially to overall childhood stunting (20%) than previously thought.[12]

The consequences of stunting, especially in the first 1,000 days of life, have been extensively described and are briefly discussed here. The consequences of stunted growth and development are typically grouped into three categories: (1) health, (2) developmental, and (3) economic.

Health Consequences

Short-term health repercussions include higher risks of mortality and morbidities. A stunted child is at increased risk of dying from infectious diseases, in particular diarrheal disease, acute respiratory infection, and malaria.[13] *The Lancet* series estimated that stunting is an underlying cause for between 14.7% and 17% of childhood deaths among children under 5 years of age.[9] There is a "vicious cycle" in the nutrition-infection relationship. A malnourished child has compromised immunity—both innate (e.g., compromised epithelial barriers) and adaptive immune (e.g., reduced number and function of T cells) systems—to fight infection. In turn, a child with an infection may have reduced appetite, increased **catabolism**, and redirected use of energy and nutrients from growth to fighting the infection. In repeated diarrheal disease particularly, the intestinal villi may be flattened and absorption impaired, a phenomenon sometimes referred to as **environmental enteropathy**.

If the child survives, there are long-term health consequences associated with stunting. Stunting occurring early in life results in reduced adult stature that may carry forward into the next generation. Offspring of women of short stature are at risk for low birth weight and being born SGA.[11,14] Some studies have also shown that mothers who are stunted are at increased risk of perinatal mortality, arising from obstructed labor, asphyxia, and infection.[15,16] Evidence is less clear on the relationship between maternal short stature and in utero growth restriction and chronic disease–related outcomes, such as diabetes or hypertension, though these relationships continue to be explored in the field of developmental origins of disease.[17]

Developmental Consequences

In part because developmental stunting is less well defined, harder to measure, and lacking the precise metric of HAZ <–2, stunted cognitive development is often characterized as an outcome or consequence in association with poor growth. While likely better characterized as a consequence of chronic malnutrition and poverty, deficits in cognitive development co-occur with linear growth stunting. Malnutrition negatively affects development, interacting with poor stimulation, diminished social interaction, and poverty more broadly.

An estimated 250 million young children (43%) in LMIC are at risk of not meeting their developmental potential.[18]

Developmental impairments are evident across all domains and manifest throughout the life span. During childhood, evidence shows stunted growth is associated with reduced cognition, language development, and socioemotional and motor development particularly. Micronutrient deficiencies that result in poor growth are similarly known to influence brain development. These nutrients include zinc, iron, iodine, choline, and vitamin B_{12}, among others.[19] As an example, iron is needed for synthesis of myelin and the neurotransmitter dopamine, playing a crucial role in signaling and processing speed. Iron deficiency has been shown to negatively impact motor and language development. It is widely established that iodine deficiency during pregnancy and early childhood has serious consequences on offspring, resulting in cretinism in the most extreme cases but more pervasively in its mild form of developmental delays. Choline is a less well-known nutrient, participating in vital one carbon pathways and playing important roles in cell membrane integrity in the brain. Importantly, choline is also necessary for synthesis of the neurotransmitter acetylcholine.

Longer-term consequences of early stunted growth and development have also been demonstrated through reduced school performance, psychological functioning in adolescence, and economic productivity.[20-22] However, the more direct implications of stunted development during different phases of the life cycle beyond the first 1,000 days have been somewhat limited. It is known that nutrition affects neuronal performance through all phases, from infancy through aging. In early and mid-childhood, there is ongoing synapse production and pruning while waves of higher cognitive development dependent on nutrition continue through adolescence.[23] Into adulthood, evidence suggests the ongoing importance of nutrients for neuroplasticity, behavior, and antiaging effects.

Economic Consequences

Studies have examined the longer-term consequences of stunting on economic productivity and human capital into adulthood. One analysis using five birth cohort studies from Brazil, Guatemala, India, the Philippines, and South Africa showed a protective effect from higher birth weight, faster linear growth on schooling completed, adult height, and chronic disease risk factors.[22] In Guatemala, nutritional supplementation early in life was shown to improve intellectual functioning.[21]

Causes of Stunting: Proximal to Distal Determinants

The global nutrition community has long drawn from the UNICEF framework to identify multilevel causes of malnutrition (figure 11.6).[24] The framework was first introduced in 1990 in the context of a UNICEF policy review and strategy to address maternal and child nutrition. It was ahead of its time in the application of the public health multidisciplinary approach and in its illustration of "causes of causes." The enduring use of the framework also suggests universality of the causes of malnutrition. At the top of framework are the proximal causes of diet and disease, which arise from the three household- and community-level drivers of food insecurity, inadequate care, and health services and the environment. The base of the framework captures macro-level determinants such as institutions, and political and economic structures that shape the distribution of resources within a society. Over the years, there have been iterations and adaptions to context and the changing epidemiology of malnutrition, with the most recent *Lancet* series introducing a framework that builds from the UNICEF to also include **nutrition-specific** and **nutrition-sensitive interventions** (table 11.1).[25]

The WHO, with nutrition and health communications experts, recently developed a framework dedicated to stunted growth and development determinants (figure 11.7).[26] Similar to past frameworks, it represents multilevel causes from proximal to distal but leverages other visual features including color and the sphere shape to illustrate the transdisciplinary nature of the

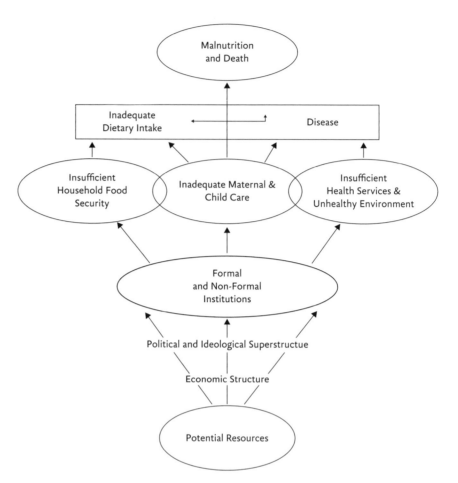

Figure 11.6. UNICEF Conceptual Framework 1990. *Source:* UNICEF. "Strategy for Improved Nutrition of Children & Women in Developing Countries." UNICEF Policy Review. 1990-1.

stunting problem. For example, the water and sanitation system determinant in the outer sphere is represented in blue and shows overlap with healthcare and agriculture systems, leading to infection, food and water safety factors and, ultimately, stunted growth and development. The WHO infographic draws from a review synthesizing the latest evidence for causes of stunting in LMIC.[27] Here, we cover key drivers of stunting drawing from this transdisciplinary WHO framework but also in consideration for advances in public health nutrition science. We begin with a discussion of the most proximate causes and work our way to the distal drivers of stunting.

Biological Determinants

In the era of precision medicine, the field of public health is also beginning to draw on scientific advances in genomics, metabolomics, and microbiology more broadly to better understand mechanistic causes of stunting. Sir Francis Galton was likely the first to explore genetic determinants of

Table 11.1. Key Practices, Services, and Policy Interventions for Preventing and Treating Stunting and Other Forms of Undernutrition and Overweight and Obesity throughout the Life Cycle

Adolescence to pregnancy	Birth	0–5 months	6–23 months	24–59 months
		Nutrition-Specific Interventions		
Food fortification including salt iodization	*Delayed cord clamping	*Exclusive breastfeeding counseling and lay support on breastfeeding through community-based and facility-based contacts	*Timely, adequate, safe, and appropriate complimentary feeding	Counseling and nutrition advice to women of reproductive age/adults
Iron and folic acid or multiple micronutrient supplementation for pregnant women	*Initiation of breastfeeding within one hour (including colostrum)	*Control of the marketing of breastmilk substitutes	*Continued breastfeeding Control of the marketing of breastmilk substitutes	Communication for behavioral and social change to prevent childhood obesity
Intermittent (weekly) iron and folic acid supplementation for reproductive-age women	*Appropriate infant feeding practices and anti-retroviral therapy for HIV-exposed infants	*Appropriate infant feeding practices and anti-retroviral therapy for HIV-exposed infants	*Appropriate infant feeding practices and anti-retroviral therapy for HIV-exposed infants	*Vitamin A supplementation Management of SAM (and moderate acute malnutrition)
Fortified food supplements for undernourished mothers		Vitamin A supplementation in first 8 weeks after delivery	*Micronutrient supplementation, including vitamin A, zinc treatment for diarrhea	*Food fortification, including salt iodization
Nutrition counseling for improved dietary intake during pregnancy		Use of fortified foods, micronutrients supplementation, and home fortification with multiple micronutrients for undernourished women	*Management of SAM Food fortification with multiple micronutrients	*Zinc supplementation with oral rehydration salts for diarrhea treatment and management
			*Zinc supplementation with oral rehydration salts for diarrhea treatment and management	

(continued)

Table 11.1. (continued)

Adolescence to pregnancy	Birth	0-5 months	6-23 months	24-59 months
		Nutrition-Sensitive Approaches		
Improved availability, access, and use of locally available foods	Kangaroo care	Maternity protection in the workplace	Handwashing with soap and improved water and sanitation practices	Handwashing with soap and improved water and sanitation practices
	Support for birth registration and strengthening of civil-registration systems			
Increased access to primary and secondary education for girls		Early childhood development: responsive care	Early childhood stimulation and education	Provision of healthy foods in schools
Adolescent health services that provide access to contraceptives and care			Improved use of locally available foods for infants (improved food access and dietary diversification)	Nutrition and physical education in school
Promotion of handwashing with soap and improved water and sanitation practices			Deworming for children	Deworming for school-age children
Antenatal care, including HIV testing & deworming Intermitting preventive treatment and promotion of insecticide-treated bed nets for pregnant women in high malaria areas			Prevention and treatment of infection disease	Prevention and treatment of infectious disease
Social protection and safety nets targeting vulnerable women			Early childhood development: responsive care	Early childhood development: child to child and school readiness
Promotion of increased age at marriage and reduced gender discrimination and gender-based violence				
Parenting and life skills for early childhood development				

Source: Adapted from 2013 *Lancet* Series on Maternal and Child Nutrition.

STUNTED GROWTH AND DEVELOPMENT

—

Context, Causes and Consequences

—

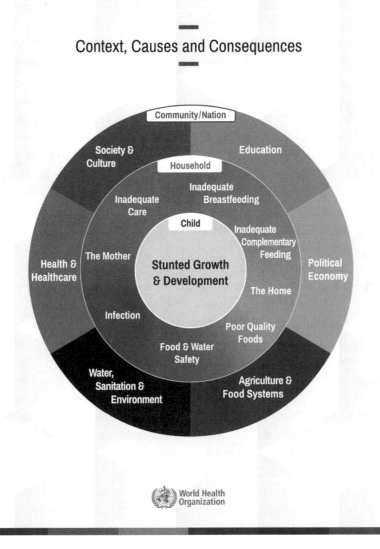

Figure 11.7. WHO Stunted Growth and Development Framework. *Source:* "Stunted Growth and Development: Context, Causes and Consequences." World Health Organization, 2017; p. 1. http://www.who.int/nutrition/childhood_stunting_framework_leaflet_en.pdf?ua=1.

height using mid-parental height to predict child height, in 1886.[28] Data from the WHO Multicentre Growth Reference Study described above recently showed that an average of 16% of between-child variability could be explained by mid-parental height.[3] Accumulated evidence suggests that in populations that experience optimal conditions for growth, genetics may determine up to 80% of height. However, in contexts where negative environmental factors play a greater role, genetics account for a much smaller proportion of the overall variation in height.[29]

Genome-wide association studies provide insight into the specific genes that may influence human growth in stature. The Genetic Investigation of Anthropometric Traits (GIANT) study examined individuals of European descent and identified variations in 180 genes that drive height variability.[30] These variations are all clustered in sections of the genome that code for metabolites involved in pathways related to bone growth and hormone.[29] Interestingly, these 180 genes explained only a mere 10% of height variance in the sample. This finding suggests there is plasticity in stature and perhaps an evolutionary advantage to height being controlled by more than one gene.

Metabolomics studies investigate connections between metabolites (the end products of metabolic pathways) and biological outcomes. With regard to stunting, results of metabolomics studies point to multiple biological factors influencing growth. These factors include nutrients, hormones, and other bioactive metabolites participating in growth pathways. Studies investigating associations between specific metabolites and growth have shown stunting to be associated with reduced serum concentrations of essential, conditionally essential, and non-essential amino acids sphingolipids, and choline.[31,32] Studies examining bone growth reveal the crucial contributions of paracrine and endocrine factors. Insulin-like growth factors, bone morphogenetic proteins, thyroid hormone, among others modulate chondrogenesis and other growth processes at epiphyseal growth plates.[31,33]

In light of findings from metabolomics studies, some trials have been designed specifically to test interventions that may influence growth through key metabolic pathways. For example, a rigorously designed randomized controlled trial (RCT) tested the efficacy of egg nutrition during infancy. Eggs were selected for the intervention because they are highly concentrated sources of key nutrients involved in infant growth, such as choline, B_{12}, vitamin A, and essential amino acids. Children in the intervention group received one egg per day for six months. At the completion of the trial, stunting was reduced by 47% within the intervention group, with an effect size of 0.63. Metabolomics analyses of children in the study revealed biomarkers of choline, docosahexanoic acid (DHA), and histidine positively mediated the effect of eggs on linear growth among children consuming eggs.[34,35]

Child-Level Determinants

We transition to "above the skin" determinants of stunting, moving into the child-level sphere. The proximal factors of diet and infection are addressed here, drawing upon both the UNICEF[24] (1990) and WHO[4] (2013) frameworks. Breastfeeding practices are widely known to influence child growth and development beginning in the immediate postpartum period through 2 years of life. WHO recommends three optimal breastfeeding behaviors: (1) early initiation of breastfeeding (within 1 hour or the first day of life); (2) exclusive breastfeeding (for six months); and (3) continued breastfeeding during the complementary feeding period (through 2 years of age). While these recommendations target LMIC, there is a strong evidence base for the importance of breastfeeding in all contexts on a wide range of health outcomes. In the first days of life, the first "milk," called colostrum, provides crucial passive immunity and micronutrients. Early initiation (on the first day of life) ensures this nutrition, establishes the practice, and reduces the risks of morbidity and neonatal mortality.[36]

Exclusive breastfeeding, defined as breastmilk only, is recommended for the first six months of life, though some debate exists for whether this should be four to six months. Predominant (breastmilk with water or other liquids) or partial breastfeeding (breastmilk with solids and liquids) increases the risk of stunting as well as infectious diseases and mortality. The early introduction of foods or other liquids can compromise the integrity of the gastrointestinal tract, enabling invasion of pathogens and expose the child to contaminated food or water before the immune system is ready. Despite progress in promoting exclusive breastfeeding globally, only 37% of infants less than 6 months of age were found to be exclusively breastfeeding in a recent review of data from 153 countries.[37] In addition to the link to child growth through nutrition and infection pathways, breastfeeding is also associated with improved cognition and child development. A systematic review showed an increase of 3 IQ points associated with breastfeeding after adjusting for confounding factors.[38]

Another important component of diet during the first 1,000 days of life is complementary feeding. **Complementary feeding** refers to the life cycle phase when a child transitions from exclusive breastfeeding to the family diet—usually consisting of soft, semi-soft, or solid foods (of varying textures and higher nutritional quality) with continued breastfeeding. Growth faltering is highly likely during the complementary feeding period from 6-24 months due to challenges in access to high-quality complementary foods, a lack of awareness and understanding for the complex set of good complementary feeding practices, and increased risk of infection. In contrast to the breastfeeding period that has a limited set of WHO recommended practices, complementary feeding guidelines are multiple and context specific. In 2003, WHO and PAHO published a set of 10 recommended complementary feeding practices (table 11.2).[39] The evidence base in support of these practices varies considerably. WHO is currently conducting systematic reviews and convening technical experts to update the guidelines with new evidence and the changing landscape of nutrition globally.

Dietary diversity and quality are two factors that have emerged as critical for stunting prevention during the complementary feeding period. Dietary

Table 11.2. Guiding Principles for Complementary Feeding of the Breastfed Child

1. Duration of exclusive breastfeeding and age of introduction of complementary foods	Practice exclusive breastfeeding from birth to 6 months of age, and introduce complementary foods at 6 months of age (180 days) while continuing to breastfeed.
2. Maintenance of breastfeeding	Continue frequent, on-demand breastfeeding until 2 years of age or beyond.
3. Responsive feeding	Practice responsive feeding, applying the principles of psychosocial care. Specifically: (a) feed infants directly and assist older children when they feed themselves, being sensitive to their hunger and satiety cues; (b) feed slowly and patiently, and encourage children to eat, but do not force them; (c) if children refuse many foods, experiment with different food combinations, tastes, textures, and methods of encouragement; (e) minimize distractions during meals if the child loses interest easily; and (f) remember that feeding times are periods of learning and love—talk to children during feeding, with eye-to-eye contact.
4. Safe preparation and storage of complementary foods	Practice good hygiene and proper food handling by (a) washing caregivers' and children's hands before food preparation and eating, (b) storing foods safely and serving foods immediately after preparation, (c) using clean utensils to prepare and serve food, (d) using clean cups and bowls when feeding children, and (e) avoiding the use of feeding bottles, which are difficult to keep clean.
5. Amount of complementary foods needed	Start at 6 months of age with small amounts of food and increase the quantity as the child gets older, while maintaining frequent breastfeeding. The energy needs from complementary foods for infants with "average" breastmilk intake in developing countries are approximately 200 kcal per day at 6-8 months of age, 300 kcal per day at 9-11 months of age, and 550 kcal per day at 12-23 months of age. In industrialized countries these estimates differ somewhat (130, 310, and 580 kcal/d at 6-8, 9-11, and 12-23 months, respectively) because of differences in average breastmilk intake.
6. Food consistency	Gradually increase food consistency and variety as the infant gets older, adapting to the infant's requirements and abilities. Infants can eat pureed, mashed, and semisolid foods beginning at 6 months. By 8 months most infants can also eat "finger foods" (snacks that can be eaten by children alone). By 12 months, most children can eat the same types of foods as consumed by the rest of the family (keeping in mind the need for nutrient-dense foods, as explained in #8 below). Avoid foods that may cause choking (i.e., items that have a shape and/or consistency that may cause them to become lodged in the trachea, such as nuts, grapes, and raw carrots).
7. Meal frequency and energy density	Increase the number of times that the child is fed complementary foods as he or she gets older. The appropriate number of feedings depends on the energy density of the local foods and the usual amounts consumed at each feeding. For the average healthy breastfed infant, meals of complementary foods should be provided 2 or 3 times per day at 6-8 months of age and 3 or 4 times per day at 9-11 and 12-24 months of age, with additional nutritious snacks (such as a piece of fruit or bread or chapatti with nut paste) offered 1 or 2 times per day, as desired. Snacks are defined as foods eaten between meals—usually self-fed, convenient, and easy to prepare. If energy density or amount of food per meal is low, or the child is no longer breastfed, more frequent meals may be required.

8. Nutrient content of complementary foods	Feed a variety of foods to ensure that nutrient needs are met. Meat, poultry, fish, or eggs should be eaten daily, or as often as possible. Vegetarian diets cannot meet nutrient needs at this age unless nutrient supplements or fortified products are used (see #9 below). Vitamin A–rich fruits and vegetables should be eaten daily. Provide diets with adequate fat content. Avoid giving drinks with low nutrient value, such as tea, coffee, and sugary drinks such as soda. Limit the amount of juice offered so as to avoid displacing more nutrient-rich foods.
9. Use of vitamin–mineral supplements or fortified products for infant and mother	Use fortified complementary foods or vitamin–mineral supplements for the infant, as needed. In some populations, breastfeeding mothers may also need vitamin–mineral supplements or fortified products, both for their own health and to ensure normal concentrations of certain nutrients (particularly vitamins) in their breastmilk. (Such products may also be beneficial for prepregnant and pregnant women.)
10. Feeding during and after illness	Increase fluid intake during illness, including more frequent breastfeeding, and encourage the child to eat soft, varied, appetizing, favorite foods. After illness, give food more often than usual and encourage the child to eat more.

Source: Adapted from Annex 11—*Guiding Principles for Complementary Feeding of the Breastfed Child*. Infant Feeding in Emergencies, Module 2, Version 1.0 for Health and Nutrition Workers in Emergency Situations. ENN, IBFAN, Terre des hommes, UNHCR, UNICEF, WFP, WHO. 2004. http://helid.digicollection.org/en/d/Js8230e/4.11.html.

diversity refers to the variety of different food types consumed, while dietary quality refers to the nutrient content of foods. A young child has a small gastric capacity and therefore requires more frequent feeding than older children or adults; but importantly, foods should deliver nutrients efficiently, rather than just supply empty calories. Animal-source foods are known to provide several important nutrients in highly bioavailable matrices. For example, vitamin A in animal-source foods comes in the form of retinol absorbed at considerably higher rates (12–24 times higher) that the plant form of carotenoids such as beta carotene. Other nutrients similarly more bioavailable in animal-source foods compared to plant-based foods include iron, zinc, choline, vitamin B_{12}, essential fatty acids, among others. Unfortunately, animal-source foods are usually more expensive and therefore less accessible to vulnerable populations most at risk for stunting. One potential solution to this (as detailed below) is to promote and support more affordable and sustainable animal-source foods, such as eggs and milk.

Another critical child-level determinant of stunting is *infection.* Multiple types of infection may contribute to poor growth and development, mediated through different inflammation and symptomatic mechanisms. Malnutrition during infection may arise from suppressed appetite and reduced dietary intakes. There may also be altered metabolism or poor absorption of nutrients in some infections. Enteric disease (diseases affecting the intestines, such as diarrhea) is the infection most commonly associated with stunting early in life.[40] A child is at highest risk for diarrheal disease in LMIC during the complementary feeding period, from 6-24 months. There are increased pathogen exposures from the introduction of food and drinks beyond breastmilk that may be contaminated. The greater risk, however, arises from increased mobility and the fecal-oral route of transmission. A child begins to crawl and explore during this phase and puts objects in his or her mouth—often in environments that may not be hygienic, increasing risk of infection.

The type and duration of diarrheal infection can matter for its contribution to stunting. For example, persistent diarrhea lasting 14 or more days places a child at higher risk for malnutrition and mortality if a child is already malnourished. The MAL-ED study was a multisite longitudinal cohort study designed to investigate interactions between enteric disease and nutrition and the impact on child development. Using surveillance data from eight sites in Asia, Africa, and South America, the study demonstrated a changing epidemiology of diarrhea.[41] In the first year of life, they found norovirus GII, rotavirus, *Campylobacter* spp., and *Cryptosporidium* spp. to be the most frequent organisms causing diarrhea. In the second year of life, major pathogens were *Campylobacter* spp., norovirus GII, rotavirus, astrovirus, and *Shigella* spp. Importantly, this study also showed high pathogen detection in the non-diarrheal stools, meaning that children may be fighting an infection even when diarrhea is not present. Subclinical infection can also contribute significantly to stunting and malnutrition.

Environmental enteropathy is a condition in which the microvilli of the small intestine are flattened and permeable through repeated bouts of infection, leading to poor absorption of nutrition and ultimately malnutrition. Finally, diarrheal infection is associated with zinc deficiency, which is also linked to linear growth and in chronic deficiency, stunting. In addition to oral rehydration solution (ORS), WHO recommends zinc supplementation for the treatment of acute diarrhea.[42]

There are other infections that show synergistic effects with malnutrition and stunting. A child who is stunted has higher odds of dying from diarrhea, but also from pneumonia, malaria, and measles.[43] Acute respiratory infection remains a leading cause of disease burden globally, and again, through inflammatory mechanisms of reduced appetite and altered metabolism it may cause or exacerbate undernutrition. Other diseases such as helminth infection and malaria also increase the risk of anemia and contribute to the infection-undernutrition cycle.[44]

Household-Level Determinants

The next sphere of stunting determinants is the household. The socioeconomic, environmental, and behavioral conditions of the child's home can support or undermine optimal growth and development. To begin, the mother's nutritional status is known to be highly correlated with her offspring. Early life and in utero events and factors can have lasting impacts on growth trajectories and are related to longer-term stunting outcomes. One study showed that being born SGA, an indicator of fetal growth restriction, vastly increased the odds of stunting for a child between 12 and 60 months of age, both for children born at term (OR 2.43 [95% CI, 2.22, 2.66]) and those born preterm (OR 4.51 [95% CI, 3.42, 5.93]).[14] Another important study showed that fetal growth restriction was the leading risk factor in 137 developing countries for stunting among children at the close of the first 1,000 days, 24-35 months.[45]

One of the primary causes of fetal growth restriction is a result of inadequate maternal nutrition or nutritional status. Thus, the mother's nutritional status is integral to stunting prevention. Attention to maternal nutritional status should begin even before conception, for example, with folate supplementation. The World Health Organization recommends iron-folic acid supplementation in pregnant women throughout pregnancy to reduce the risk of low birth weight, maternal anemia, and preterm birth.[46] Globally, countries have protocols for iron-folic acid supplementation during pregnancy to mitigate the risks for low birth weight and anemia for mother and child. Generally, offspring nutrition is protected preferentially during pregnancy and lactation, sometimes to the detriment of the mother. However, nutritional deficiencies and poor growth for the child will result if the mother is malnourished. Adolescent pregnancies and short birth spacing are both risk factors for fetal growth restriction and low birth weight. A teenage mother is still growing herself, so there is competition for nutrients.[47]

With insufficient time between births, a mother is unable to replenish her nutrient reserves. Adolescence is increasingly being viewed as a "second window of opportunity" (the first window being the first 1,000 days) to improve malnutrition of girls themselves and potentially the next generation.[48-50] More recent evidence also shows associations between maternal hypertension during pregnancy[51,52] and increased risk of fetal growth restriction and preterm birth, two key factors associated with child growth. In an effort to reduce gestational hypertension, WHO recommends calcium supplementation among populations with low dietary calcium.

The home environment is also a key driver in stunting. This might include such factors as intra-household food allocation and gender dynamics (e.g., males eat before females in the household). Relatedly, there may be suboptimal caregiver practices and inadequate stimulation and interaction with the child. There is evidence demonstrating the synergies between early learning, responsive caregiving, and nutrition for growth and development.[18] Responsive feeding is among the complementary feeding guidelines promoted by WHO. Black and Aboud have conceptualized this as a four-step process: (1) the caregiver creates a routine, structure, expectations, and emotional context that promote interaction; (2) the child responds and signals to the caregiver; (3) the caregiver responds promptly in a manner that is emotionally supportive, contingent, and developmentally appropriate; and (4) the child experiences predictable responses.[52]

Caregiver education, particularly maternal education, is a widely established determinant of stunting. The pathways to stunting from education level are many, including caregiver behaviors, knowledge about nutrition and adequate diets, income and livelihoods, among others.

Finally, household poverty is one of the most important determinants of stunting worldwide, as evidenced by the vast differences in risk for stunting according to household wealth quintile, discussed earlier in this chapter.[14] Poverty has long been associated with food and nutrition insecurity. Families may not be able to afford higher-quality foods, such as animal-source foods, that promote growth and development. Additionally, families who are poor may not be able to afford sanitary conditions or materials for cognitive stimulation. Even more nuanced, income and food prices have been linked to particular nutrient deficiencies in vitamin A, B_{12}, iron, zinc, among others.[53]

Community- and Societal-Level Determinants

Moving outside the child's home to the community level and even more broadly, the societal level, there are several important determinants of stunting. These contextual factors could largely be considered as "systems," operating in complex and interrelated ways. Originating first in the discipline of engineering and now practiced by social scientists and others, **systems science** is a field developed to assess and model these systems across different public health problems.[54] The goal is often to identify critical leverage points within the system that might ultimately impact the outcome of interest. One could apply system dynamic modeling of a community's food system to examine the factors influencing child nutrition (figure 11.8).[55] Food and agriculture systems particularly are recognized to underlie stunting. The factors begin at the level of food production and extend through food processing and markets—locally, nationally, and internationally. However, despite the obvious links to malnutrition, "nutrition-sensitive" agriculture programming as discussed below does not include specific nutrition objectives. Food availability through production should include a diverse range of foods, or crops and livestock, that generate income to purchase higher-quality foods. Small livestock production has been held up as an important driver of stunting alleviation, both through direct consumption by children of the animal-source foods or through the sale of livestock for building income and wealth.

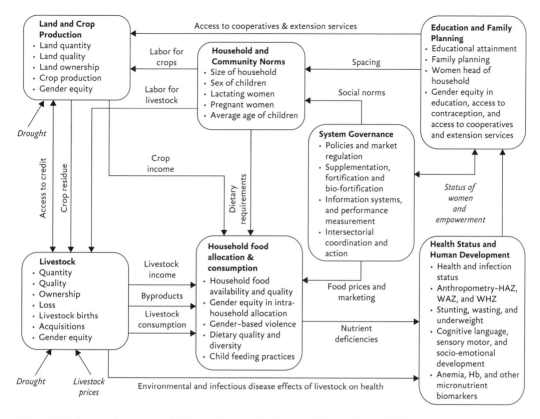

Figure 11.8. System dynamic model: Animal source foods and child nutrition in Ethiopia.

In many contexts, the food system is resulting in production and sale of ultra-processed foods that are similarly contributing to hidden hunger, overweight/obesity, and stunting.[56]

Other crucial systems that influence nutrition include education, sanitation, and health care.[27] As previously discussed, caregiver education is a consistent determinant of child nutritional status. There are multiple pathways through which education impacts nutrition, such as improved livelihoods and thus, access to higher-quality foods, or modified health behaviors through knowledge.[57] Some education programs have targeted girls to address gender disparities, reduce adolescent pregnancies, and reach future caregivers. Sanitation systems are also vital for reducing fecal contamination in the community. This is especially the case in contexts where open defecation remains a widespread practice. Some programs targeting household hygiene or water quality may have limited impacts unless sanitation systems are simultaneously maintained to address contamination at the community level. Finally, the health care system is widely recognized to play an important role in stunting. Access to both prevention and treatment services can mitigate infection-related causes of malnutrition.

At the same time, social, political, and environmental factors are among the basic causes of malnutrition as outlined in both the original UNICEF framework and the 2013 *Lancet* framework. Social factors might include culture, beliefs, and norms around diets, for example, or other determinants such as women's status in the household. Demographic trends such as urbanization have been associated with an increased risk of stunting.[58] Food prices and trade policy or marketing regulations can impact population nutrition, while employment and financial opportunities may serve to uphold or impede nutrition progress. Political instability is an important contributor to hunger and malnutrition, as exemplified in recent humanitarian crises such as in Yemen or Afghanistan.[59,60] Finally, climate conditions can ultimately contribute to food insecurity and stunting. For example, extreme weather events such as drought or floods may impact food production or increase infection in a population, leading to malnutrition.

The Solutions
Definitions and Stakeholders

Solutions to address stunting may be classified across different realms of action: (1) policies, (2) programing and (3) research. *Programming* refers to intervention projects aimed at improving child growth and sometimes multiple other objectives. *Policy* may be standards or principles, with official approval, that guide and regulate nutrition activities at global, national, or local levels. There might also be internal policies for agencies directing their own operations. *Research* is systematic investigation with a view toward generating evidence and facts. It may be laboratory-based "bench" science, epidemiological data analyses, observational field trials, or intervention studies such as RCTs. If designed well, program and policy evaluations, as described in chapter 6, can serve as research to inform modifications or adaptations to existing programs or suggest entirely new program and policies in the future.

Actors in nutrition programming, policy, and research in LMIC may be grouped as multilaterals, bilaterals, government agencies (public sectors), nongovernmental organizations (NGOs), community-based organizations (CBOs), social enterprises, private sector, and education or research institutions. Multilateral agencies are formed between multiple governments and include groups such as UNICEF or the World Bank. Bilaterals operate from one government to another, such as the United States Agency for International Development (USAID) or the Canadian International Development Agency (CIDA). Generally, the largest stakeholders in nutrition programming in a country are found in the public sector in different government agencies and operating at varying administrative levels. NGOs, both international and national, are also key players in nutrition programming. Helen Keller International, CARE, and Save the Children have been actively engaged in nutrition activities for many years. There are also many CBOs, generally considerably smaller in size and resources, for programming. A relatively new classification of stakeholders in nutrition is social entrepreneurs, who apply a business model for a social development outcome such as child growth and nutrition. An example of this stakeholder might be those organizations in the "PlumpyField" network, such as Edesia and Meds & Food for Kids in Haiti, producing fortified peanut butter pastes for sale by development organizations but with the motive to alleviate malnutrition. Research stakeholders might include universities or research institutes sometimes referred to as think tanks. The final set of stakeholders includes the donors who fund programming, policy, and research.

Policy, Programming, and Research Solutions
Policies

Policies aimed at stunting mitigation are usually subsumed in larger, overall nutrition guidelines. At the global level, there are two sets of policies that have served as standards and guidelines for upholding young child nutrition: (1) *Global Strategy for Infant and Young Child Feeding*;[61] and (2) the *Guiding Principles for Complementary Feeding of the Breastfed Child*,[38] and *Guiding Principles for Feeding Non-Breastfed Children 6-24 Months of Age*.[62] Experts from around the world were convened to develop the documents and come to a consensus around content. Both documents will be updated in the coming years. There are also global policies or standards that relate to specific components of the stunting problem such as food safety, *Codex Alimentarius* (FAO, WHO) or surveillance and measurement of child growth, and *WHO Growth Standards* (2006).[63] These policy types are often mirrored at national and local levels. Governments might have an overarching policy such as the *National Plans of Action for Nutrition* that emerged from the International Conference on Nutrition in 1992, and they might also have policies in specific areas of nutrition such as food safety or infant feeding guidelines. There are local policies and institutional policies as well that exist to guide and regulate action for promoting child growth and development. For example, in 2010, the Haitian government developed and adopted the country's own National Food Security and Nutrition Plan, followed by the implementation of the National School Feeding Policy and Strategy in 2016.

Programming

Nutrition programs can be grouped into categories as well and, like policies, these program types are found at varying administrative levels—global, national, and local. In the most recent *Lancet* Series on Maternal and Child Nutrition, two broad categories of programs and approaches were delineated: *nutrition-specific* and *nutrition-sensitive*. The categories refer to the level of determinants targeted by various interventions. As illustrated in the framework, *nutrition-specific* approaches address more proximal factors, while distal factors are addressed in *nutrition-sensitive* programs (table 11.1).[25] There are a larger number of studies investigating the effects of nutrition-specific interventions in part because these intervention types are easier to test in RCTs or using other experimental designs. Specifically targeting stunting, most programs focus on the complementary feeding period. Most common program types include single or multiple nutrient supplementation; food fortification during preharvest (biofortification) or in processing (salt iodization or fortified peanut butter pastes), food-based approaches (promotion or provision of animal-source foods, diet diversification), **WASH (water, sanitation, and hygiene)**, and agriculture or development programs (small livestock development or conditional cash transfers).

Research

There is surprisingly minimal evidence for interventions that can significantly reduce stunting. This may be due to the multifactorial nature of the problem and need for integrated approaches. In the second *Lancet* series, released in 2013, investigators compiled research findings from around the world to compare the efficacy of different interventions. For stunting reduction, the evidence came from education and supplementation trials conducted during the complementary feeding period of 6–24 months. Using data from 16 RCTs and quasi-experimental studies of provision of a complementary food with or without education in food-insecure settings, investigators quantified an average effect size of 0.39 increase in HAZ with a nonsignificant stunting reduction.[64]

There have been numerous trials examining single-nutrient supplementation (vitamin A, iron, and zinc) or multiple micronutrient supplementation. These studies have improved micronutrient status and reduced anemia but have had minimal effects on linear growth. Lipid-based nutrient supplements, or fortified peanut butter pastes, were recently tested across several different contexts. Some trials demonstrated significant increases in linear growth and stunting reductions (in Ghana and Burkina Faso)[65,66] while others did not (in Malawi).[67] More promising results were shown in a trial in Ecuador, testing one egg per day for six months introduced early in the complementary feeding period, increasing linear growth by 0.63 LAZ and reducing stunting by 47%.[35] Evidence from recent WASH trials have also been disappointing in terms of growth outcomes for young children.[68] In view of the complex nature of stunting, there is a need to test integrated approaches that begin in pregnancy and continue through the complementary feeding period. Additionally, recent calls to action suggest the need for interventions focused on improving maternal nutrition status during the preconception period in an effort to break the intergenerational cycle of malnutrition.

Conclusion

In the UN Decade of Action on Nutrition, it is incumbent on the global community to end hunger and eradicate malnutrition worldwide.[4] Efforts should be mobilized to confront the complex array of factors causing stunted growth and development, from cells to society. Maternal nutritional status, both preconception and during pregnancy, as well as breastfeeding practices should be supported as early determinants of stunting. Access to high-quality, diverse diets is also critical with particular attention given to animal-source foods during the complementary feeding period. Concerted efforts are needed to mitigate infection risk through improved WASH, access to health care, and other strategies. At the community and societal levels, nutrition goals should be integral to education, agriculture development, and poverty alleviation programs. Ultimately, populations globally have the right to be food secure with the opportunity to grow and develop to their fullest potential.

Review Questions

1. Who is affected by stunting (age, socioeconomic status, regional distributions, etc.)? How can programs and policies better target these populations?
2. What are some of the key determinants or factors that contribute to childhood stunting? In what ways do these factors interact with one another to contribute to the problem?
3. What are the implications of stunted growth and development for a child, household, community, and society?
4. What measures would you use to fully capture the spectrum of stunting determinants in a community?
5. Why is it challenging to develop and implement integrated programs that address the multifactorial nature of stunting?
6. How would you develop a program to address the problem of stunting in Martha's community of Tingo Pucara? Which stakeholders should be involved? What nutrition-specific or nutrition-sensitive approaches might you use?
7. The first nutrition goal of the World Health Assembly, to reduce stunting by 40% by 2025, will not be met if trends continue. What programming, policy, and research strategies are needed to shift this trajectory and better ensure the global community meets this target?

References

1. Jelliffe, Derrick Brian. 1966. "The Assessment of Nutritional Status in the Community." WHO Monograph Series no. 53. Geneva, Switzerland: World Health Organization.

2. Onis, Mercedes de, Cutberto Garza, Cesar G. Victora, Maharaj K. Bhan, and Kaare R. Norum. 2004. "The WHO Multicentre Growth Reference Study (MGRS):

Rationale, Planning and Implementation." *Food and Nutrition Bulletin* 25 (supplement 1): S3–84.

3. Garza, Cutberto, Elaine Borghi, Adelheid W. Onyango, and Mercedes de Onis. 2013. "Parental Height and Child Growth from Birth to 2 Years in the WHO Multicentre Growth Reference Study." *Maternal & Child Nutrition* 9 (September): 58–68. https://doi.org/10.1111/mcn.12085.

4. United Nations General Assembly. Resolution adopted by the General Assembly on 1 April 2016. 70/259 United Nations Decade of Action on Nutrition (2016–2025). https://www.un.org/en/ga/search/view_doc.asp?symbol=A/RES/70/259.

5. Onis, Mercedes de, Kathryn G. Dewey, Elaine Borghi, Adelheid W. Onyango, Monika Blössner, Bernadette Daelmans, Ellen Piwoz, et al. 2013. "The World Health Organization's Global Target for Reducing Childhood Stunting by 2025: Rationale and Proposed Actions." *Maternal & Child Nutrition* 9 (September): 6–26. https://doi.org/10.1111/mcn.12075.

6. "Levels and Trends in Child Malnutrition: Joint Child Malnutrition Estimates." 2017. UNICEF, WHO, The World Bank Group.

7. Freire, Wilma, Maria Ramirez Luzuriaga, Philippe Belmont, M.-J. Mendieta, M. K. Silva-Jaramillo, N. Romero, Klever Saenz, et al. 2013. *Tomo I: Encuesta Nacional de Salud y Nutrición de La Población Ecuatoriana de 0 a 59 Años. ENSANUT-ECU 2012.*

8. Soria Carrillo, Angela Rocio, and Alejandro Robert Vaca Almeida. 2012. "Determinants of Chronic Malnutrition in Children Under Five Years in the Province of Cotopaxi." Universidad Central del Ecuador Facultad de Ciencias Econóicas.

9. Black, Robert E., Cesar G. Victora, Susan P. Walker, Zulfiqar A. Bhutta, Parul Christian, Mercedes De Onis, Majid Ezzati, et al. 2013. "Maternal and Child Undernutrition and Overweight in Low-Income and Middle-Income Countries." *The Lancet* 382 (9890): 427–51. https://doi.org/10.1016/S0140-6736(13)60937-X.

10. Wamani, Henry, Anne Nordrehaug Åstrøm, Stefan Peterson, James K Tumwine, and Thorkild Tylleskär. 2007. "Boys Are More Stunted than Girls in Sub-Saharan Africa: A Meta-Analysis of 16 Demographic and Health Surveys." *BMC Pediatrics* 7 (1): 17. https://doi.org/10.1186/1471-2431-7-17.

11. Victora, Cesar G., Mercedes De Onis, Pedro C. Hallal, Monika Blossner, and Roger Shrimpton. 2010. "Worldwide Timing of Growth Faltering: Revisiting Implications for Interventions." *Pediatrics* 125 (3): e473–80. https://doi.org/10.1542/peds.2009-1519.

12. Christian, Parul, Sun Eun Lee, Moira Donahue Angel, Linda S. Adair, Shams E. Arifeen, Per Ashorn, Fernando C. Barros, et al. 2013. "Risk of Childhood Undernutrition Related to Small-for-Gestational Age and Preterm Birth in Low- and Middle-Income Countries." *International Journal of Epidemiology* 42 (5): 1340–55. https://doi.org/10.1093/ije/dyt109.

13. Olofin, Ibironke, Christine M. McDonald, Majid Ezzati, Seth Flaxman, Robert E. Black, Wafaie W. Fawzi, Laura E. Caulfield, and Goodarz Danaei. 2013. "Associations of Suboptimal Growth with All-Cause and Cause-Specific Mortality in Children under Five Years: A Pooled Analysis of Ten Prospective Studies."

Edited by Andrea S. Wiley. *PLoS ONE* 8 (5): e64636. https://doi.org/10.1371/journal .pone.0064636.

14. Victora, Cesar G, Linda Adair, Caroline Fall, Pedro C Hallal, Reynaldo Martorell, Linda Richter, and Harshpal Singh Sachdev. 2008. "Maternal and Child Undernutrition: Consequences for Adult Health and Human Capital." *The Lancet* 371 (9609): 340–57. https://doi.org/10.1016/S0140-6736(07)61692-4.

15. Özaltin, Emre, Kenneth Hill, and S. V. Subramanian. 2010. "Association of Maternal Stature With Offspring Mortality, Underweight, and Stunting in Low- to Middle-Income Countries." *JAMA* 303 (15): 1507. https://doi.org/10.1001 /jama.2010.450.

16. Lawn, Joy E., Simon Cousens, Gary L. Darmstadt, Vinod Paul, and Jose Martines. 2004. "Why Are 4 Million Newborn Babies Dying Every Year?" *The Lancet* 364 (9450): 2020. https://doi.org/10.1016/S0140-6736(04)17511-9.

17. Heindel, Jerrold J., and Laura N. Vandenberg. 2015. "Developmental Origins of Health and Disease." *Current Opinion in Pediatrics* 27 (2): 248–53. https://doi.org /10.1097/MOP.0000000000000191.

18. Black, Maureen M., Susan P. Walker, Lia C. H. Fernald, Christopher T. Andersen, Ann M. DiGirolamo, Chunling Lu, Dana C. McCoy, et al. 2017. "Early Childhood Development Coming of Age: Science through the Life Course." *The Lancet* 389 (10064): 77–90. https://doi.org/10.1016/S0140-6736(16)31389-7.

19. Georgieff, Michael K. 2007. "Nutrition and the Developing Brain: Nutrient Priorities and Measurement." *American Journal of Clinical Nutrition* 85 (2): 614S– 620S. https://doi.org/10.1093/ajcn/85.2.614S.

20. Walker, Susan P., Susan M. Chang, Christine A. Powell, Emily Simonoff, and Sally M. Grantham-McGregor. 2006. "Effects of Psychosocial Stimulation and Dietary Supplementation in Early Childhood on Psychosocial Functioning in Late Adolescence: Follow-up of Randomised Controlled Trial." *BMJ* 333 (7566): 472. https://doi.org/10.1136/bmj.38897.555208.2F.

21. Stein, Aryeh D., Meng Wang, Ann DiGirolamo, Ruben Grajeda, Usha Ramakrishnan, Manuel Ramirez-Zea, Kathryn Yount, et al. 2008. "Nutritional Supplementation in Early Childhood, Schooling, and Intellectual Functioning in Adulthood: A Prospective Study in Guatemala." *Archives of Pediatrics & Adolescent Medicine* 162 (7): 612. https://doi.org/10.1001/archpedi.162.7 .612.

22. Adair, Linda S., Caroline H. D. Fall, Clive Osmond, Aryeh D. Stein, Reynaldo Martorell, Manuel Ramirez-Zea, Harshpal Singh Sachdev, et al. 2013. "Associations of Linear Growth and Relative Weight Gain during Early Life with Adult Health and Human Capital in Countries of Low and Middle Income: Findings from Five Birth Cohort Studies." *The Lancet* 382 (9891): 525–34. https://doi .org/10.1016/S0140-6736(13)60103-8.

23. Prado, Elizabeth L., and Kathryn G. Dewey. 2014. "Nutrition and Brain Development in Early Life." *Nutrition Reviews* 72 (4): 267–84. https://doi.org/10 .1111/nure.12102.

24. UNICEF. 1990. "Strategy for Improved Nutrition of Children and Women in Developing Countries." New York: United Nations Children's Fund. https://doi.org /10.1007/BF02810402.

25. "UNICEF's Approach to Scaling Up Nutrition for Mothers and Children." 2015. New York: Program Division, United Nations Children's Fund.

26. "The Healthy Growth Project: The Conceptual Framework." 2014. Geneva, Switzerland: World Health Organization. http://www.who.int/nutrition/healthy growthproj/en/index1.html.

27. Stewart, Christine P., Lora Iannotti, Kathryn G. Dewey, Kim F. Michaelsen, and Adelheid W. Onyango. 2013. "Contextualising Complementary Feeding in a Broader Framework for Stunting Prevention." *Maternal & Child Nutrition* 9 (September): 27-45. https://doi.org/10.1111/mcn.12088.

28. Galton, Francis. 1886. "Regression Towards Mediocrity in Hereditary Stature." *The Journal of the Anthropological Institute of Great Britain and Ireland* 5: 329-48. https://doi.org/10.2307/2841583.

29. Perola, Markus, Sampo Sammalisto, Tero Hiekkalinna, Nick G. Martin, Peter M. Visscher, Grant W. Montgomery, Beben Benyamin, et al. 2007. "Combined Genome Scans for Body Stature in 6,602 European Twins: Evidence for Common Caucasian Loci." *PLoS Genetics* 3 (6): e97. https://doi.org/10.1371/journal .pgen.0030097.

30. Lango Allen, Hana, Karol Estrada, Guillaume Lettre, Sonja Berndt, Michael N. Weedon, Fernando Rivadeneira, Cristen J. Willer, et al. 2010. "Hundreds of Variants Clustered in Genomic Loci and Biological Pathways Affect Human Height." *Nature* 467 (7317): 832-38. https://doi.org/10.1038/nature09410.

31. Semba, Richard D., Pingbo Zhang, Marta Gonzalez-Freire, Ruin Moaddel, Indi Trehan, Kenneth M. Maleta, M. Isabel Ordiz, et al. 2016. "The Association of Serum Choline with Linear Growth Failure in Young Children from Rural Malawi." *The American Journal of Clinical Nutrition* 104 (1): 191-97. https://doi.org/10 .3945/ajcn.115.129684.

32. Semba, Richard D., Michelle Shardell, Fayrouz A. Sakr Ashour, Ruin Moaddel, Indi Trehan, Kenneth M. Maleta, M. Isabel Ordiz, et al. 2016. "Child Stunting Is Associated with Low Circulating Essential Amino Acids." *EBioMedicine* 6 (April): 246-52. https://doi.org/10.1016/j.ebiom.2016.02.030.

33. Iannotti, Lora L., Chessa K. Lutter, William F. Waters, Carlos Andres Gallegos Riofrío, Carla Malo, Gregory Reinhart, Ana Palacios, et al. 2017. "Eggs Early in Complementary Feeding Increase Choline Pathway Biomarkers and DHA: A Randomized Controlled Trial in Ecuador." *The American Journal of Clinical Nutrition* 106 (6): 1482-89. https://doi.org/10.3945/ajcn.117.160515.

34. Iannotti, Lora L., Chessa K. Lutter, Christine P. Stewart, Carlos Andres Gallegos Riofrío, Carla Malo, Gregory Reinhart, Ana Palacios, et al. 2017. "Eggs in Early Complementary Feeding and Child Growth: A Randomized Controlled Trial." *Pediatrics* 140 (1): e20163459. https://doi.org/10.1542/peds.2016-3459.

35. Lui, J. C., O. Nilsson, and J. Baron. 2014. "Recent Insights into the Regulation of the Growth Plate." *Journal of Molecular Endocrinology* 53 (1): T1-9. https://doi .org/10.1530/JME-14-0022.

36. Edmond, K. M., C. Zandoh, M. A. Quigley, S. Amenga-Etego, S. Owusu-Agyei, and B. R. Kirkwood. 2006. "Delayed Breastfeeding Initiation Increases Risk of Neonatal Mortality." *Pediatrics* 117 (3): e380-86. https://doi.org/10.1542/peds .2005-1496.

37. Victora, Cesar G., Rajiv Bahl, Aluísio J. D. Barros, Giovanny V. A. França, Susan Horton, Julia Krasevec, Simon Murch, et al. 2016. "Breastfeeding in the 21st Century: Epidemiology, Mechanisms, and Lifelong Effect." *The Lancet* 387 (10017): 475–90. https://doi.org/10.1016/S0140-6736(15)01024-7.

38. Horta, Bernardo L., Bahl Rajiv, Jose Carlos Martines, Cesar G. Victora, and World Health Organization. 2007. "Evidence of the Long-Term Effects of Breastfeeding: Systematic Reviews and Meta-Analyses." Geneva, Switzerland: World Health Organization, Department of Child and Adolescent Health and Development.

39. Dewey, Kathryn, Pan American Health Organization, and World Health Organization. 2003. *Guiding Principles for Complementary Feeding of the Breastfed Child.* Washington, DC: World Health Organization, Division of Health Promotion and Protection.

40. Checkley, William, Gillian Buckley, Robert H. Gilman, Ana M. O. Assis, Richard L. Guerrant, Saul S. Morris, Kåre Mølbak, et al. 2008. "Multi-Country Analysis of the Effects of Diarrhoea on Childhood Stunting." *International Journal of Epidemiology* 37 (4): 816–30. https://doi.org/10.1093/ije/dyn099.

41. Platts-Mills, James A., Sudhir Babji, Ladaporn Bodhidatta, Jean Gratz, Rashidul Haque, Alexandre Havt, Benjamin J. J. McCormick, et al. 2015. "Pathogen-Specific Burdens of Community Diarrhoea in Developing Countries: A Multisite Birth Cohort Study (MAL-ED)." *The Lancet Global Health* 3 (9): e564–75. https://doi.org/10.1016/S2214-109X(15)00151-5.

42. "Zinc Supplementation in the Management of Diarrhoea." 2017. E-Library of Evidence for Nutrition Actions (ELENA). World Health Organization. 2017. http://www.who.int/elena/titles/zinc_diarrhoea/en/.

43. Black, Robert E., Lindsay H. Allen, Zulfiqar A. Bhutta, Laura E. Caulfield, Mercedes de Onis, Majid Ezzati, Colin Mathers, et al. 2008. "Maternal and Child Undernutrition: Global and Regional Exposures and Health Consequences." *The Lancet* 371 (9608): 243–60. https://doi.org/10.1016/S0140-6736(07)61690-0.

44. "The Global Prevalence of Anaemia in 2011." 2015. Geneva, Switzerland: World Health Organization.

45. Danaei, Goodarz, Kathryn G. Andrews, Christopher R. Sudfeld, Günther Fink, Dana Charles McCoy, Evan Peet, Ayesha Sania, et al. 2016. "Risk Factors for Childhood Stunting in 137 Developing Countries: A Comparative Risk Assessment Analysis at Global, Regional, and Country Levels." Edited by James K. Tumwine. *PLOS Medicine* 13 (11): e1002164. https://doi.org/10.1371/journal.pmed.1002164.

46. "Daily Iron and Folic Acid Supplementation during Pregnancy." E-Library of Evidence for Nutrition Actions (ELENA). Geneva, Switzerland: World Health Organization. http://www.who.int/elena/titles/daily_iron_pregnancy/en/.

47. Rah, Jee H., Parul Christian, Abu Ahmed Shamim, Ummeh T. Arju, Alain B. Labrique, and Mahbubur Rashid. 2008. "Pregnancy and Lactation Hinder Growth and Nutritional Status of Adolescent Girls in Rural Bangladesh." *The Journal of Nutrition* 138 (8): 1505–11. https://doi.org/10.1093/jn/138.8.1505.

48. Srinivas, S. K., A. G. Edlow, P. M. Neff, M. D. Sammel, C. M. Andrela, and M. A. Elovitz. 2009. "Rethinking IUGR in Preeclampsia: Dependent or Independent

of Maternal Hypertension?" *Journal of Perinatology* 29 (10): 680-84. https://doi.org/10.1038/jp.2009.83.

49. Duley, Lelia. 2009. "The Global Impact of Pre-Eclampsia and Eclampsia." *Seminars in Perinatology* 33 (3): 130-37. https://doi.org/10.1053/j.semperi.2009.02.010.

50. "Calcium Supplementation during Pregnancy to Reduce the Risk of Pre-Eclampsia." 2017. E-Library of Evidence for Nutrition Actions (ELENA). Geneva, Switzerland: World Health Organization. http://www.who.int/elena/titles/calcium_pregnancy/en/.

51. Thangaratinam, S., E. Rogozinska, K. Jolly, S. Glinkowski, T. Roseboom, J. W. Tomlinson, R. Kunz, et al. 2012. "Effects of Interventions in Pregnancy on Maternal Weight and Obstetric Outcomes: Meta-Analysis of Randomised Evidence." *BMJ* 344 (may16 4): e2088-e2088. https://doi.org/10.1136/bmj.e2088.

52. Black, Maureen M., and Frances E. Aboud. 2011. "Responsive Feeding Is Embedded in a Theoretical Framework of Responsive Parenting." *The Journal of Nutrition* 141 (3): 490-94. https://doi.org/10.3945/jn.110.129973.

53. Iannotti, Lora L., Miguel Robles, Helena Pachón, and Cristina Chiarella. 2012. "Food Prices and Poverty Negatively Affect Micronutrient Intakes in Guatemala." *The Journal of Nutrition* 142 (8): 1568-76. https://doi.org/10.3945/jn.111.157321.

54. Hovmand, Peter S. 2014. *Community Based System Dynamics*. New York: Springer. https://doi.org/10.1007/978-1-4614-8763-0.

55. Ionnati, Lora, and Peter Hovmand. n.d. "Conceptual Model of the Animal Source Food System's Impact on Child Health."

56. Monteiro, Carlos A., J. C. Moubarac, Geoffrey Cannon, Shu Wen Ng, and Barry Popkin. 2013. "Ultra-processed Products Are Becoming Dominant in the Global Food System." *Obesity Reviews* 14 (S2): 21-28. https://doi.org/10.1111/obr.12107.

57. Bhutta, Zulfiqar A., Tahmeed Ahmed, Robert E. Black, Simon Cousens, Kathryn Dewey, Elsa Giugliani, Batool A. Haider, et al. 2008. "What Works? Interventions for Maternal and Child Undernutrition and Survival." *The Lancet* 371 (9610): 417-40. https://doi.org/10.1016/S0140-6736(07)61693-6.

58. Garrett, James L., and Marie T. Ruel. 2005. "Stunted Child–Overweight Mother Pairs: Prevalence and Association with Economic Development and Urbanization." *Food and Nutrition Bulletin* 26 (2): 209-21. https://doi.org/10.1177/156482650502600205.

59. World Food Programme. n.d. "Yemen Emergency." https://www.wfp.org/emergencies/yemen/.

60. "Afghanistan." n.d. World Food Programme. http://www1.wfp.org/countries/afghanistan.

61. World Health Organization, and UNICEF. 2003. "Global Strategy for Infant and Young Child Feeding." Geneva, Switzerland: World Health Organization.

62. World Health Organization. 2005. "Guiding Principles for Feeding Non-Breastfed Children 6-24 Months of Age." Geneva, Switzerland: World Health Organization, Department of Child and Adolescent Health and Development.

63. WHO Multicentre Growth Reference Study Group. 2006. "WHO Child Growth Standards: Methods and Development." Geneva, Switzerland: World Health Organization.

64. Bhutta, Zulfiqar A., Jai K. Das, Arjumand Rizvi, Michelle F. Gaffey, Neff Walker, Susan Horton, Patrick Webb, et al. 2013. "Evidence-Based Interventions for Improvement of Maternal and Child Nutrition: What Can Be Done and at What Cost?" *The Lancet* 382 (9890): 452–77. https://doi.org/10.1016/S0140-6736(13)60996-4.

65. Adu-Afarwuah, Seth, Anna Lartey, Harriet Okronipa, Per Ashorn, Janet M Peerson, Mary Arimond, Ulla Ashorn, Mamane Zeilani, et al. 2016. "Small-Quantity, Lipid-Based Nutrient Supplements Provided to Women during Pregnancy and 6 Mo Postpartum and to Their Infants from 6 Mo of Age Increase the Mean Attained Length of 18-Mo-Old Children in Semi-Urban Ghana: A Randomized Controlled Trial." *American Journal of Clinical Nutrition* 104 (3): 797–808. https://doi.org/10.3945/ajcn.116.134692.

66. Hess, Sonja Y., Souheila Abbeddou, Elizabeth Yakes Jimenez, Jérôme W. Somé, Stephen A. Vosti, Zinéwendé P. Ouédraogo, Rosemonde M. Guissou, et al. 2015. "Small-Quantity Lipid-Based Nutrient Supplements, Regardless of Their Zinc Content, Increase Growth and Reduce the Prevalence of Stunting and Wasting in Young Burkinabe Children: A Cluster-Randomized Trial." Edited by James G. Beeson. *PLoS One* 10 (3): e0122242. https://doi.org/10.1371/journal.pone.0122242.

67. Maleta, Kenneth M., John Phuka, Lotta Alho, Yin Bun Cheung, Kathryn G. Dewey, Ulla Ashorn, Nozgechi Phiri, et al. 2015. "Provision of 10–40 g/d Lipid-Based Nutrient Supplements from 6 to 18 Months of Age Does Not Prevent Linear Growth Faltering in Malawi." *Journal of Nutrition* 145 (8): 1909–15. https://doi.org/10.3945/jn.114.208181.

68. Arnold, Benjamin F., Clair Null, Stephen P. Luby, Leanne Unicomb, Christine P. Stewart, Kathryn G. Dewey, Tahmeed Ahmed, et al. 2013. "Cluster-Randomised Controlled Trials of Individual and Combined Water, Sanitation, Hygiene and Nutritional Interventions in Rural Bangladesh and Kenya: The WASH Benefits Study Design and Rationale." *BMJ Open* 3 (8): e003476. https://doi.org/10.1136/bmjopen-2013-003476.

PART THREE

Influences on Nutrition

12

Environmental Determinants of Nutrition-Related Health in High-Income Countries: Focus on the Neighborhood Food Environment

Kimberly B. Morland

LEARNING OBJECTIVES

- Describe the theoretical pathways by which our food environments can influence dietary intake and nutrition-related chronic diseases
- Describe the scientific evidence for the associations between food environments and dietary intake
- Understand different study designs used to evaluate the relationship between the food environment and dietary intake

Case Study: Restricted Local Food Environments in the United States—First-Person Perspectives from Residents of Brooklyn Neighborhoods

"I'm tired of eating this food—rotten vegetables, rotten fruit, with high prices—and getting sick. I've gotten food poisoning before, and I'm tired of getting sick. You know they're repackaging food and they're very slick; they put all the good vegetables on the top, and all the bad stuff on the bottom or in the middle. They try to fool the customers."

"Our local store has rotten meat—I have seen meat that is actually green. Meat isn't supposed to be green. And they have it out for display! It's like we're worse than dogs; it's sickening. One time I bought their chicken, and it was slimy to the touch, and it was rotten. I'm sure the owners wouldn't eat it. And I don't understand—is it just because this is East New York, or a low-income, black community? What happened to the Health Department inspectors that are supposed to inspect these stores?"

"The supermarkets around here are horrible. I like hummus, and none of the supermarkets here carry hummus. I usually get my co-workers that have health food stores in their neighborhood to bring it to me. I like health food, but to stores in my neighborhood, fruit is considered health food."

"When my family was young, I used to go to neighborhoods in Queens to shop because the food was so healthy—and we didn't get sick that often. But why should I have to go to Queens when I live in East New York? And, especially in this neighborhood, we just bury our heads in the sand. We need to confront these issues. We need to think about others, not only about ourselves."

"The politicians here wouldn't eat half of the food that's available to us."

Our food choices are influenced by the contexts in which we live. These contexts include a broad array of factors at different levels. At the country level, our context is shaped by economic development, levels of income inequality, as well as economic, political, and food systems, to name a few.[1] At the local level, our contexts can be shaped by local institutions such as schools, workplaces, or health care systems. The Institute for Medicine has also recognized the "messaging environment," including advertising, as an important environmental factor that likely influences food choice. Additionally, our residential neighborhoods are an important component of the context or environments in which we live. Our local neighborhood context can also modify the extent to which we experience the broader environmental context. For instance, living in a neighborhood devoid of parks, playgrounds, and conveniently located healthy food, or one saturated with conveniently located unhealthy food, can make it difficult to eat healthfully or participate in physical activity. Our individual circumstances can additionally modify how we experience our local and broader environments. Living in a neighborhood with conveniently located healthy food may not affect our intake if we cannot afford that food (the prices of which are shaped by the larger economic and political systems).

Clearly, there are many potential environmental determinants of our food intake. However, perhaps the most widely studied of these determinants in the United States is the neighborhood food environment. For this reason, this chapter will focus primarily on what is known about how our neighborhood food environments are associated with our dietary intake and nutrition-related chronic disease.

The influence of individual-level factors, such as nutrition knowledge, is well accepted as a predictor of an individual's dietary choices. More recently, research suggests that our local food environments, including conveniently located food, may also be influential in our dietary choices. Although much of this literature has been conducted within the United States, issues regarding access to healthy food options have been investigated in Europe, Australia, Japan, and Canada. This area of public health nutrition relies heavily on examining the placement of food retailers in relation to other neighborhood characteristics, dietary behaviors, or health outcomes.[2] To appreciate the concept of *conveniently located food*, one must first understand how food retailers locate their stores in high-income countries and the historical context of the food policies that contributed to the food retail market as it is currently structured.

Briefly, the food retail market is embedded in a larger food industry, where food retailers make profit-driven decisions about the products to be sold and their prices, as well as the best locations to place their stores. Using the United States as an example, the modern food retailer utilizes mass merchandising, defined as stimulating a high inventory turnover with a small net profit

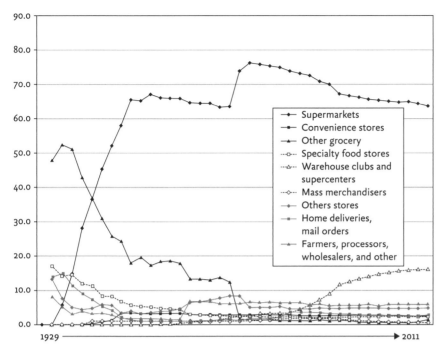

Figure 12.1. Proportion of food sales by type of food retailer: USA 1926–2011. *Source:* USDA ERS. *Local Food Environments: Food Access in America.* Kimberly Morland (Ed). "Introduction." Copyright 2015.

margin in order to make a profit. The development of large grocery stores (e.g., supermarkets, see figure 12.1) over the past century has allowed retailers to offset the lower profit margin of one type of food with the higher margins of many other products sold. For example, the introduction of processed nonperishable foods has impacted the profitability for food retailers because it allows grocers to increase their stock without being concerned about perishability, unlike the risk involved in stocking fresh foods, such as fruit and vegetables. A typical supermarket sells roughly 38,000 different items that generate revenue from a relatively small profit margin.[3,4] Relatively little is written in the public health literature about how economic and racial characteristics of neighborhood residents affect the location of commercial establishments. Of all food retailer types, supermarkets hold the greatest proportion of food sales in the United States.[5]

At least in the United States, this trend coincides with the migration patterns of the white middle class toward suburbs during the 1960s, which was spurred by US federal loan programs that made homeownership affordable.[6] The development of suburban residential areas also allowed for larger commercial footprints to build new food stores. Hence, the policies that supported this pattern of growth also inadvertently supported a disinvestment of commercial entities within inner cities.[7,8] As just one example, the loss of large grocery stores within urban areas between 1980 and 1990 was documented in a report that investigated 21 American cities and highlighted food delivery distribution problems in the United States—in other words, a disparity in access to food for some Americans.[9] More recent investigations continue to document disparities in the placement of large-scale food stores, such as supermarkets, by either the wealth and/or the racial composition of residents, wherein neighborhoods with lower incomes or with a larger proportion of their population being black or Hispanic/Latino have systematically lower access to healthy food options.[10-19] Some of these studies have shown that the lack of healthy food options is driven by presence or absence of supermarkets within urban centers.[11,15,18-21] Still other studies have documented disparities in the availability of selected healthy foods options independent of supermarket presence, where those differences have been associated with the demographics of residents and geographic factors such as urbanization.[22-26] Many researchers have suggested that supermarkets tend to have lower prices compared to medium-size grocery stores and small stores; however, until recently the few studies that had empirically examined this had inconsistent findings.[15,19,27-29] This burgeoning concern, however, led to a Congressional report from the US Department of Agriculture (USDA) titled, "Access to Affordable and Nutritious Foods: Measuring and Understanding Food Deserts and Their Consequences,"[30] which found:

- food costs are lower within supermarkets compared to smaller stores;
- 11.5 million low-income Americans live more than a mile away from a supermarket; and
- low-income households are more likely to utilize available supercenters, due to lower prices.

Dietary Intake: A Health Behavior

Before examining the environmental determinants of nutrition-related health, it is important to appreciate that dietary intake is a very complicated behavior. There are numerous factors that contribute to this complication. First, dietary intake is a unique, mandatory health behavior (i.e., one must eat to survive) that is typically repeated multiple times a day. Since many foods are unhealthy when eaten in excess, we are challenged to make changes to this mandatory daily behavior through exchanging less-healthy food for more-healthy food. Second, it has been estimated that we make an average of 200 food-related decisions each day, and these decisions are processed in a series of interrelated thoughts and feelings that can be influenced by other factors, such as cognitive issues, food preferences, and hunger.[31-33] Each eating event can be described with a series of decisions described in figure 12.2.[4] Third, at best, dietary decisions are made by individuals who can assess the relationship between their dietary choices and impact on disease risk.

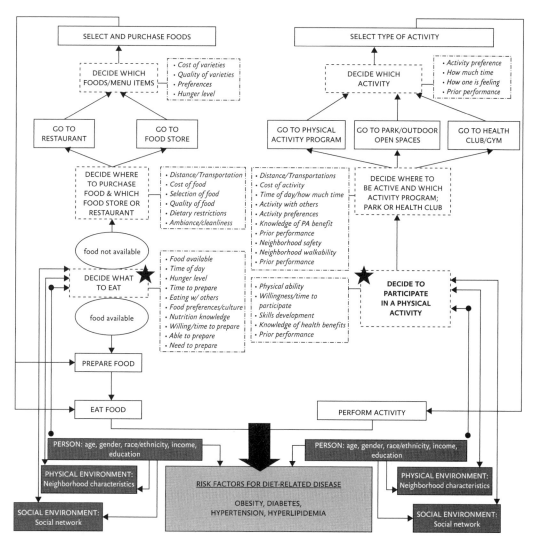

Figure 12.2. The decision tree influencing dietary intake and diet-related diseases.
Source: Reprinted with permission from *Local Food Environments: Food Access in America.*
Kimberly Morland (Ed). "Introduction." Copyright 2015.

Although an individual may make those decisions multiple times per day, for public health scientists, it is the long-term effect of "usual" dietary intake that is hypothesized to influence the occurrence of diet-related diseases. Because dietary intake is an intermediate between the local food environment and diet-related health outcomes, all concerns related to measuring diet are important in the studies that measure the impact of environmental determinants of nutrition-related diseases.

Health Behavior Theory, Dietary Intake, and Food Environments

Many of the traditional health behavior theories do not explicitly consider how our environment might influence our health behaviors. For example, the **knowledge-attitude-behavior model (KABM)** postulates that, as a person accumulates knowledge, attitudes begin to change and, in turn, as attitudes shift and develop, behavior change is increasingly likely to occur. The **health belief model** adds to the principal behind KABM but contributes the idea that an individual must use knowledge to perceive risks or benefits before a behavior change will occur. Both models focus on individuals' knowledge and have been the cornerstone of health education campaigns to increase fruit and vegetable consumption, such as the widely disseminated "5-a-day" campaign. As the evidence of the disparities in the placement of healthy food retailers has grown, public health investigators have considered existing health behavior models as potential frameworks for evaluating how the placement of food retailers (e.g., supermarkets, fast-food restaurants) may affect dietary choices and subsequent risk for diet-related diseases.[34-36]

While social cognitive theory (SCT) stresses that whether an individual has high self-efficacy with regard to achieving a changed dietary behavior is fostered by the modeling and reinforcement of that behavior, the model also posits that the availability of the necessary environmental resources (e.g., the convenient availability of healthy foods) is also an important determinant of behavior.[37,38] However, behavioral interventions that use this model often focus on self-efficacy without consideration of the environmental support.[34] To date, researchers interested in considering the physical environment as a causal factor related to health behaviors have looked toward the socio-ecological model or the **ecological model (EM)**. The EM suggests that proximal factors affecting behavior change (such as a response to a stimuli as described in behavioral learning theory or perceived benefit as described in the health belief model) need to be considered within the environments where people live, work, and play. The ecological model posits that an individual's behaviors are affected by a series of inter-related systems including: (1) a micro-system (e.g., family and peers), (2) an exo-system (e.g., social and health service; food stores), and (3) a macro-system (e.g., culture, legislation).[37] This theory has been used effectively to show that both neighborhood aesthetics and the convenience of physical activity facilities are important environmental factors associated with greater physical activity.[39]

The use of the ecological model to guide neighborhood food environmental interventions proves to be more difficult.[40] Unlike city parks, food retailing is entirely privately owned in high-income countries. Consequently, unlike local or state parks that can have physical attributes changed by government agencies, local jurisdictions have no legal authority to impose any modifications to the products sold and have limited influence on the prices (i.e., taxes) that are set by retailers. Some influence on the placement of a food retailer's stores might be accomplished by zoning restriction, however in general there is no federal legislation that ensures all Americans have the same convenient access to foods. In the United States, the Farm Bill, which governs commodity foods and the many USDA nutrition programs, is an important vehicle for legislation around many public health nutrition issues; but it creates no authority or oversight over food retailers' private business practices. Legislators have only recently begun to attempt to utilize aspects of the Farm Bill to regulate foods that can be sold in private businesses (e.g., such as minimum stocking requirements for stores that accept WIC and SNAP benefits).[41]

Identifying the most applicable behavioral theory is further complicated in studies aiming to measure the effect of the environmental determinants on nutrition-related health, primarily because these studies aim to assess a series of behavioral changes that happen sequentially. For example, the relationship between opening a new store and improved dietary intake is measurable by the following sequence of individual behaviors: (1) the adoption of the new store, (2) change in purchasing patterns within the new store, and (3) change in dietary intake. The **transtheoretical model** (also called stages of change) proposes a person moves through a series of five states before a new behavior is fully adopted (e.g., an individual moves from precontemplative to contemplative, then to planning, action, and finally maintenance of a given behavior). However, the amount of time it takes to move through these stages is unclear and most certainly will vary for different behaviors. Using this model to try and understand how the local food environment may impact food consumption, one can reasonably assume that the introduction of a new food store would first set a resident into a precontemplative state, whereby they would have to consider whether or not it was to their benefit to change his or her existing food shopping behavior (e.g., start shopping at the new food store). This can be illustrated with the opening of the community-owned and operated food store in East New York.[42] Although the neighborhood is otherwise a food desert, the surrounding community did not flood the front door of the cooperative on opening day, or the day after, for that matter. Sales records were certainly a testament to the slow adoption of the store as a regular source of groceries for most cooperative members. But critical feedback from a community member offered insight into other reasons for the slow adoption—namely, community skepticism that the new food store would stay in business, because most businesses historically failed in that neighborhood.[43] The point here is that, without uncovering and addressing this issue directly, the residents may have remained in a precontemplative period thus preventing the success of the intervention.

Food Environment and Dietary Intake

Interest in the potential role of the food environment on food intake has grown tremendously over the last 10-15 years; many studies and multiple systematic reviews have assessed this relationship. The vast majority of studies on the relationship between food environments and dietary intake have been cross-sectional observational studies; however, in more recent years, a handful of longitudinal observational studies have emerged, as well as some quasi-experimental studies. We will briefly summarize the evidence to date, beginning with the smaller body of quasi-experimental evidence and then examining what we have learned so far from the observational evidence.

Experimental Evidence

Truly experimental evidence on how the neighborhood food environment impacts dietary intake is not currently available since it is difficult, if not impossible, to randomly assign individuals to different types of food environments and then follow them long enough to detect any potential changes in their diets. However, researchers have been able to study the impact of new supermarket openings on dietary intake for residents living nearby using quasi-experimental study designs. Over a decade ago, Cummins et al.[44] conducted a longitudinal study in the United Kingdom comparing fruit and vegetable consumption of 412 households before and after the opening of a supermarket and concluded there was no association between the presence of supermarkets and fruit and vegetable consumption 10 months post-intervention. More recently, four similar studies have been conducted in the United States. For example, using a quasi-experimental design, Sadler et al. conducted a longitudinal study of 352 US adults who were the primary shoppers for their households. Ten months after the store opened, no association was detected between the opening of the new supermarket and changes in fruit and vegetable consumption among study participants.[45] The authors of this study hypothesized that the price point of the new store may have been too high for residents to switch to shopping there. A quasi-experimental study of a new supermarket in a Philadelphia neighborhood found an improved sense of healthy food availability but no change in diet or body mass index (BMI). A quasi-experimental study in New York City found similar results, with no change in healthy food intake. A similar study in Pittsburgh had slightly more encouraging findings—it found an improvement in diet; however, this improvement was not associated with shopping at the new supermarket. Researchers found increases in income and health in the neighborhood that received the supermarket compared to the comparison neighborhood, but it is unclear whether these changes can be attributed to the supermarket or to other factors simultaneously occurring in the neighborhood.[46]

Recalling the discussion of the stages of change model as it relates to the hypothesized pathways by which supermarkets are thought to affect behavior, with these studies, it is assumed the participants will move through the precontemplative to action stages for (a) adopting a new store, (b) making changes in food purchases of each type of fruit and vegetable, and (c) consuming each type of fruit and vegetable. Follow-up from these studies ranged from several months to one year. It is possible that it would take longer for residents to move from precontemplative to action in each of these sequential behaviors.

Observational Evidence

While there are only a handful of quasi-experimental studies, the relationship between the food environment and dietary intake has been studied extensively using observational cross-sectional data. Researchers conducting these studies have grappled with many issues, including the measurement of diet, as well as the conceptual challenges related to determining which aspects of dietary intake would likely be affected by the local food environment (and how to measure those aspects). In addition, investigators have also had to make decisions regarding how to define and measure the local food environments—for example, which food outlets to measure (supermarkets, grocery stores, small corner markets, convenience stores, fast-food and other types of restaurants) and at what geographical unit (e.g., distance to the closest, density within a specified geographical unit [census track, 1-mile buffer, ZIP code, county, etc.]). Finally, other factors may be involved in food purchasing, such as income and transportation, which should also be considered as influencing factors in these evaluations.

Studies that have investigated the relationship between the local food environments of residents have been conducted in the United States, Australia, United Kingdom, Canada, and Japan. Caspi et al. provides a summary of findings from 38 studies conducted between 1991 and 2011.[47] The review includes studies that measured associations between diet and the following: (1) perceived food environment; (2) store presence/density; (3) distance/travel time; and/or (4) in-store measures, such as product availability, price, and quality. Many studies have found positive associations between local food environments and various aspects of diet. However, there is little consistency across studies about what aspects of diet are susceptible to the influences of the local environment for food. Below we summarize studies that have assessed the relationship between food environments and fruit and/or vegetable intake and fast-food intake, since these are two of the more commonly examined outcomes.

Fruits and/or Vegetables

A seminal study conducted in four states of the United States showed that there was a 32% higher intake of fruit and vegetable servings per week for black Americans for each additional supermarket located in his or her neighborhood.[48] Other studies have corroborated these findings, concluding: (a) the proximity to a supermarket or large grocery store is positively associated with fruit and vegetable intake;[49-51] (b) distance and access to a supermarket and fruit intake are inversely associated in both rural and urban areas of the United States;[52-54] and (c) studies have documented these associations among adults, adolescents, and children.[55-62] For example, an inverse relationship between distance to supermarkets and meeting the recommendation of five or more servings of fruits and vegetables per day was documented at the county level across the United States using the Behavioral Risk Factor Surveillance System.[54] Zenk evaluated the relationship between the presence of large grocery stores in Detroit, Michigan, and found supermarket availability was positively associated with fruit and vegetable intake.[49] More recent studies in the United Stated have focused on objective versus perceived access to recommended foods, as well as food store density. These studies have not shown perceived measurements of food convenience to be associated with intake.[55,63]

In countries outside of the United States, fewer investigators have found associations between local food environments and dietary intake, suggesting that perhaps these high-income countries may have policies or practices that affect food distribution differently than in the United States.[44,64-70] Additionally, there are also US-based studies that have not shown associations. For example, Beydoun focused solely on the influence of price on fruit and vegetable consumption and did not find an association between price and dietary intake,[64] whereas Powell found that young adults living in neighborhoods with higher-priced fruits and vegetables had lower intakes of those foods.[61] Christian et al. used global positioning tracking data of 121 US adults over a three-day period, linking the GPS data to dietary survey data, and found nonsignificant associations between the food environment and intake of fruits and vegetables, whole grains, or added sugar.[65] This new method of measuring the local food environment and small sample size may explain the null findings. Another US-based study did not find any associations between the availability of healthy foods in the stores where women shopped (assessed using the in-store tool called the Nutrition Environment Measures Survey in Stores [NEMS-S]) and their fruit and vegetable intake.[55] The 186 women in the study sample ate four servings of fruit and vegetables per day on average, which is nearly the recommended number of servings per day. Additionally, the study population was drawn from women enrolled in a weight loss intervention study, who might have been highly motivated to eat fruits and vegetables during the study, so, in addition to this study reflecting only the stores where the women chose to shop, these null findings could be due to the nature of the study (i.e., being embedded in a weight loss study).

There are few examples of longitudinal studies measuring the impact of the local food environment on diet. One study was conducted using a longitudinal cardiovascular US-based cohort (CARDIA study), where diet was measured among young adults (aged 18-30 years old) multiple times over a 15-year study.[71] The authors added to the CARDIA study by using commercially available databases to determine the availability of fast-food chains, su-permarkets, or grocery stores during the same time period and used Geo-graphical Information Systems (GIS) to measure the density of supermarkets and other food stores within a series of distances from the respondents' homes. The cohort was followed over time and individual socioeconomic variables were controlled for in analyses of the relationship between the local food environment and dietary outcomes. It was concluded that al-though some association was detected for men, there was little evidence supporting a causal relationship between neighborhood availability of su-permarket and meeting fruit and vegetable recommendations. However, this study is also limited by the use of historical records to quantify the lo-cal food environment[72] and use of statistical methods that were inconsistent with existing studies, then making comparisons to the current literature challenging.

Fast-Food Consumption

Whereas studies that have investigated the environmental determinants of fruit and vegetable consumption have focused on the availability of this food group within food stores primarily, the investigation of fast food from fast-food vendors has also been investigated. It is worth pointing out that the decision pathway for eating described in figure 12.2 includes a pointed deci-sion of where to purchase food. Away-from-home food preparation has be-come increasingly popular in the United States, with an estimate that 75% of Americans eat outside of their homes at least once a week.[73] The food in-dustry has responded to this growing need for eating outside of the home, with the number of full- and limited-service restaurants in the last decade increasing substantially.[74] For example, it has been estimated that in the United States, foods purchased at fast-food restaurants account for a signifi-cant proportion of daily energy in children.[75] It has also been documented that fast-food consumption is associated with higher BMI[76,77] and metabolic disorders.[78,79] The hypothesis that the availability of fast-food vendors may promote increased consumption of food from these retailers is consistent with the supermarket and fruit and vegetable research. Numerous studies have measured the availability of fast-food restaurants using GIS to either produce density measurements (e.g., number of fast-food restaurants per area) or distance measurements (e.g., distance to nearest fast-food restaurant). One large study in California showed that higher residential density of fast-food restaurants was associated with higher fast-food consumption.[57] However, other investigators have had difficulty replicating that finding, concluding there is little evidence of the dietary impact of the residential proximity to these types of food vendors.[48,80-83] Other investigators have considered al-ternative measurements of fast-food availability, including perception of accessibility—which has shown some associations in the expected direction (e.g., higher perceived accessibility related to higher consumption)[82,84] and fast-food price index.[85]

Researchers have included other outcomes of dietary intake in their research, including meeting dietary recommendations for fat consumption and sodium, overall diet quality as assessed by the healthy eating index, as well as other specific food groups such as milk, meat, and whole grains. However, these outcomes are sparse in the literature and therefore it is difficult to assess the reproducibility of findings. Moreover, these dietary outcomes are not specific to one type of food vendor, making the causal relationship between the local food environments and diet more difficult to determine in these evaluations.

Food Environment and Obesity and Other Diet-Related Diseases

Since dietary intake is known to affect obesity and other chronic diseases, studies of the food environment have also been interested in assessing whether food environments are associated with these chronic disease outcomes. Regarding the relationship between the food environment and diet-related diseases, obesity has been studied most extensively. In large epidemiologic studies, assessment of weight status is easier and cheaper than assessment of dietary intake, which may contribute to why so many studies have examined the relationship between food environments and obesity. Over 50 studies have recently been reviewed for the relationship between weight and aspects of local food environments.[86-89] Authors conclude that the evidence in the United States is mixed regarding the relationship between obesity and food environments. A second recent systematic review included 71 studies and additionally examined study quality.[90] This review found that the vast majority of studies were cross-sectional and of low quality. It also found predominantly null relationships (e.g., no relationship between food environment and obesity). However, of all the non-null relationships, there was some indication that supermarkets were associated with lower prevalence of obesity among adults whereas fast-food restaurants were associated with higher prevalence of obesity for adults and for children living in low-income neighborhoods.[90] A recent longitudinal study studied the effects of a change in food environment for participants who moved to a new residence and found a modest but statistically significant weight loss for those with improved food environments (i.e., an increase in supermarkets in their new neighborhoods).[91]

Overall, the evidence for a direct relationship between local food environments and obesity is not very compelling. The entire body of literature has included study populations of children and adults, racial and ethnic minorities, and people with low socioeconomic backgrounds. Some investigators attribute findings that are null or not in the expected direction to weak study design and methodological limitations.[88,90,91] These authors have argued that many factors related to the food and physical activity environments should be considered in tandem in order to best understand the effects of the neighborhood environment on health outcomes. Furthermore, the body of literature describing the influence of food environments on diet and health is primarily focused on residential environments and not various other sites that could affect individuals' food choices. Tseng and colleagues sought to create an index of neighborhood factors that promote obesity in disadvantaged areas of Victoria, Australia, comprising walkability, food environment, and physical activity environment.[92] Even here, the authors found that "obesity-promoting" neighborhoods were not associated with BMI, nor were any of these three components associated with BMI individually. Studies evaluating the relationship between local food environments and other diet-related diseases (e.g., diabetes, blood pressure, blood cholesterol) are sparse.[78,79,89]

Other Environmental Exposures and Nutrition-Related Outcomes

The health effects of neighborhood characteristics other than food environments have also been considered. Decreases in area-level food prices over time have been associated with increases in BMI.[93] Multilevel analyses have endeavored to understand the interactions between food insecurity, residents' perceptions of their environments and their barriers to healthy eating, neighborhood safety, and property values.

Additionally, neighborhood economic circumstances have been associated with obesity, above and beyond individual socioeconomic position. Specifically, neighborhoods with higher levels of economic deprivation and lower built environment amenities, such as sidewalks and parks and playgrounds, have been associated with higher levels of childhood obesity.[94] In the seminal Moving to Opportunities study, which randomized participants to move from high-poverty neighborhoods to low-poverty neighborhoods, the group randomized to the low-poverty neighborhoods had lower risk of grade II and grade III obesity and diabetes 10 years after randomization.[95]

Finally, other types of interventions to the food environment (broadly considered) have focused on the modification of foods, messaging, or prices within existing retail environments, such as: (a) changes to food labeling; (b) regulatory changes, such as city bans on *trans* fats in restaurants or changes to public school lunch programs; or (c) economic incentives and disincentives, such as subsidies or taxation.[86,96,97] For example, alterations to school lunch policies have resulted in positive changes in dietary quality of foods served and dietary consumption among children.[96,98] Also, citywide policies restricting *trans* fats in restaurants have resulted in decreased *trans* fats in purchases made at fast-food restaurants in New York City[97] and have been associated with decreases in heart attacks.[99] These studies have met with greater success, possibly because investigators had direct control over the targeted aspect of the food environment in their research, and/or because populations affected would have to go to greater lengths to avoid being influenced by the policy or intervention. For example, students would have to actively opt out of receiving and consuming the healthier lunches or travel far distances to find food cooked with *trans* fats. In other words, these might be more controlled studies and/or they could represent more effective mechanisms for inducing difficult behavior change. Other policy interventions to the food environment are discussed in more detail in chapter 14.

Conclusion

Similar to the studies that aim to show an association between the local food environments and diet, the research that aims to show a more distal relationship with health outcomes are also in need of behavioral theories and realistic causal mechanisms to guide this science.[100] Health outcomes are rarely promoted by a single cause, and this is certainly true for obesity, diabetes, hypertension, and other diseases—all of which are hypothesized to be influenced by the local food environment (whether in the occurrence and/or management of the disease). The underpinnings of these studies reasonably assume that the relationship between the local food environment and disease is mediated through dietary intake, yet this relationship has not been demonstrated for all groups of people. Therefore, it is unlikely that the local food environment would affect diet-related health outcomes universally.

Perhaps this is the very point of this growing body of research; which is to say some groups of people are more sensitive to the effect of conveniently available food. Recall the 200 dietary decisions made daily and the factors involved in each of those decisions depicted in figure 12.2. As researchers and practitioners, it is customary to assume that each of those decisions are met with clear intention, such that a resulting poor diet falls directly on the shoulders of the person making those decisions. This growing body of research over the past two decades has given people living in varying levels of food deserts a voice to respond to that assertion. For some groups of people, such as the ones quoted at the beginning of this chapter, the types of foods conveniently available to them matter a great deal. Does this sensitive subpopulation shop outside of their immediate neighborhood for food? Yes. Do they do that because the healthy foods they desire are not available to them locally? Yes. Would this behavior affect our ability as researchers to detect an association between local food environments and dietary intake? Yes. Does this mean it is adequate to have disparities in local food environments in high-income countries?

Researchers continue to conduct studies aiming to measure the relationship between local food environments, diets, and diet-related diseases. However, nearly two decades into forming this public health literature, investigators continue to use secondary datasets, follow cross-sectional designs, and recycle the same research questions. It may be time to modify the research questions. One approach would be to focus clearly on the behavior of interest—dietary intake (a complicated and mandatory behavior). For example, using behavioral theory and a decision tree (such as the one described in figure 12.2), investigators can ask how an individual's use of the local food environment fits into each of those iterative decisions. More detailed qualitative work, such as a grocery shopping tag-along study that was conducted to observe food purchasing patterns of urban older adults, may be needed.[101] This contextual work may allow researchers and nutritionists to better understand the complicated steps involved in obtaining food for some groups of people that may be more susceptible to their local food environments. Qualitative work may offer a formative perspective to inform where changes in local food environments may have the greatest impact. For example, using mixed methods, investigators can begin to improve their research questions by aiming to understand the mechanistic influence of conveniently available foods and begin to target group(s) of people that are most vulnerable to its influence.

The fact is, the quantitative methods used to date to determine the environmental determinants of dietary behaviors and outcomes may be too blunt, and the research questions may simply be too broad. Researchers have agreed that there are disparities in local food environments. But assessing how those disparities may influence a health behavior that is mandatorily repeated multiple times per day requires a precise tool that can probe numerous points along the decision tree. Investigators have called for better research methods, usually referring to study designs; however, neighborhood-level interventions are perhaps premature without identifying the point of intervention and the groups of people to target. Arguably, we need smaller, mixed-methods studies that are informed by behavioral theories to better understand *how* the local food environment influences dietary intake. Until this relationship is fully understood, it will be difficult to effectively produce public health prevention programs centered around this environmental determinant in order to prevent diet-related diseases.

In the meantime, government agencies like the USDA will continue to monitor areas for disparities in access to food, while states like Pennsylvania will continue broad approaches in reducing disparities between local food environments with hopes to be implementing primary prevention for diet-related diseases.[30,100]

Review Questions

1. Describe the limitations in determining the causal relationship between the convenient availability of healthy foods and individuals' diets.
2. Use Google Maps to measure the distance from your home to the food stores where you purchase most of your groceries. How far is it? What type of

transportation do you use? How many other food stores do you pass before you get to your store? Does this store have all of the foods you need? If not, what do you do? Are you satisfied with the quality and prices? If not, what do you do?

3. Identify the nearest geographic area to your residential neighborhood where 50% of the population are living below the poverty line (in the United States, you can use US Census data: https://www.census.gov/quickfacts/fact/table /PST045217). Select an address from this area and use Goggle Maps to select the nearest grocery store to that address. Visit that grocery store. Compare it to your grocery store by answering these questions: Are the types of products similar? Are the prices similar? Evaluate the quality of the produce. Would you shop at this store? How far would someone living in this neighborhood have to travel to shop at your grocery store?

Acknowledgments

Thanks to Corrine Munoz-Plaza, MPH, at CMP Consulting for providing the qualitative quotes on page 271 and Susan Filomena at the Icahn School of Medicine at Mount Sinai for assisting in the preparation of this chapter.

References

1. Swinburn, Boyd A., Gary Sacks, Kevin D. Hall, Klim McPherson, Diane T. Finegood, Marjory L. Moodie, and Steven L. Gortmaker. 2011. "The Global Obesity Pandemic: Shaped by Global Drivers and Local Environments." *The Lancet* 378 (9793): 804–14. https://doi.org/10.1016/S0140-6736.

2. US Department of Agriculture (USDA), and Economic Research Service. n.d. "Food at Home: Total Expenditure Table 2." http://www.ers.usda.gov/data -products/food-expenditures.aspx#26634.

3. Food Marketing Institute. 2010. http://www.fmi.org.

4. Morland, Kimberly B. 2015. "Introduction." In *Local Food Environments: Food Access in America*, edited by Kimberly B. Morland, 1st ed. Boca Raton, FL: CRC Press, Taylor & Francis Group.

5. US Census Bureau, and the Bureau of Labor Statistics. n.d. "USDA ERS AER-575." Washington, DC.

6. Helper, Rose. 1970. *Racial Policies and Practices of Real Estate Brokers*. Minneapolis: University of Minnesota Press.

7. US House of Representatives Select Committee on Hunger. 1992. "Urban Grocery Gap." Washington, DC.

8. US House of Representatives Select Committee on Hunger. 1987. *Obtaining Food: Shopping Constraints on the Poor*. Washington, DC.

9. Cotterill, Ronald W., and Andrew W. Franklin. 1995. "The Urban Grocery Store Gap." Issue Paper 08. University of Connecticut, Department of Agricultural and Resource Economics, Charles J. Zwick Center for Food and Resource Policy.

10. Filomena, Susan, Kathleen Scanlin, and Kimberly B. Morland. 2013. "Brooklyn, New York Foodscape 2007–2011: A Five-Year Analysis of Stability in Food Retail Environments." *International Journal of Behavioral Nutrition and Physical Activity* 10 (1): 46. https://doi.org/10.1186/1479-5868-10-46.

11. Morland, Kimberly, and Susan Filomena. 2007. "Disparities in the Availability of Fruits and Vegetables between Racially Segregated Urban Neighbourhoods." *Public Health Nutrition* 10 (12). https://doi.org/10.1017/S1368980007000079.

12. Moore, Latetia V., and Ana V. Diez Roux. 2006. "Associations of Neighborhood Characteristics with the Location and Type of Food Stores." *American Journal of Public Health* 96 (2): 325-31. https://doi.org/10.2105/AJPH.2004.058040.

13. Morland, Kimberly, Steve Wing, Ana Diez Roux, and Charles Poole. 2002. "Neighborhood Characteristics Associated with the Location of Food Stores and Food Service Places." *American Journal of Preventive Medicine* 22 (1): 23-29. http://www.ncbi.nlm.nih.gov/pubmed/11777675.

14. Powell, Lisa M., Sandy Slater, Donka Mirtcheva, Yanjun Bao, and Frank J. Chaloupka. 2007. "Food Store Availability and Neighborhood Characteristics in the United States." *Preventive Medicine* 44 (3): 189-95. https://doi.org/10.1016/j.ypmed.2006.08.008.

15. Block, Daniel, and Joanne Kouba. 2006. "A Comparison of the Availability and Affordability of a Market Basket in Two Communities in the Chicago Area." *Public Health Nutrition* 9 (7): 837-45. http://www.ncbi.nlm.nih.gov/pubmed/17010248.

16. Zenk, Shannon N., Amy J. Schulz, Barbara A. Israel, Sherman A. James, Shuming Bao, and Mark L. Wilson. 2005. "Neighborhood Racial Composition, Neighborhood Poverty, and the Spatial Accessibility of Supermarkets in Metropolitan Detroit." *American Journal of Public Health* 95 (4): 660-67. https://doi.org/10.2105/AJPH.2004.042150.

17. Sharkey, Joseph R., and Scott Horel. 2008. "Neighborhood Socioeconomic Deprivation and Minority Composition Are Associated with Better Potential Spatial Access to the Ground-Truthed Food Environment in a Large Rural Area." *The Journal of Nutrition* 138 (3): 620-27. https://doi.org/10.1093/jn/138.3.620.

18. Alwitt, Linda F., and Thomas D. Donley. 1997. "Retail Stores in Poor Urban Neighborhoods." *Journal of Consumer Affairs* 31 (1): 139-64. https://doi.org/10.1111/j.1745-6606.1997.tb00830.x.

19. Jetter, Karen M., and Diana L. Cassady. 2006. "The Availability and Cost of Healthier Food Alternatives." *American Journal of Preventive Medicine* 30 (1): 38-44. https://doi.org/10.1016/j.amepre.2005.08.039.

20. Baker, Elizabeth A, Mario Schootman, Ellen Barnidge, and Cheryl Kelly. 2006. "The Role of Race and Poverty in Access to Foods That Enable Individuals to Adhere to Dietary Guidelines." *Preventing Chronic Disease* 3 (3): A76. https://doi.org/10.1152/ajpgi.1992.263.1.G75.

21. Sloane, David C., Allison L. Diamant, LaVonna B. Lewis, Antronette K. Yancey, Gwendolyn Flynn, Lori Miller Nascimento, William J. McCarthy, et al. 2003. "Improving the Nutritional Resource Environment for Healthy Living through Community-Based Participatory Research." *Journal of General Internal Medicine* 18 (7): 568-75. https://doi.org/10.1046/j.1525-1497.2003.21022.x.

22. Horowitz, Carol R., Kathryn A. Colson, Paul L. Hebert, and Kristie Lancaster. 2004. "Barriers to Buying Healthy Foods for People with Diabetes: Evidence of Environmental Disparities." *American Journal of Public Health* 94 (9): 1549-54. http://www.ncbi.nlm.nih.gov/pubmed/15333313.

23. Hosler, Akiko S., Deepa Varadarajulu, Adrienne E. Ronsani, Bonnie L. Fredrick, and Brian D. Fisher. 2006. "Low-Fat Milk and High-Fiber Bread Availability in Food Stores in Urban and Rural Communities." *Journal of Public Health Management and Practice:* 12 (6): 556-62. http://www.ncbi.nlm.nih.gov/pubmed/17041304.

24. Lewis, LaVonna Blair, David C. Sloane, Lori Miller Nascimento, Allison L. Diamant, Joyce Jones Guinyard, Antronette K. Yancey, and Gwendolyn Flynn. 2005. "African Americans' Access to Healthy Food Options in South Los Angeles Restaurants." *American Journal of Public Health* 95 (4): 668-73. https://doi.org/10.2105/AJPH.2004.050260.

25. Fisher, Brian D., and David S. Strogatz. 1999. "Community Measures of Low-Fat Milk Consumption: Comparing Store Shelves with Households." *American Journal of Public Health* 89 (2): 235-37. https://doi.org/10.2105/AJPH.89.2.235.

26. Algert, Susan J., Aditya Agrawal, and Douglas S. Lewis. 2006. "Disparities in Access to Fresh Produce in Low-Income Neighborhoods in Los Angeles." *American Journal of Preventive Medicine* 30 (5): 365-70. https://doi.org/10.1016/j.amepre.2006.01.009.

27. Chung, Chanjin, and Samuel L. Myers. 1999. "Do the Poor Pay More for Food? An Analysis of Grocery Store Availability and Food Price Disparities." *Journal of Consumer Affairs* 33 (2): 276-96. https://doi.org/10.1111/j.1745-6606.1999.tb00071.x.

28. Cole, Shaun, Susan Filomena, and Kimberly Morland. 2010. "Analysis of Fruit and Vegetable Cost and Quality Among Racially Segregated Neighborhoods in Brooklyn, New York." *Journal of Hunger & Environmental Nutrition* 5 (2): 202-15. https://doi.org/10.1080/19320241003800250.

29. Hayes, Lashawn Richburg. 2000. "Are Prices Higher for the Poor in New York City?" *Journal of Consumer Policy* 23 (2): 127-52. https://doi.org/10.1023/A:1006421500820.

30. US Department of Agriculture (USDA). 2009. "Access to Affordable and Nutritious Food: Measuring and Understanding Food Deserts and Their Consequences. Report to Congress." http://www.ers.usda.gov/media/242675/ap036_1.pdf.

31. Wansink, Brian, and Jeffery Sobal. 2007. "Mindless Eating: The 200 Daily Food Decisions We Overlook." *Environment and Behavior* 39 (1): 106-23. https://doi.org/10.1177/0013916506295573.

32. Adam, Tanja C., and Elissa S. Epel. 2007. "Stress, Eating and the Reward System." *Physiology & Behavior* 91 (4): 449-58. https://doi.org/10.1016/j.physbeh.2007.04.011.

33. Epel, Elissa S., Janet Tomiyama, and Mary F. Dallman. 2012. "Stress and Reward: Neural Networks, Eating and Obesity." In *Food and Addiction: A Comprehensive Handbook*, edited by Kelly D. Brownell and Mark S. Gold. New York: Oxford University Press.

34. Baranowski, Tom, Karen W. Cullen, Theresa Nicklas, Deborah Thompson, and Janice Baranowski. 2003. "Are Current Health Behavioral Change Models Helpful in Guiding Prevention of Weight Gain Efforts?" *Obesity Research* 11 (S10): 23S-43S. https://doi.org/10.1038/oby.2003.222.

35. Armitage, Christopher J., and Mark Conner. 2000. "Social Cognition Models and Health Behaviour: A Structured Review." *Psychology & Health* 15 (2): 173-89. https://doi.org/10.1080/08870440008400299.

36. Wetter, Annie C., Jeanne P. Goldberg, Abby C. King, Madeleine Sigman-Grant, Roberta Baer, Evelyn Crayton, Carol Devine, et al. 2009. "How and Why Do Individuals Make Food and Physical Activity Choices?" *Nutrition Reviews* 59 (3): S11-20. https://doi.org/10.1111/j.1753-4887.2001.tb06981.x.

37. Baranowski, Tom, Cheryl L. Perry, and Guy S. Parcel. 2002. "How Individuals, Environments, and Health Behavior Interact: Social Cognitive Theory." In *Health Behavior and Health Education: Theory Research and Practice*, edited by Karen Glanz, Barbara K. Rimer, and K. Viswanath, 3rd ed., 246-79. San Francisco, CA: Jossey-Bass.

38. Contento, Isobel, George I. Balch, Yvonne L. Bronner, L. A. Lytle, S. K. Maloney, C. M. Olson, and S. Sharaga Swadener. 1995. "The Effectiveness of Nutrition Education and Implications for Nutrition Education Policy, Programs, and Research: A Review of Research." *Journal of Nutrition Education* 27 (6): 284-418.

39. Sallis, J. F., T. L. McKenzie, J. E. Alcaraz, B. Kolody, N. Faucette, and M. F. Hovell. 1997. "The Effects of a 2-Year Physical Education Program (SPARK) on Physical Activity and Fitness in Elementary School Students. Sports, Play and Active Recreation for Kids." *American Journal of Public Health* 87 (8): 1328-34. http://www.ncbi.nlm.nih.gov/pubmed/9279269.

40. MacIntyre, Sally, and Anne Ellaway. 2000. "Ecological Approaches: Rediscovering the Role of the Physical and Social Environment." In *Social Epidemiology*, edited by Lisa F. Berkman, Ichiro Kawachi, and Maria Glymour, 2nd ed., 332-48. London: Oxford University Press.

41. Spark, Arlene. 2015. "U.S. Agricultural Policies and the U.S. Food Industry." In *Local Food Environments: Food Access in America*, edited by Kimberly B. Morland, 1st ed. Boca Raton, FL: CRC Press, Taylor & Francis Group.

42. Morland, Kimberly B. 2010. "An Evaluation of a Neighborhood-Level Intervention to a Local Food Environment." *American Journal of Preventive Medicine* 39 (6): e31-38. https://doi.org/10.1016/j.amepre.2010.08.006.

43. Personal Communication ENY Food Co-Op (6/19/2006).

44. Cummins, Steven, Mark Petticrew, Cassie Higgins, Anne Findlay, and Leigh Sparks. 2005. "Large Scale Food Retailing as an Intervention for Diet and Health: Quasi-Experimental Evaluation of a Natural Experiment." *Journal of Epidemiology and Community Health* 59 (12): 1035 LP-1040. http://jech.bmj.com/content/59/12/1035.abstract.

45. Sadler, Richard, Jason Gilliland, and Godwin Arku. 2013. "A Food Retail-Based Intervention on Food Security and Consumption." *International Journal of Environmental Research and Public Health* 10 (8): 3325-46. https://doi.org/10.3390/ijerph10083325.

46. Richardson, Andrea S., Madhumita Ghosh-Dastidar, Robin Beckman, Karen R. Flórez, Amy DeSantis, Rebecca L. Collins, and Tamara Dubowitz. 2017. "Can the Introduction of a Full-Service Supermarket in a Food Desert Improve Residents' Economic Status and Health?" *Annals of Epidemiology* 27 (12): 771-76. https://doi.org/10.1016/j.annepidem.2017.10.011.

47. Caspi, Caitlin E., Glorian Sorensen, S. V. Subramanian, and Ichiro Kawachi. 2012. "The Local Food Environment and Diet: A Systematic Review." *Health & Place* 18 (5): 1172-87. https://doi.org/10.1016/j.healthplace.2012.05.006.

48. Morland, Kimberly, Steve Wing, and Ana Diez Roux. 2002. "The Contextual Effect of the Local Food Environment on Residents' Diets: The Atherosclerosis Risk in Communities Study." *American Journal of Public Health* 92 (11): 1761–67. http://www.ncbi.nlm.nih.gov/pubmed/12406805.

49. Zenk, Shannon N., Laurie L. Lachance, Amy J. Schulz, Graciela Mentz, Srimathi Kannan, and William Ridella. 2009. "Neighborhood Retail Food Environment and Fruit and Vegetable Intake in a Multiethnic Urban Population." *American Journal of Health Promotion* 23 (4): 255–64. https://doi.org/10.4278/ajhp.071204127.

50. Casagrande, Sarah Stark, Melicia C. Whitt-Glover, Kristie J. Lancaster, Angela M. Odoms-Young, and Tiffany L. Gary. 2009. "Built Environment and Health Behaviors Among African Americans." *American Journal of Preventive Medicine* 36 (2): 174–81. https://doi.org/10.1016/j.amepre.2008.09.037.

51. Zenk, Shannon N., Amy J. Schulz, Teretha Hollis-Neely, Richard T. Campbell, Nellie Holmes, Gloria Watkins, Robin Nwankwo, and Angela Odoms-Young. 2005. "Fruit and Vegetable Intake in African Americans." *American Journal of Preventive Medicine* 29 (1): 1–9. https://doi.org/10.1016/j.amepre.2005.03.002.

52. Sharkey, Joseph R., Cassandra M. Johnson, and Wesley R. Dean. 2010. "Food Access and Perceptions of the Community and Household Food Environment as Correlates of Fruit and Vegetable Intake among Rural Seniors." *BMC Geriatrics* 10 (1): 32. https://doi.org/10.1186/1471-2318-10-32.

53. Rose, Donald, and Rickelle Richards. 2004. "Food Store Access and Household Fruit and Vegetable Use among Participants in the US Food Stamp Program." *Public Health Nutrition* 7 (08). https://doi.org/10.1079/PHN2004648.

54. Michimi, Akihiko, and Michael C. Wimberly. 2010. "Associations of Supermarket Accessibility with Obesity and Fruit and Vegetable Consumption in the Conterminous United States." *International Journal of Health Geographics* 9 (1): 49. https://doi.org/10.1186/1476-072X-9-49.

55. Gustafson, Alison A., Joseph Sharkey, Carmen D. Samuel-Hodge, Jesse Jones-Smith, Mary Cordon Folds, Jianwen Cai, and Alice S. Ammerman. 2011. "Perceived and Objective Measures of the Food Store Environment and the Association with Weight and Diet among Low-Income Women in North Carolina." *Public Health Nutrition* 14 (6): 1032–38. https://doi.org/10.1017/S1368980011000115.

56. Jago, Russell, Tom Baranowski, Janice C Baranowski, Karen W Cullen, and Debbe Thompson. 2007. "Distance to Food Stores & Adolescent Male Fruit and Vegetable Consumption: Mediation Effects." *International Journal of Behavioral Nutrition and Physical Activity* 4 (1): 35. https://doi.org/10.1186/1479-5868-4-35.

57. Hattori, Aiko, Ruopeng An, and Roland Sturm. 2013. "Neighborhood Food Outlets, Diet, and Obesity Among California Adults, 2007 and 2009." *Preventing Chronic Disease* 10 (March): 120123. https://doi.org/10.5888/pcd10.120123.

58. An, Ruopeng, and Roland Sturm. 2012. "School and Residential Neighborhood Food Environment and Diet Among California Youth." *American Journal of Preventive Medicine* 42 (2): 129–35. https://doi.org/10.1016/j.amepre.2011.10.012.

59. Izumi, Betty T., Shannon N. Zenk, Amy J. Schulz, Graciela B. Mentz, and Christine Wilson. 2011. "Associations between Neighborhood Availability and Individual Consumption of Dark-Green and Orange Vegetables among Ethnically

Diverse Adults in Detroit." *Journal of the American Dietetic Association* 111 (2): 274-79. https://doi.org/10.1016/j.jada.2010.10.044.

60. Bodor, J. Nicholas, Donald Rose, Thomas A. Farley, Christopher Swalm, and Susanne K. Scott. 2008. "Neighbourhood Fruit and Vegetable Availability and Consumption: The Role of Small Food Stores in an Urban Environment." *Public Health Nutrition* 11 (4). https://doi.org/10.1017/S1368980007000493.

61. Powell, Lisa M., Zhenxiang Zhao, and Youfa Wang. 2009. "Food Prices and Fruit and Vegetable Consumption among Young American Adults." *Health & Place* 15 (4): 1064-70. https://doi.org/10.1016/j.healthplace.2009.05.002.

62. Timperio, Anna, Kylie Ball, Rebecca Roberts, Karen Campbell, Nick Andrianopoulos, and David Crawford. 2008. "Children's Fruit and Vegetable Intake: Associations with the Neighbourhood Food Environment." *Preventive Medicine* 46 (4): 331-35. https://doi.org/10.1016/j.ypmed.2007.11.011.

63. Ollberding, Nicholas J., Claudio R. Nigg, Karly S. Geller, Caroline C. Horwath, Rob W. Motl, and Rod K. Dishman. 2012. "Food Outlet Accessibility and Fruit and Vegetable Consumption." *American Journal of Health Promotion* 26 (6): 366-70. https://doi.org/10.4278/ajhp.101215-ARB-401.

64. Beydoun, May A., Lisa M. Powell, and Youfa Wang. 2008. "The Association of Fast Food, Fruit and Vegetable Prices with Dietary Intakes among US Adults: Is There Modification by Family Income?" *Social Science & Medicine* 66 (11): 2218-29. https://doi.org/10.1016/j.socscimed.2008.01.018.

65. Christian, W. Jay. 2012. "Using Geospatial Technologies to Explore Activity-Based Retail Food Environments." *Spatial and Spatio-Temporal Epidemiology* 3 (4): 287-95. https://doi.org/10.1016/j.sste.2012.09.001.

66. Pearce, J., R. Hiscock, T. Blakely, and K. Witten. 2008. "The Contextual Effects of Neighbourhood Access to Supermarkets and Convenience Stores on Individual Fruit and Vegetable Consumption." *Journal of Epidemiology & Community Health* 62 (3): 198-201. https://doi.org/10.1136/jech.2006.059196.

67. Thornton, L. E., D. A. Crawford, and K. Ball. 2010. "Neighbourhood-Socioeconomic Variation in Women's Diet: The Role of Nutrition Environments." *European Journal of Clinical Nutrition* 64 (12): 1423-32. https://doi.org/10.1038/ejcn.2010.174.

68. Pearson, Tim, Jean Russell, Michael J. Campbell, and Margo E. Barker. 2005. "Do 'Food Deserts' Influence Fruit and Vegetable Consumption?—A Cross-Sectional Study." *Appetite* 45 (2): 195-97. https://doi.org/10.1016/j.appet.2005.04.003.

69. Williams, Lauren, Kylie Ball, and David Crawford. 2010. "Why Do Some Socioeconomically Disadvantaged Women Eat Better than Others? An Investigation of the Personal, Social and Environmental Correlates of Fruit and Vegetable Consumption." *Appetite* 55 (3): 441-46. https://doi.org/10.1016/j.appet.2010.08.004.

70. Fuller, Daniel, Steven Cummins, and Stephen A. Matthews. 2013. "Does Transportation Mode Modify Associations between Distance to Food Store, Fruit and Vegetable Consumption, and BMI in Low-Income Neighborhoods?" *American Journal of Clinical Nutrition* 97 (1): 167-72. https://doi.org/10.3945/ajcn.112.036392.

71. Boone-Heinonen, Janne. 2011. "Fast Food Restaurants and Food Stores." *Archives of Internal Medicine* 171 (13): 1162. https://doi.org/10.1001/archinternmed.2011.283.

72. Lehmann, Yael. 2012. "Supermarkets: Components of Causality for Healthy Diets." *Archives of Internal Medicine* 172 (2): 195. https://doi.org/10.1001/archinte.172.2.195-b.

73. Stewart, Hayden, Noel Blisard, and Dean Jolliffe. 2006. "Let's Eat Out: Americans Weigh Taste, Convenience, and Nutrition." *Economic Information Bulletin* no. 19. Economic Research Service, US Department of Agriculture.

74. US Department of Agriculture (USDA), and Economic Research Service. 2012. "The Demand for Disaggregated Food-Away-From-Home and Food-at-Home Products in the United States." http://www.ers.usda.gov/publications/err-economic-research-report/err139.aspx.

75. Poti, Jennifer M., and Barry M. Popkin. 2011. "Trends in Energy Intake among US Children by Eating Location and Food Source, 1977-2006." *Journal of the American Dietetic Association* 111 (8): 1156-64. https://doi.org/10.1016/j.jada.2011.05.007.

76. Duffey, Kiyah J., Penny Gordon-Larsen, David R. Jacobs, O. Dale Williams, and Barry M. Popkin. 2007. "Differential Associations of Fast Food and Restaurant Food Consumption with 3-y Change in Body Mass Index: The Coronary Artery Risk Development in Young Adults Study." *American Journal of Clinical Nutrition* 85 (1): 201-8. https://doi.org/10.1093/ajcn/85.1.201.

77. French, S. A., L. Harnack, and R. W. Jeffery. 2000. "Fast Food Restaurant Use among Women in the Pound of Prevention Study: Dietary, Behavioral and Demographic Correlates." *International Journal of Obesity and Related Metabolic Disorders* 24 (10): 1353-59. http://www.ncbi.nlm.nih.gov/pubmed/11093299.

78. Duffey, Kiyah J., Penny Gordon-Larsen, Lyn M. Steffen, David R. Jacobs, and Barry M. Popkin. 2009. "Regular Consumption from Fast Food Establishments Relative to Other Restaurants Is Differentially Associated with Metabolic Outcomes in Young Adults." *Journal of Nutrition* 139 (11): 2113-18. https://doi.org/10.3945/jn.109.109520.

79. Pereira, Mark A., Alex I. Kartashov, Cara B. Ebbeling, Linda Van Horn, Martha L. Slattery, David R. Jacobs, and David S. Ludwig. 2005. "Fast-Food Habits, Weight Gain, and Insulin Resistance (the CARDIA Study): 15-Year Prospective Analysis." *The Lancet* 365 (9453): 36-42. https://doi.org/10.1016/S0140-6736(04)17663-0.

80. Turrell, Gavin, and Katrina Giskes. 2008. "Socioeconomic Disadvantage and the Purchase of Takeaway Food: A Multilevel Analysis." *Appetite* 51 (1): 69-81. https://doi.org/10.1016/j.appet.2007.12.002.

81. Thornton, Lukar E., Rebecca J. Bentley, and Anne M. Kavanagh. 2009. "Fast Food Purchasing and Access to Fast Food Restaurants: A Multilevel Analysis of VicLANES." *International Journal of Behavioral Nutrition and Physical Activity* 6 (1): 28. https://doi.org/10.1186/1479-5868-6-28.

82. Moore, L. V., A. V. Diez Roux, J. A. Nettleton, D. R. Jacobs, and M. Franco. 2009. "Fast-Food Consumption, Diet Quality, and Neighborhood Exposure to Fast Food: The Multi-Ethnic Study of Atherosclerosis." *American Journal of Epidemiology* 170 (1): 29-36. https://doi.org/10.1093/aje/kwp090.

83. Paquet, Catherine, Mark Daniel, Bärbel Knäuper, Lise Gauvin, Yan Kestens, and Laurette Dubé. 2010. "Interactive Effects of Reward Sensitivity and Residential Fast-Food Restaurant Exposure on Fast-Food Consumption." *The American Journal of Clinical Nutrition* 91 (3): 771-76. https://doi.org/10.3945/ajcn.2009.28648.

84. Inglis, V., K. Ball, and D. Crawford. 2008. "Socioeconomic Variations in Women's Diets: What Is the Role of Perceptions of the Local Food Environment?" *Journal of Epidemiology & Community Health* 62 (3): 191–97. https://doi.org/10.1136 /jech.2006.059253.

85. Beydoun, May A., Lisa M. Powell, Xiaoli Chen, and Youfa Wang. 2011. "Food Prices Are Associated with Dietary Quality, Fast Food Consumption, and Body Mass Index among US Children and Adolescents." *The Journal of Nutrition* 141 (2): 304–11. https://doi.org/10.3945/jn.110.132613.

86. Mayne, S. L., A. H. Auchincloss, and Y. L. Michael. 2015. "Impact of Policy and Built Environment Changes on Obesity-Related Outcomes: A Systematic Review of Naturally Occurring Experiments." *Obesity Reviews* 16 (5): 362–75. https://doi.org/10.1111/obr.12269.

87. Gamba, Ryan J., Joseph Schuchter, Candace Rutt, and Edmund Y. W. Seto. 2015. "Measuring the Food Environment and Its Effects on Obesity in the United States: A Systematic Review of Methods and Results." *Journal of Community Health* 40 (3): 464–75. https://doi.org/10.1007/s10900-014-9958-z.

88. Gordon-Larsen, Penny. 2014. "Food Availability/Convenience and Obesity." *Advances in Nutrition* 5 (6): 809–17. https://doi.org/10.3945/an.114.007070.

89. Zenk, Shannon N., Esther Thatcher, Margarita Reina, and Angela M. Odoms-Young. 2015. "Local Food Environments and Diet Related Health Outcomes: A Systematic Review of Local Food Environments, Body Weight and Other Diet Related Outcomes." In *Local Food Environments: Food Access in America*, edited by Kimberly B. Morland, 1st ed. Boca Raton, FL: CRC Press, Taylor & Francis Group.

90. Cobb, Laura K., Lawrence J. Appel, Manuel Franco, Jessica C. Jones-Smith, Alana Nur, and Cheryl A. M. Anderson. 2015. "The Relationship of the Local Food Environment with Obesity: A Systematic Review of Methods, Study Quality, and Results." *Obesity* 23 (7): 1331–44. https://doi.org/10.1002/oby.21118.

91. Laraia, Barbara A., Janelle M. Downing, Y. Tara Zhang, William H. Dow, Maggi Kelly, Samuel D. Blanchard, Nancy Adler, et al. 2017. "Food Environment and Weight Change: Does Residential Mobility Matter?" *American Journal of Epidemiology* 185 (9): 743–50. https://doi.org/10.1093/aje/kww167.

92. Tseng, Marilyn, Lukar E. Thornton, Karen E. Lamb, Kylie Ball, and David Crawford. 2014. "Is Neighbourhood Obesogenicity Associated with Body Mass Index in Women? Application of an Obesogenicity Index in Socioeconomically Disadvantaged Neighbourhoods." *Health & Place* 30 (November): 20–27. https://doi .org/10.1016/j.healthplace.2014.07.012.

93. Xu, Xin, Jayachandran N. Variyam, Zhenxiang Zhao, and Frank J. Chaloupka. 2014. "Relative Food Prices and Obesity in U.S. Metropolitan Areas: 1976–2001." Edited by C. Mary Schooling. *PLoS ONE* 9 (12): e114707. https://doi.org /10.1371/journal.pone.0114707.

94. Singh, Gopal K., Mohammad Siahpush, and Michael D. Kogan. 2010. "Neighborhood Socioeconomic Conditions, Built Environments, and Childhood Obesity." *Health Affairs* 29 (3): 503–12. https://doi.org/10.1377/hlthaff.2009.0730.

95. Ludwig, Jens, Lisa Sanbonmatsu, Lisa Gennetian, Emma Adam, Greg J. Duncan, Lawrence F. Katz, Ronald C. Kessler, et al. 2011. "Neighborhoods,

Obesity, and Diabetes—A Randomized Social Experiment." *New England Journal of Medicine* 365 (16): 1509-19. https://doi.org/10.1056/NEJMsa1103216.

96. Mullally, Megan L., Jennifer P. Taylor, Stefan Kuhle, Janet Bryanton, Kimberley J. Hernandez, Debbie L. MacLellan, Mary L. McKenna, et al. 2010. "A Province-Wide School Nutrition Policy and Food Consumption in Elementary School Children in Prince Edward Island." *Canadian Journal of Public Health* 101 (1): 40-43. http://www.ncbi.nlm.nih.gov/pubmed/20364537.

97. Angell, Sonia Y., Laura K. Cobb, Christine J. Curtis, Kevin J. Konty, and Lynn D. Silver. 2012. "Change in Trans Fatty Acid Content of Fast-Food Purchases Associated with New York City's Restaurant Regulation." *Annals of Internal Medicine* 157 (2): 81. https://doi.org/10.7326/0003-4819-157-2-201207170-00004.

98. Johnson, Donna B., Mary Podrabsky, Anita Rocha, and Jennifer J. Otten. 2016. "Effect of the Healthy Hunger-Free Kids Act on the Nutritional Quality of Meals Selected by Students and School Lunch Participation Rates." *JAMA Pediatrics* 170 (1): e153918. https://doi.org/10.1001/jamapediatrics.2015.3918.

99. Brandt, Eric J., Rebecca Myerson, Marcelo Coca Perraillon, and Tamar S. Polonsky. 2017. "Hospital Admissions for Myocardial Infarction and Stroke Before and After the Trans-Fatty Acid Restrictions in New York." *JAMA Cardiology* 2 (6): 627. https://doi.org/10.1001/jamacardio.2017.0491.

100. Lehmann, Yael, April White, Jordan Tucker, and Allison Karpyn. 2015. "State-Level Interventions: Pennsylvania's Fresh Food Financing Initiative." In *Local Food Environments: Food Access in America*, edited by Kimberly B. Morland, 1st ed., 273-95. Boca Raton, FL: CRC Press, Taylor & Francis Group.

101. Munoz-Plaza, Corrine E., Kimberly B. Morland, Jennifer A. Pierre, Arlene Spark, Susan E. Filomena, and Philip Noyes. 2013. "Navigating the Urban Food Environment: Challenges and Resilience of Community-Dwelling Older Adults." *Journal of Nutrition Education and Behavior* 45 (4): 322-31. https://doi.org/10.1016/j.jneb.2013.01.015.

13

Underlying Determinants of and Solutions for Malnutrition in Low- and Middle-Income Countries

Marie L. Spiker, Scott B. Ickes, and Jessica Fanzo

LEARNING OBJECTIVES

- Describe the purpose of the Sustainable Development Goals and understand systems approaches to nutrition
- Define the concept of nutrition-sensitive approaches and provide examples from sectors such as agriculture, education, and social safety nets that tackle underlying determinants of malnutrition
- Discuss challenges of implementing nutrition-sensitive approaches and measuring progress to address malnutrition in all its forms

Case Study: Double Burden of Malnutrition in Egypt

Egypt is struggling with the double burden of malnutrition: 21% of children under the age of 5 are stunted, 8% are wasted, and 15% are overweight.[1] This reflects a decline in childhood stunting (down from 35% in 1988), yet the current rates are 20% higher than expected for a country with Egypt's GDP.[2] These trends also reflect a rapid increase in overweight; 85% of adult women are overweight or obese, compared to 58% in 1992.[1] The double burden is present not only at a national scale but also at the household and individual levels: in 2014, 34% of children who were stunted were *also* overweight.[2]

What kind of underlying determinants account for Egypt's declining yet stubbornly high rates of undernutrition and rising rates of overweight and obesity? Egypt has seen marked improvements in its health systems infrastructure over the past few decades, but some things lag behind. Whereas urban residents have almost universal access to improved toilet facilities, 14% of rural residents lack access.[1] Rural areas are more likely to see childhood stunting, whereas urban residents are more likely to be overweight,[1] have diets higher in fat,[3] and consume more convenience foods.[4] Egyptian diets are trending toward more fats, meat, and dairy.[3] Convenience foods such as sugary cakes and cookies are commonly given to children under 2, and these foods have even been found to be perceived as "ideal" complementary foods by some caregivers.[4]

Nutrition in Egypt is also interwoven with larger issues of equity, stability, and agricultural production. Egypt is ranked at 134 out of 144 countries on the Global Gender Gap Index.[5] Only 25% of women participate in the labor force compared to 80% of men, and women's literacy rates lag 15%

behind men's.[5] This is important in light of the fact that the children of women with higher educational attainment are less likely to be stunted.[1] When the global price of staple grains spiked in 2007-2008, soaring prices for bread in Egypt prompted riots that were interlinked with underlying political unrest in what was known as the Arab Spring. Like many countries, food prices in Egypt are influenced by global trends. Egypt imports the majority of its food supply, and the country's dependence on the River Nile for agricultural irrigation poses some unique susceptibilities to climate change.

Addressing both undernutrition and overweight in Egypt will require multisectoral approaches that address many of the "building blocks" described in this chapter—food production, systems infrastructure, health systems, equity and inclusion, and peace and stability. Any approach will also need to be context specific, as Egypt displays remarkable heterogeneity across its geographic and social contexts.

Addressing Underlying Determinants of Nutrition in LMICs Requires Systems Approaches
The Sustainable Development Goals (SDGs)

The **Sustainable Development Goals**—the SDGs—call on the world to approach development differently—that is, to see development across the goals as part of an *integrated whole* and that each goal, working in tandem with the other goals, is essential in order to achieve meaningful, impactful development (figure 13.1). The goals call for all people to work collectively and to do so in a *universal way*, one that ensures no one is left behind on the path toward sustainable development. Nutrition is central to this path. The main architects of the SDGs intended to create a universal agenda and roadmap that was relevant for every country, in contrast to the Millennium Development Goals, which focused on countries dealing with absolute poverty. With this grand agenda, the SDGs also bring significant implications for how to achieve nutrition for everyone.

The SDGs focus on areas such as climate change and natural resources, economic growth, peace, infrastructure, education, and women's empowerment. Many of these areas serve as core underlying determinants of sound nutrition, or are impacted by nutrition. Additionally, two of the SDG targets directly relate to nutrition: SDG 2.2 and SDG 3.4, as box 13.1 illustrates.

Addressing Nutrition-Related SDGs Requires Systems Thinking

Many systems, sectors, disciplines, and actors must come together if the world is to address the multiple burdens of malnutrition. As stated in a letter to *The Lancet* about the SDGs, "system[s] thinking requires a change in mindset: recognizing that the whole is greater than the sum of its parts and contrasting with a traditional, reductionist approach."[6] This allows for a different way of interlinking, analyzing, and solving challenges that moves away

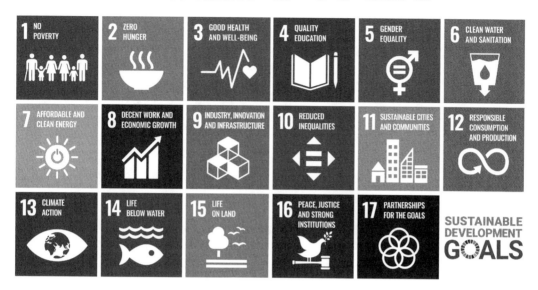

Figure 13.1. Sustainable Development Goals.

from traditional problem-solving in which a complex system is divided into smaller, more digestible parts in isolation.

A **system** can be defined as a network of interconnected parts that operate toward a purpose.[7] The characteristic of interconnectedness is key: changing one part of the system affects other parts. Systems can be categorized by their complexity. A **simple system**, for example, may have just a few elements, and the relationship between those elements may be stable and predictable. An example of a relatively simple system is an automobile: when you press the gas pedal, a throttle valve opens to allows air into the engine. In this way, the gas pedal and the engine are connected in a (hopefully!) predictable way. On the other hand, a **complex system** may have many elements, and the relationships between these elements may be unknown, unpredictable, or they may adapt over time. For example, body weight is not influenced by a single element such as caloric intake; the effect of caloric intake on body weight may be influenced by hormonal signals and changes in the body's metabolic processes over time, and these factors may be further influenced by human behavior and other environmental factors. Table 13.1 shows additional characteristics of complex systems, with examples that draw from the chapter. Using **systems thinking** to address nutrition in low- and middle-income countries (LMICs) involves acknowledging that different components of the system are interconnected and leveraging the interconnectedness of the components rather than ignoring it (see box 13.2).

Box 13.1. Selected SDGs Directly Related to Nutrition

2.2: By 2030, end all forms of malnutrition, including achieving, by 2025, the internationally agreed targets on stunting and wasting in children under 5 years of age, and address the nutritional needs of adolescent girls, pregnant and lactating women, and older persons

- **2.2.1:** Prevalence of stunting (height for age <−2 standard deviation from the median of

the World Health Organization [WHO] Child Growth Standards) among children under 5 years of age

- **2.2.2:** Prevalence of malnutrition (weight for height >+2 or <−2 standard deviation from the median of the WHO Child Growth Standards) among children under 5 years of age, by type (wasting and overweight)

3.4: By 2030, reduce by one-third premature mortality from noncommunicable diseases through prevention and treatment and promote mental health and well-being

- **3.4.1:** Mortality rate attributed to cardiovascular disease, cancer, diabetes, or chronic respiratory disease

Table 13.1. Characteristics of Complex Systems

Characteristic of complex systems	Description	Example
Bidirectional feedback	Two components may affect one another	Undernutrition makes children more susceptible to infectious disease, and infection makes children more susceptible to undernutrition.
Time-delayed responses	Some impacts may not be felt immediately	Exposures to undernutrition during gestation or early life can increase the likelihood of obesity or chronic disease in later life.
Nonlinear relationships	A small change in the system may produce disproportionately large effects	Multiple interventions may produce outcomes that are greater than the sum of their parts. For example, combining micronutrient supplementation with psychosocial stimulation may have synergistic effects on children's cognitive development.
Convergence	Many routes may lead to the same outcome	There is not just one reason that a household could experience increased income; possible sources of income generation include trading high-value agricultural crops or participating in a social safety net program.
Divergence	One route may produce many outcomes	In households where livestock is kept separate from living quarters, raising chickens could help nutritional status through intake of animal-source foods or income generation. But in households where livestock is not separate from living quarters, children's exposure to *Campylobacter* could increase risk of environmental enteric dysfunction and impaired growth.

Box 13.2. Addressing Obesity in LMICs Requires Systems Thinking

Obesity poses a major challenge to the health systems of low- and middle-income countries (LMICs) that are simultaneously struggling with undernutrition and infectious disease. Obesity is an example of a health problem that is created by complex systems and underlying drivers and that requires systems thinking to solve.[38,39] Using systems thinking to address obesity in LMICs means acknowledging the underlying factors that drive obesity, planning interventions that work at multiple levels, and being aware of unintended consequences that may result from single interventions. Although individual-level factors such as knowledge and individual behavior are important, interventions that focus solely on individuals are unlikely to be successful in the absence of efforts to also address societal shifts toward sedentary work and leisure, built environments and food environments, and the larger social and economic factors that shape the architecture of consumers' choices within these environments.

Take, for example, the issue of young children in LMICs consuming packaged convenience foods. These foods are highly palatable, socially desirable, rich in calories and sugar, and largely devoid of the micronutrients frequently lacking in the diets of low-income populations. The convenience of these foods appeals to families with less time to prepare food, such as families with women entering the workforce. These foods are also typically cheaper than nutrient-rich, perishable foods such as fruits, vegetables, and animal-source foods, owing to their shelf stability; this is especially important in rural areas, where fresh seasonal fruits and vegetables are less likely to survive transport without cold storage. Interventions to decrease consumption of packaged convenience foods among youth can include efforts to change individual choice, but they should also address the relative price and accessibility of more nutritious options, factors that increase the desirability of these foods (such as food advertising

targeted toward children), and the underlying conditions that affect food-related behaviors and physical activity (such as employment and neighborhood safety and walkability).

It is difficult to characterize food environments in LMICs as they vary by setting, but there are a number of common challenges. Many LMICs are experiencing patterns of rapid urbanization. Many families leaving rural areas are discontinuing agricultural livelihoods, and in urban areas they are more likely to engage in sedentary occupations.[40] Urbanization also means that women are more likely to enter the formal workforce, which may change their caregiving behaviors. Easy access to convenience foods is one manifestation of rapidly changing food systems in LMICs. LMICs are seeing a rapid proliferation of modern retail outlets rather than traditional markets, increased availability of processed foods, and a trend away from preparing food at home.[41] What is unique and concerning about LMICs is that these changes are still taking place in settings with high rates of micronutrient deficiencies and impaired physical growth, which some characterize as the triple burden of obesity, micronutrient deficiency, and undernourishment.[42]

Addressing obesity in LMICs requires a range of systems-oriented interventions. It should be noted that when intervening on underlying causes, it can be more challenging to demonstrate impact. For example, whereas a sugar-sweetened beverage (SSB) tax (a more proximal intervention) can be studied to assess whether increased prices decrease SSB purchases, for a more distal intervention like investing in urban planning to promote neighborhood safety and walkability, it can be challenging to attribute changes in health outcomes to the intervention. However, this should not be a reason to disengage from the work, but rather it should reinforce the need for research methods, including those from systems science, that are designed to embrace the complexity of the issue.

The Importance of Nutrition-Sensitive Approaches
What Are Nutrition-Sensitive Approaches?

Nutrition-sensitive approaches are approaches that attempt to address the underlying determinants of malnutrition, such as those listed in figure 13.2. Figure 13.2 is an adaptation of the classic UNICEF model of the determinants of undernutrition and undernutrition-related mortality. This rendition depicts the key immediate and underlying causes of malnutrition at the household level as in the UNICEF model. But, whereas the original UNICEF model then depicts "basic causes" such as country-level conditions that shape household conditions, we have substituted "the SDG building blocks" (which are discussed in depth later in the chapter) to provide more specificity about what conditions can be addressed in order to support improved underlying household determinants. Both interventions on the underlying determinants and on the building blocks can be thought of as nutrition-sensitive approaches. Nutrition-sensitive approaches have indirect causal associations with reductions in malnutrition, meaning they impact malnutrition indirectly through mediating mechanisms, rather than directly impacting malnutrition. These approaches include interventions on agriculture and food systems; water, sanitation, and hygiene (WASH); social protection; women's

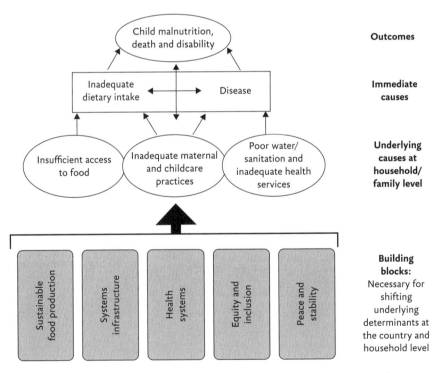

Figure 13.2. Conceptual diagram. *Source:* Adapted from the UNICEF Conceptual Framework[11] and the 2017 Global Nutrition Report.[12]

empowerment; and early childhood development programs. Nutrition-sensitive approaches can serve as delivery platforms for nutrition-specific interventions, which are focused on the more immediate causes of malnutrition shown in figure 13.2, such as inadequate dietary intake or infectious disease. Yet, little research has identified the ways in which individual interventions contribute or interact with larger multisectoral collaborations, nor has it examined the most efficient and systematic measurements to evaluate outcomes when nutrition-specific and nutrition-sensitive approaches are considered as a "package."[8]

Nutrition-sensitive interventions are vital because it is estimated that if nutrition-specific interventions were scaled up to 90% in the 36 countries with the highest burden of stunting, only 20% of stunting would be addressed.[9] In countries that have more successfully addressed undernutrition, much of the reductions have come from nutrition-sensitive approaches. An analysis of stunting rates in 116 countries between 1970 and 2012 showed that key drivers of stunting reductions were safe water access, sanitation, women's education, gender equality, and the quantity and quality of the food supply.[10]

Below we briefly discuss some of the pathways through which nutrition-sensitive approaches can impact malnutrition outcomes.

Ways That Nutrition-Sensitive Approaches Can Address Undernutrition

Given the importance of addressing underlying determinants of undernutrition, what do nutrition-sensitive approaches look like?

Agriculture

It is clear that agriculture and nutrition are linked: in order for nutritious foods to be consumed, they must first be cultivated, distributed through supply chains, and made available for purchase at an affordable price. Food producers in many LMICs are predominantly smallholder farmers with limited financial capital.[13] When it comes to food producers, there are two main pathways through which agriculture can impact nutrition: producers can grow a greater quantity and diversity of foods for their own consumption, and they can grow a greater quantity and diversity of foods to generate income through trade or exchange. Some interventions for **homestead food production**—in which participants are given resources and training to create or improve existing systems of household crop production, animal husbandry, or aquaculture—have shown improvements in outcomes such as dietary diversity, consumption of animal-source foods, and income.[14] Homestead food production is not the only way to intervene at the level of agriculture; equally important are efforts to improve the micronutrient content of the food supply through biofortification (i.e., selectively breeding for crops with greater micronutrient content)[15] and to strengthen the supply chains through which food is distributed.[16,17]

Improving Health through Water, Sanitation, and Hygiene (WASH)

Childhood infection and undernourishment are linked in a vicious cycle: as discussed in chapter 9, infection exacerbates undernutrition, and children who are undernourished are more susceptible to infectious disease and may take longer to recover.[18] In the past decade, a new direction in child nutrition research has examined the interplay between improving infant and young child feeding and the WASH environment to address a condition known as environmental enteric dysfunction.[19] Environmental enteric dysfunction is a condition of subclinical infection hypothesized to be associated with chronic exposure to poor sanitary environments. A key mechanism by which children develop environmental enteric dysfunction is that many infants and young children in low-resource, rural settings are frequently in contact with soil that has been contaminated with fecal microbes from livestock, and children of this age engage in exploratory mouthing behaviors as part of their sensorimotor development.[20] Some interventions have sought to improve household WASH conditions by improving access to clean water, providing physical infrastructure such as latrines, and promoting maternal hand washing and sanitary food preparation. These interventions may decrease levels of fecal contamination in the larger household environment, but decreasing levels of fecal contamination in areas immediately surrounding children—including their hands—is more challenging. The concept of "baby WASH" describes targeted efforts to reduce the ingestion of fecal microbes by children under 2 years of age,[21] and baby WASH interventions are now being integrated with early childhood development interventions.

It is estimated that environmental enteric dysfunction may contribute substantially to the child stunting burden through increasing gut permeability to infections and by contributing to chronic inflammation and decreased nutrient absorption, all of which may impair growth.[22] Approximately one-tenth of the world's population lives in conditions of extreme poverty in which conditions of poor sanitation and hygiene are prevalent,[23] and children are more likely to experience environmental enteric dysfunction during critical periods of physical and cognitive growth. Some data suggest that in addition to undernutrition, childhood stunting and repeated gut infections also place individuals at an increased risk for obesity in later life.[24]

Education and Early Child Development

Higher educational attainment for girls is linked with delayed first marriage, lower fertility rates, and greater empowerment, all of which have the potential to improve the nutritional status of infants, girls, and women.[25] There are many ways that higher parental educational attainment can lead to positive nutritional outcomes for children—education can enable higher potential for household income, higher levels of nutritional knowledge, and better performance of protective caregiver behaviors such as ensuring that children receive immunizations and micronutrient supplementation.[26]

In addition to the educational status of caregivers, the educational experience of children is also important, especially during periods of early childhood development. The first 1,000 days of life (conception through 2 years of age) is an especially important period for physical and cognitive development. Intervention studies have demonstrated that when children receive both nutrition interventions and increased psychosocial stimulation—referring to physical, sensory, and emotional input through play and other activities—they see synergistic benefits for both physical and cognitive development.[27]

Social Safety Nets

There is a strong, well-documented link between poverty and undernutrition. When households have enough resources, they are able to live in improved sanitary conditions, achieve higher educational attainment, access health services, and purchase nutrient-rich foods (which may be more expensive than starchy staples or convenience foods).[28] **Social safety net programs** are programs intended to provide basic goods, services, or care to individuals in need in order to protect against poverty and hardship. In the context of nutrition, the most relevant social safety nets might be programs that provide cash or food to low-income households. Programs that transfer food can take many forms, including school feeding programs or distributing rations of micronutrient-fortified foods (such as corn–soy blends) during emergency situations. Programs that transfer cash can take the form of subsidizing the cost of food (such as India's National Food Security Program, in which eligible households can purchased staple grains at subsidized prices), unconditional cash transfers, and conditional cash transfers. With conditional cash transfers, benefits are not received unless certain criteria are met; for example, a family may have to agree to immunize children or enroll children in school. In general, while cash transfer programs have been shown to have a consistently positive impact on some determinants of childhood nutrition such as dietary diversity and the physical and mental health of caregivers, outcomes related to improvements in child growth have been mixed.[28,29] Conditional and unconditional cash transfer programs are discussed at length in chapter 16.

Challenges of Nutrition-Sensitive Approaches

Even though the majority of reductions in undernutrition are associated with observed changes in underlying causes such as poverty, education, and sanitation, implementing nutrition-sensitive approaches does not always guarantee that there will be quick, measurable improvements in nutritional status. There are two major challenges: measurement and implementation.

Nutrition-sensitive approaches pose several measurement challenges. One measurement challenge is the choice of outcome. Stunting—height-for-age more than 2 standard deviations below the WHO Child Growth Standards median—has been chosen as an indicator of chronic undernutrition. It is difficult to shift population-level rates of stunting within the course of a single intervention, and given the multigenerational influence of maternal stunting on children's nutritional status, it can be difficult to achieve full growth potential within a single generation.[30] Additionally, efforts to reduce stunting may be most effective during the first thousand days of life—conception through 2 years of age—as this is a critical window for growth and development (although efforts outside of this window can also have an impact).[31] We could choose more proximal indicators that are likely to be more responsive to interventions, such as dietary diversity or protective behaviors (e.g., responsive feeding). But more proximal indicators may not always translate into impact. For example, a homestead food production intervention may improve dietary diversity; but if the increased dietary diversity is not also linked to improvements in child growth and other health outcomes, has the intervention created true health impact?

Another measurement challenge of nutrition-sensitive approaches is the complexity of causal pathways. The previous section described different categories of nutrition-sensitive approaches, and these interventions are highly interlinked. For example, if a family has increased income—either from selling high-value agricultural products or benefitting from a social safety net program—they may be able to build a concrete floor, which may reduce children's exposure to enteric infection. This synergistic impact of nutrition-sensitive approaches is a positive, but it also poses a measurement challenge; in this example, would a positive outcome be attributed to the income, the high-value agricultural products, the social safety net program, or the concrete floor? Does it matter whether the net increase in income is stemming from high-value agricultural products or a social safety net program?

One of the key challenges of implementing nutrition-sensitive approaches is that it is difficult to intervene in ways that truly alter underlying conditions. Although many observational studies have found associations between poor sanitary conditions and nutritional status, experimental studies in which communities are randomized to receive interventions for improved WASH conditions in Bangladesh,[32] Kenya,[33] and Uganda[34] have struggled to demonstrate that the WASH interventions improve nutritional status. This does *not* mean that WASH truly has no impact on nutrition; rather, it reflects the difficulty of creating meaningful improvement WASH conditions in ways that produce substantial reductions in environmental enteric dysfunction and impaired growth. WASH interventions raise an important question: if the nature of common interventions does not meaningfully alter underlying conditions that lead to environmental enteric dysfunction in children, what *would* meaningfully alter these underlying conditions? Some would argue that broader efforts to alleviate poverty would more effectively enable people to improve their standard of living, but broad-based poverty alleviation efforts are also challenging to implement. One such example was the Millennium Villages Project, which worked in 10 countries in sub-Saharan Africa to help rural areas achieve economic development through simultaneous interventions in infrastructure, entrepreneurial opportunities, education, agriculture, and health—an attempt at a multisectoral approach to development. While the villages saw improvements in agriculture and maternal health, they did not achieve all desired outcomes, such as improvements in poverty and malnutrition. The Millennium Villages Project is an example of not only the potential of such multisectoral interventions but the immense challenges of implementing them.[35]

Another challenge of implementing nutrition-sensitive approaches is that they are highly context specific. Between any two settings, there is huge variation in the underlying nutritional challenges and in how an intervention would play out given those challenges. For example, a social safety net program that provided food and conditional cash transfers to rural communities in Mexico resulted in both positive changes (e.g., improved dietary quality at the household level) and unfavorable changes—participants who were overweight or obese at the beginning of the program showed an increase in their caloric consumption because the program's in-kind transfers included many energy-dense, nutrient-poor foods.[36]

A further challenge of implementation is that some interventions involve tradeoffs with other interventions. For example, the presence of animals poses a tradeoff: although livestock can be a source of income (if they are sold) or micronutrients (if animal-source foods are consumed), they also create an environment that increases the risk of environmental enteric dysfunction, as described in the section on WASH interventions above. Raising chickens, for example, is frequently promoted as part of homestead food production interventions, but chickens are a prime source of *Campylobacter*, which is linked to environmental enteric dysfunction.[37]

It should be noted that for most of the nutrition-sensitive approaches described in this chapter, results have displayed remarkable heterogeneity in their impact across a range of outcomes. For example, homestead food production interventions have shown mixed results in terms of their ability to improve dietary intake, micronutrient status, and growth. The context of the intervention matters: in settings where health systems infrastructure is weak and the burden of infectious disease is high, even the most rigorously implemented agricultural strategies will find it difficult to improve nutritional status.[14] Heterogeneous results do not indicate that an intervention is not worth doing, but they reinforce that it is important to carefully document research methods and findings to inform adaptations to other contexts.

Nutrition and the Building Blocks of the SDGs

This section walks through each of the SDG building blocks in figure 13.1. The building blocks reflect specific conditions that can be addressed in order to improve the underlying household determinants of malnutrition. How do we ensure that the SDGs are meaningful for nutrition? First, we must have integrated action. In the Global Nutrition Report, a standalone, independent report that is published every year on the global status of nutrition, a roadmap was created to demonstrate integrated action using the SDGs as a framework.[12] Each SDG was accounted for by asking: How can nutrition action help achieve this goal? And how does each goal influence nutrition?

The report outlined five areas where there are shared SDG agendas with nutrition. These five areas are depicted as "building blocks" in figure 13.1. First, nutrition can help deliver on more sustainable food production, which includes climate change objectives and more species diversity on land and seas. Second is the infrastructure agenda. Nutrition can improve the "gray matter infrastructure," or brainpower, that builds knowledge-based economies vital for national futures. As discussed in chapter 11, the chronic undernutrition that results in physical growth stunting also contributes to developmental stunting, which impacts nations' human capital. We also need systems infrastructure such as technological systems, roads, sanitation, and electricity to deliver services including food, water, and energy to both rural and urban places. Third, the health agenda is indivisible from nutrition. Moreover, better nutrition would reduce the burden on health systems. Yet health systems could do much more to prevent and treat undernutrition and diet-related noncommunicable diseases including interventions such as exclusive breastfeeding promotion or the management of cardiovascular disease. Fourth, addressing poverty, quality education, gender equality, and decent work will further move the world toward equity and inclusion and will influence nutrition through a variety of pathways, such as impacts on family planning and reproductive health, increased incomes for food purchasing and knowledge about healthy eating, and greater participation of women in nutritional decision-making. Fifth, nutrition is essential for peace and stability, and vice versa. The impacts of conflicts and social unrest on undernutrition are increasing.[38] Investing in food security and the fair distribution of natural resources is critical for both nutrition resiliency and reduced fragility.

Sustainable Food Production

With an expected global population of 10.5 billion by the year 2050, it is essential that we produce food in a way that truly sustains us, now and into the future. Food production includes crops, animal agriculture, and aquaculture.

Do we produce enough food to feed the world now? According to FAO Food Balance Sheets,[39] we produce enough food globally to provide an average of 2,884 calories and 81 grams of protein per person per day, excluding some losses and nonfood uses such as livestock feed and biofuel. Though this global average production surpasses the daily needs of a typical adult, it is clear that the food we produce is not allocated in ways that prevent undernutrition and micronutrient deficiency in all populations. Food is not distributed equally between countries (e.g., per capita caloric availability is 3,768 kcal/day in Austria, compared to 1,930 kcal/day in Zambia), nor is it distributed equally within countries. Furthermore, it is not just about the number of calories available; the quality of the food supply—including whether food is safe from foodborne illness, free of mycotoxins and other contaminants, and rich in diverse food sources of micronutrients—is also important. For example, 65% of protein intake originates from plant sources and 35% from animal sources worldwide, but these proportions are nearly reversed in the United States;[40] whereas plant-based protein sources are rich in fiber and beneficial phytochemicals, for many micronutrients of public health concern (such as iron and zinc), animal sources provide greater density and bio-availability.[41]

In addition to the fact that our current global population is not served well, the ways we produce food now may threaten our future ability to do so. **Sustainability**, in broad terms, refers to the capacity to meet current goals without compromising future capacity. There are a number of ways that current methods of food production, in both high-income countries and LMICs, are unsustainable. In terms of agricultural production, major issues include expanding agricultural land use,[42] soil erosion,[43] and dependence on synthetic fertilizers sourced from finite resources. As an example of the latter, nutrients commonly applied to soil to enhance fertility include nitrogen, phosphate, and potassium. Although the global supply of nitrogen is basically unlimited in its atmospheric form, "fixing" atmospheric nitrogen to convert it into ammonia—the form that plants can utilize—is done through the Haber Bosch process, which relies on hydrogen derived from finite resources such as fossil fuels.[44] Additionally, phosphorous is derived from phosphate rock, which is another finite resource.[44]

Complementary to terrestrial food production are marine resources, which include fish, mollusks, crustaceans, algae, and aquatic plants such as seaweed. The global stock of capture fisheries (which refers to wild-caught fish) peaked in 1996 and has since gradually declined,[39] and aquaculture (breeding in controlled environments) provides more than half of the global supply of fish for human consumption.[45] There is remarkable heterogeneity in aquacultural species and practices. Issues that influence the sustainability of marine resources include overfishing, pollution, and ocean acidification, which results from increased atmospheric carbon dioxide. Also relevant is the choice of fish feed—using small, wild-caught fish is not sustainable given the growing global demand for fish, yet switching to crop-based feed ingredients such as soy has the potential to place further strain on agricultural resources.[46]

Many of these issues are likely to be exacerbated by climate change. **Climate change** entails shifts in global climate patterns linked to solar output or altered atmospheric composition; increased levels of greenhouse gases (including carbon dioxide, methane, nitrous oxide, and fluorinated gases) contribute to atmospheric warming, which affects ocean temperatures, sea level, precipitation patterns, and extreme weather events. As a result of climate change, access to food may be limited due to conflict over scarce land and water resources.[47] Food prices may increase due to volatility in food production resulting from unpredictable climate patterns.[48] The protein and micronutrient content of certain staple grains may decline given increased atmospheric carbon dioxide.[49] Susceptibility to infectious disease, which is linked to undernutrition, may be heightened due to changes in precipitation patterns, displacement, and crowding.[50] Aquaculture may be impacted by direct physical effects of climate change (e.g., changes in sea level and ocean temperatures) and biological responses to these physical effects (e.g., changes in the locations and abundance of different species and pathogens).

For current food production systems to be sustainable, they also need to be resilient to the short- and long-term impacts of climate change. **Resilience** is the capacity of a system to withstand and adapt to disturbances over time. Of the poorest billion global residents, 75% live in rural areas and depend on agricultural livelihoods.[51] In Asia and Africa, average farm size is quite small, and so many of these more vulnerable producers are smallholder farmers. In addition to producing food for themselves, these residents produce food for the rest of us. Ways of improving the resilience of smallholder farmers include breeding seeds that are resilient to drought or flood, increasing the biodiversity of food production, and using effective water management practices. Many of these efforts fall under the category of **climate-smart agriculture**, which describes agricultural approaches that aim to increase agricultural productivity in ways that reduce or remove greenhouse gas emissions and build resilience to climate change.[52]

Systems Infrastructure

Providing healthy, nutritious food to a growing population that increasingly lives in urban environments is another major public health nutrition challenge. Currently, 54% of the world's population live in cities. By 2045, the number of people living in cities is expected to increase by 2 billion.[53] The rapid growth in **urbanization** is concentrated in low- and middle-income countries, which are home to over 80% of the 550 and growing "megacities" around the world with over 1 million residents. While living in urban environments is often associated with some health benefits, such as better access to health care and improved water, nutrition and physical activity patterns can be compromised, and living in urban environments is associated with increased risk of chronic diseases in some LMIC contexts.[54,55] Beyond the increased access to convenience foods described above, urbanization is associated with reduced consumption of fruits and vegetables and whole grains, and a greater consumption of sugar-sweetened beverages.[56]

A leading challenge to nutritional health in urban environments is the reliable provision of adequate and reliable **WASH infrastructure** (water, sanitation, and hygiene). Over the past 30 years, substantial improvements in WASH have been made. Between 1990 and 2015, the world saw more than a 15 percentage point increase (from 76% to 91%) in the number of people with access to an improved water source.[57] While access to an improved water source is lower in rural areas, the rate of increase in access has been faster in these areas.[57] It is clear that improving infrastructure for WASH is critical for nutrition, but as noted above, efforts to demonstrate marked improvements in child growth have thus far proven challenging. The task of scaling up WASH interventions is also challenged by the need for a high level of community participation in a breadth of sanitary practices to substantially reduce exposure to sanitation-related environmental pathogens.[58]

Beyond food production and safety through clean environments lies the need to improve the efficiency of the food system by minimizing **food loss and waste**. On a global scale, approximately one-third of all food that is produced is wasted.[59] In industrialized nations, food loss and waste are concentrated at the retail and consumer end of the supply chain. For example, food wasted at the retail and consumer levels of the supply chain in the United States contains an amount of iron equivalent to the recommended iron intake for two-thirds of the adult population.[60] In LMICs most losses occur earlier in the supply chain due to weak infrastructure for on-farm storage, food processing, and distribution.[61,62] The high rates of postharvest loss in LMICs reflect underlying challenges of rural development; if small farmers lack the resources to store food on farm for later consumption or trade it at markets, this not only exacerbates postharvest losses but it also hinders income generation and food security. Postharvest loss is disproportionately high for fruits and vegetables, which are not only perishable but also rich in micronutrients. Food loss and waste in LMICs not only makes it more difficult to meet nutritional needs, but it also has environmental impacts—when food is not consumed, the finite natural resources used to produce it are also wasted.[63]

Health Systems

Malnutrition can serve as a risk factor for both communicable and noncommunicable diseases (NCDs). In turn, ill-health can put an individual at a higher risk of poor dietary intake and compromised nutritional status.[64] Strengthening health systems is essential for building a supportive environment for integrating nutrition into existing health care prevention, treatment, and services, which includes diet counseling and education, nutritional assessment and monitoring, as well as treatment and management of disease.[64,65]

A key issue for health systems is to build the capacity among health worker professionals to address the complexity of double and triple burdens of malnutrition. Very few professionals are trained on dietary education and counseling across the life span, as one example. Further, while growth monitoring may be a core part of health visits, what to do with growth results and how to intervene is not systematically practiced. Creating an institutional culture where providers value nutrition, and understand their role in integrating nutrition as part of health care, is important in order to make a dent in the complexities of malnutrition burdens.[66]

Investments in health systems should address the current disease burden that nations face. There is a shift in disease patterns from communicable to noncommunicable diseases. While the communicable and undernutrition agenda is far from over, there needs to be more significant investments toward addressing all forms of malnutrition. Currently, less than 0.1% of the overseas development assistance goes to obesity and diet-related noncommunicable diseases and 0.5% goes to undernutrition.[12,67] Treating the burdens of malnutrition is costly for health systems and households if preventative measures are no longer an option.[68] Globally, it is estimated that from 2011 to 2025, the economic burden of noncommunicable diseases will be US$7 trillion.[69]

Equity and Inclusion
Women's Agency

As primary caregivers, mothers have potential control over factors critical for child well-being, including food preparation and storage, feeding practices, psychosocial care, hygiene and health practices, and newborn care.[70] During the period of the Millennium Development Goals, the empowerment of women became a major focus of development organizations. While various definitions of empowerment exist, recent frameworks for increasing empowerment have emerged. A recent systematic review concluded that raising maternal autonomy is an important goal for improving children's nutritional status, yet gaps in the current knowledge exist, further confounded by issues with how autonomy is measured and limitations of cross-cultural comparability.[71] While definitions of empowerment constructs vary, most organizations seek to expand one or more of the following aspects of women's status: autonomy, empowerment, and agency. *Autonomy* is considered a multidimensional construct, consisting of dimensions such as the ability to make purchases and control resources, the ability to make decisions about health care or child care, and freedom from domestic violence.[72] *Empowerment* is the "expansion of assets and capabilities of poor people to participate in, negotiate with, influence, control, and hold accountable institutions that affect their lives."[73] Similarly, the concept of *agency* describes the ability to influence and have power to control one's life. Maternal agency applies this concept to mothers, describing that mothering can be an opportunity for empowerment and a venue for social change for women via the process of mothering.[74] More recently, the field of *capabilities* has been applied to health and nutrition.[75] The term captures the freedoms that individuals experience "to be and to act" and derives from the field of development economics. Related to nutrition, potential caregiver capabilities of interest are social support, psychological well-being, bodily integrity, and agency. These constructs collectively form a mother's capabilities to provision care for children, generally, and specific to nutrition.[76,77] The connections between women's agency and nutrition outcomes appear to be through at least three primary mechanisms: increased reproductive decision-making/control over the timing of pregnancies and family size; increased personal advocacy for antenatal care, delivery, and early child care; and increased participation in household purchasing.

Education

The education of girls is a major policy objective of many development organizations. Supporting the right to education has many short- and long-term benefits—especially for girls—however, the strength of associations between education and child nutrition is particularly strong. Maternal education has robust associations with child anthropometry.[78-80] However, a threshold level of education may exist for improvements in children's nutritional status to be observed. For example, in three African countries, maternal education beyond primary school was necessary to see significant reductions in child undernutrition.[81] Interventions to improve literacy and numeracy among mothers can benefit children's dietary quality and nutritional status through increasing mother's nutritional knowledge, suggesting that supporting these specific skills can help to reduce undernutrition even if formal education cannot be improved.[82-84]

Poverty Reduction

Connected to expanding education opportunities and increasing women's autonomy, higher levels of wealth, at the country-level and individual level, are associated with substantially lower levels of undernutrition. Robust demographic health survey (DHS) data—an initiative from the US Agency for International Development (USAID) to collect nationally representative data related to family planning, maternal and child health, gender, HIV/AIDS, malaria, and nutrition in over 90 countries—demonstrate the strong linear relationship between wealth quintile, children's dietary quality, and child anthropometry. Poverty can be reduced through a variety of measures and indeed, climbing out of poverty is one of the fastest methods for reducing undernutrition. While most nutrition interventions address more immediate or underlying causes of poor diet and nutritional status, some initiatives like conditional and unconditional cash transfer programs seek to improve nutritional status and to reduce poverty and to improve food security concurrently.[85] However, these programs have not been uniformly successful across contexts and they do not necessary address long-term intergenerational cycles of poverty.[86]

Peace and Stability

Conflict has devastating implications for nutrition and can be exacerbated by climate change and political unrest.[87] These events may cause people to move to find better prospects. Hundreds of thousands of internally displaced persons (IDPs) and millions of refugees, the majority of whom are children, are constantly on the move to flee violence, and thus have little access to stable food sources.

Conflicts seem to be related to both longer-term and short-term food insecurity and malnutrition. In fact, countries affected by conflict—and to a larger extent those in protracted crises and fragile situations—have made the least progress in reducing hunger, compared to countries not affected by conflict. Countries in protracted crisis also have a higher concurrence of children suffering from both wasting (acute) and stunting (chronic).[88]

Indeed, conflicts have increased in number and complexity.[38] Civil wars and fighting affect food security and nutrition both in the immediate term as well as long-term prospects through a variety of channels, such as economic recession and inflation, disturbances across agro-food value chains, disruption of livelihoods and social networks, and erosion of social services. These can affect availability and access to food, assets, and basic services, along with feeding, care, and hygiene practices.

Further understanding the complexities of conflict as an increasing driver of both chronic and acute food insecurity and malnutrition, along with their policy and programming implications, are essential in the efforts to bridge the divide between humanitarian and development action.

Conclusion

Malnutrition—in all of its forms—is driven by complex systems and will require systems thinking to address the underlying determinants. Nutrition-sensitive approaches that involve multiple sectors are critically important; although they are challenging to implement and measure, they are essential for change at the level of the fundamental building blocks of the SDGs. It is impossible to separate malnutrition from the challenges of food production, systems infrastructure, health systems, equity and inclusion, and peace and stability. The SDGs provide an integrated framework for achieving nutritional goals for all populations, but to achieve the 17 goals by 2030 integrated action by many stakeholders and innovative investment will be required.

Review Questions

1. Identify an example of a nutrition-sensitive approach that can be implemented by a single sector and an example of a nutrition-sensitive approach that requires multiple sectors to implement. Describe some of the tradeoffs of both interventions.

2. Food is certainly a determinant of nutritional status, both in terms of quantity and quality of dietary intake. But there are many other factors that influence nutritional status. What are some of the other factors, besides food, that influence nutrition in LMICs?

3. One of the most commonly reported types of nutritional outcomes is anthropometric measures, such as childhood stunting or overweight/obesity (indicated by BMI). What are some of the benefits and drawbacks of using anthropometric measures as the primary outcomes for nutrition-sensitive interventions? What other types of outcomes do you think are important to consider? What are some of the challenges of using these other outcomes?

4. Let's say there is a randomized controlled trial on homestead food production and it shows no improvement in nutritional status. Does this mean that there is no link between homestead food production and nutrition? What are some of the challenges of implementing such an intervention and measuring progress?

5. For a low- or middle-income country of your choice, identify one example for each of the building blocks as it relates to nutrition.

References

1. Egypt Ministry of Health and Population, El-Zanaty and Associates, ICF International. 2015. *Egypt Demographic and Health Survey 2014*. Cairo, Egypt and Rockville, Maryland.

2. Ghosh, S., G. Namirembe, M. Moaz, et al. 2017. "Relationship of Stunting and Overweight in Egyptian Children under Five Years of Age: Trends and Associated Risk Factors." *FASEB Journal* 31 (Suppl 1).

3. Galal, O. M. 2002. "The Nutrition Transition in Egypt: Obesity, Undernutrition and the Food Consumption Context." *Public Health Nutrition* 5 (1a): 141–48. doi:10.1079/PHN2001286.

4. Kavle, J. A., S. Mehanna, G. Saleh, et al. 2015. "Exploring Why Junk Foods Are 'Essential' Foods and How Culturally Tailored Recommendations Improved Feeding in Egyptian Children." *Maternal & Child Nutrition* 11 (3): 346–70. doi:10.1111/mcn.12165.

5. World Economic Forum. 2017. *The Global Gender Gap Report 2017.* Geneva, Switzerland: World Economic Forum.

6. Russell, E., R. C. Swanson, R. Atun, S. Nishtar, and S. Chunharas. 2014. "Systems Thinking for the Post-2015 Agenda." *The Lancet* 383 (9935): 2124-25. doi:10.1016/S0140-6736(14)61028-X.

7. Peters, D. H. 2014. "The Application of Systems Thinking in Health: Why Use Systems Thinking? *Healthy Research Policy and Systems* 12 (1): 51. doi:10.1186 /1478-4505-12-51.

8. Reinhardt, K., and J. Fanzo. 2016. "Addressing Chronic Malnutrition through Multi-sectoral, Sustainable Approaches: A Review of Causes and Consequences." *World Review of Nutrition & Dietics* 114 (August): 120-21. doi:10.1159/000441823.

9. Black, R. E., Victora C. G., Walker S. P., et al. 2013. "Maternal and Child Undernutrition and Overweight in Low-income and Middle-income Countries." *The Lancet* 382 (9890): 427-451. doi:10.1016/S0140-6736(13)60937-X.

10. Smith, L. C., and L. Haddad. 2015. "Reducing Child Undernutrition: Past Drivers and Priorities for the Post-MDG Era." *World Development* 68 (1): 180-204. doi:10.1016/j.worlddev.2014.11.014.

11. UNICEF. 1991. "Strategy for improved nutrition of children and women in developing countries." *Indian Journal of Pediatrics* 58 (1): 13-24. doi:10.1007/ BF02810402.

12. Hawkes, C., and J. Fanzo. 2017. *Global Nutrition Report 2017: Nourishing the SDGs.* New York: UNICEF.

13. Peter Hazell, Colin Poulton, Steve Wiggins, and Andrew Dorward. 2007. "The Future of Small Farms for Poverty Reduction and Growth." 2020 Discussion Paper No. 42. Washington, DC: International Food Policy Research Institute.

14. Girard, A. W., J. L. Self, C. McAuliffe, and O. Olude. 2012. "The Effects of Household Food Production Strategies on the Health and Nutrition Outcomes of Women and Young Children: A Systematic Review." *Paediatric and Perinatal Epidemiology* 26 (Suppl 1): 205-22. doi:10.1111/j.1365-3016.2012.01282.x.

15. Bouis, H. E., C. Hotz, B. McClafferty, J. V. Meenakshi, and W. H. Pfeiffer. 2011. "Biofortification: A New Tool to Reduce Micronutrient Malnutrition." *Food and Nutrition Bulletin* 32 (Suppl 1): 31-40. doi:10.1177/15648265110321S105.

16. Gómez, M. I., and K. D. Ricketts. 2013. "Food Value Chain Transformations in Developing Countries: Selected Hypotheses on Nutritional Implications." *Food Policy* 42:139-50. doi:10.1016/j.foodpol.2013.06.010.

17. Maestre, M., N. Poole, and S. Henson. 2017. "Assessing Food Value Chain Pathways, Linkages and Impacts for Better Nutrition of Vulnerable Groups." *Food Policy* 68:31-39. doi:10.1016/j.foodpol.2016.12.007.

18. Guerrant, R. L., R. B. Oriá, S. R. Moore, M. O. Oriá, and A. A. Lima. 2008. "Malnutrition as an Enteric Infectious Disease with Long-term Effects on Child Development." *Nutrition Reviews* 66 (9): 487-505. doi:10.1111/j.1753-4887.2008.00082.x.

19. Prendergast, A. J., J. H. Humphrey, K. Mutasa, et al. 2015. "Assessment of Environmental Enteric Dysfunction in the SHINE Trial: Methods and Challenges." *Clinical Infectious Diseases* 61 (suppl 7): S726-32. doi:10.1093/cid /civ848.

20. Reid, B., J. Orgle, K. Roy, C. Pongolani, M. Chileshe, and R. Stoltzfus. 2018. "Characterizing Potential Risks of Fecal-Oral Microbial Transmission for Infants and Young Children in Rural Zambia." *American Journal of Tropical Medicine and Hygiene* 98 (3): 816–23.

21. Ngure, F. M., B. M. Reid, J. H. Humphrey, M. N. Mbuya, G. Pelto, and R. J. Stoltzfus. 2014. "Water, Sanitation, and Hygiene (WASH), Environmental Enteropathy, Nutrition, and Early Child Development: Making the Links." *Annals of the New York Academy of Sciences* 1308 (1): 118–28. doi:10.1111/nyas.12330.

22. Mbuya, M. N. N., and J. H. Humphrey. 2016. "Preventing Environmental Enteric Dysfunction through Improved Water, Sanitation and Hygiene: An Opportunity for Stunting Reduction in Developing Countries." *Maternal & Child Nutrition* 12 (Suppl 1): 106–20. doi:10.1111/mcn.12220.

23. World Bank Group. 2016. *Poverty and Shared Prosperity 2016: Taking on Inequality.* doi:10.1596/978-1-4648-0958-3.

24. Guerrant, R. L., M. D. Deboer, S. R. Moore, R. J. Scharf, and A. A. M. Lima. 2013. "The Impoverished Gut: A Triple Burden of Diarrhoea, Stunting and Chronic Disease. *Nature Reviews Gastroenterology & Hepatology* 10 (4): 220–29. doi:10.1038/nrgastro.2012.239.

25. Martin, T. C. 1995. "Women's Education and Fertility: Results from 26 Demographic and Health Surveys." *Studies in Family Planning* 26 (4): 187. doi:10.2307/2137845.

26. Ruel, M. T., and H. Alderman. 2013. "Nutrition-sensitive Interventions and Programmes: How Can They Help to Accelerate Progress in Improving Maternal and Child Nutrition?" *The Lancet* 382 (9891): 536–51. doi:10.1016/S0140-6736(13)60843-0.

27. Walker, S.P., S. M. Chang, C. A. Powell, and S. M. Grantham-McGregor. 2005. "Effects of Early Childhood Psychosocial Stimulation and Nutritional Supplementation on Cognition and Education in Growth-stunted Jamaican Children: Prospective Cohort Study. *The Lancet* 366 (9499): 1804–7. doi:10.1016/S0140-6736(05)67574-5.

28. de Groot, R., T. Palermo, S. Handa, L. P. Ragno, and A. Peterman. 2017. "Cash Transfers and Child Nutrition: Pathways and Impacts." *Developmental Policy Review* 35 (5): 621–43. doi:10.1111/dpr.12255.

29. Leroy, J. L., M. Ruel, and E. Verhofstadt. 2009. "The Impact of Conditional Cash Transfer Programmes on Child Nutrition: A Review of Evidence using a Programme Theory Framework." *Journal of Development Effectiveness* 1 (2): 103–29. doi:10.1080/19439340902924043.

30. Behrman, J. R., M. C. Calderon, S. H. Preston, J. Hoddinott, R. Martorell, and A. D. Stein. 2009. "Nutritional Supplementation in Girls Influences the Growth of Their Children: Prospective Study in Guatemala." *American Journal of Clinical Nutrition* 90:1372–79. doi:10.3945/ajcn.2009.27524.INTRODUCTION.

31. Prentice, A. M., K. A. Ward, G. R. Goldberg, et al. 2013. "Critical Windows for Nutritional Interventions against Stunting." *American Journal of Clinical Nutrition* 97 (5): 911–18. doi:10.3945/ajcn.112.052332.

32. Luby, S. P., Rahman M, Arnold BF, et al. 2018. "Effects of Water Quality, Sanitation, handwashing, and nutritional interventions on Diarrhoea and Child

Growth in Rural Bangladesh: A Cluster Randomised Controlled Trial." *The Lancet Global Health* 6 (3): e302-15. doi:10.1016/S2214-109X(17)30490-4.

33. Null, C., C. P. Stewart, A. J. Pickering, et al. 2018. "Effects of Water Quality, Sanitation, Handwashing, and Nutritional Interventions on Diarrhoea and Child Growth in Rural Kenya: A Cluster-randomised Controlled Trial." *The Lancet Global Health* 6 (3): e316-29. doi:10.1016/S2214-109X(18)30005-6.

34. Muhoozi, G. K. M., P. Atukunda, L. M. Diep, et al. 2018. "Nutrition, Hygiene, and Stimulation Education to Improve Growth, Cognitive, Language, and Motor Development among Infants in Uganda: A Cluster-randomized Trial." *Maternal & Child Nutrition* 14 (2): e12527. doi:10.1111/mcn.12527/.

35. Fanzo, J. 2018. "Addressing Poverty in Rural Africa." *Nature Sustainability* 1 (6): 269-70. doi:10.1038/s41893-018-0082-4.

36. Leroy, J. L., P. Gadsden, S. Rodríguez-Ramírez, and T. G. de Cossío. 2010. "Cash and In-Kind Transfers in Poor Rural Communities in Mexico Increase Household Fruit, Vegetable, and Micronutrient Consumption but Also Lead to Excess Energy Consumption." *Journal of Nutrition* 140 (3): 612-17. doi:10.3945/jn.109.116285.

37. François, R., P. P. Yori, S. Rouhani, et al. 2018. "The Other Campylobacters: Not Innocent Bystanders in Endemic Diarrhea and Dysentery in Children in Low-income Settings." Vinetz JM, ed. *PLoS Neglected Tropical Diseases* 12 (2): e0006200. doi:10.1371/journal.pntd.0006200.

38. FAO, IFAD, UNICEF, WFP, WHO. 2017. *The State of Food Security and Nutrition in the World*. Rome: Food and Agriculture Organization of the United Nations.

39. Food and Agriculture Organization of the United Nations. FAOSTAT Statistics Database.

40. Wu, G., J. Fanzo, D. D. Miller, et al. 2014. "Production and Supply of High-quality Food Protein for Human Consumption: Sustainability, Challenges, and Innovations." *Annals of the New York Academy of Sciences* 1321 (1): 1-19. doi:10.1111/nyas.12500.

41. Allen, L. H. 2008. "To What Extent Can Food-based Approaches Improve Micronutrient Status?" *Asia Pacific Journal of Clinical Nutrition* 17 (Suppl 1): 103-5.

42. Foley, J. A., R. DeFries, G. P. Asner, et al. 2005. "Global Consequences of Land Use." *Science (80-)* 209 (5734): 570-74.

43. Montgomery, D. R. 2007. "Soil Erosion and Agricultural Sustainability." *Proceedings of the National Academy of Sciences* 104 (33): 13268-72. doi:10.1073/pnas.0611508104.

44. Dawson, C., and J. Hilton. 2011. "Fertiliser Availability in a Resource-limited World: Production and Recycling of nitrogen and phosphorus. *Food Policy* 36 (Suppl 1): S14-22. doi:10.1016/j.foodpol.2010.11.012.

45. Food and Agriculture Organization. FishStat J database. http://www.fao.org/fishery/statistics/software/fishstatj/en.

46. Fry, J. P., D. C. Love, G. K. MacDonald, et al. 2016. "Environmental Health Impacts of Feeding Crops to Farmed Fish." *Environment International* 91:201-14. doi:10.1016/j.envint.2016.02.022.

47. Barnett, J., and W. N. Adger. 2007. "Climate Change, Human Security and Violent Conflict." *Political Geography* 26 (6): 639-55. doi:10.1016/j.polgeo.2007.03.003.

48. Wheeler, T., and J. von Braun. 2013. "Climate Change Impacts on Global Food Security." *Science* 341 (6145): 508-13. doi:10.1126/science.1239402.

49. Dietterich, L. H., A. Zanobetti, I. Kloog, et al. 2015. "Impacts of Elevated Atmospheric CO2 on Nutrient Content of Important Food Crops." *Scientific Data* 2:150036. doi:10.1038/sdata.2015.36.

50. Myers, S. S., M. R. Smith, S. Guth, et al. 2017. "Climate Change and Global Food Systems: Potential Impacts on Food Security and Undernutrition." *Annual Review of Public Health* 38 (1): 259-77. doi:10.1146/annurev-publhealth-031816 -044356.

51. Olinto, P., K. Beegle, C. Sobrado, and H. Uematsu. 2013. *The State of the Poor: Where Are The Poor, Where Is Extreme Poverty Harder to End, and What Is the Current Profile of the World's Poor?* Washington, DC: World Bank.

52. Lipper, L., P. Thornton, B. M. Campbell, et al. 2014. "Climate-smart Agriculture for Food Security." *Nature Climate Change* 4 (12): 1068-72. doi:10.1038/nclimate2437.

53. The World Bank. Urban Development.

54. Allender, S., C. Foster, L. Hutchinson, and C. Arambepola. 2008. "Quantification of Urbanization in Relation to Chronic Diseases in Developing Countries: A Systematic Review." *Journal of Urban Health* 85 (6): 938-51. doi:10.1007/s11524 -008-9325-4.

55. Attard, S. M., A. G. Howard , A. H. Herring, et al. 2015. "Differential Associations of Urbanicity and Income with Physical Activity in Adults in Urbanizing China: Findings from the Population-based China Health and Nutrition Survey 1991-2009." *International Journal of Behavioral Nutrition and Physical Activity* 12 (1): 1-12. doi:10.1186/s12966-015-0321-2.

56. Ghosh-Dastidar, B, D. Cohen, G. Hunter, et al. 2014. "Distance to Store, Food Prices, and Obesity in Urban Food Deserts." *American Journal of Preventative Medicine* 47 (5): 587-95. doi:10.1016/j.amepre.2014.07.005.

57. Ritchie, H. and M. Roser. 2019. "Clean Water." Published online at Our-WorldInData.org. https://ourworldindata.org/water-access.

58. Johnston, E. A., J. Teague, and J. P. Graham. 2015. "Challenges and Opportunities Associated with Neglected Tropical Disease and Water, Sanitation and Hygiene Intersectoral Integration Programs." *BMC Public Health* 15 (1): 1-14. doi:10.1186/s12889-015-1838-7.

59. Gustavsson, J., C. Cederberg, U. Sonesson, R. van Otterdijk, and A. Maybeck. 2011. "Global Food Losses and Food Waste: Extent, Causes and Prevention." Rome: Food and Agriculture Organization of the United Nations. doi:10.1098 /rstb.2010.0126.

60. Spiker, M. L., H. A. B. Hiza, S. M. Siddiqi, and R. A. Neff. 2017. "Wasted Food, Wasted Nutrients: Nutrient Loss from Wasted Food in the United States and Comparison to Gaps in Dietary Intake." *Journal of the Academy of Nutrition and Dietetics* 117 (7): 1031-40.e22. doi:10.1016/j.jand.2017.03.015.

61. Parfitt, J., M. Barthel, and S. Macnaughton. 2010. "Food Waste within Food Supply Chains: Quantification and Potential for Change to 2050." *Philosophical Translations of the Royal Society B: Biological Sciences* 365 (1554): 3065-81. doi:10.1098 /rstb.2010.0126.

62. Rolle, R. 2006. *Postharvest Management of Fruits and Vegetables in the Asia-Pacific Region*. Tokoyo: Asian Productivity Organization; Rome: Food and Agriculture Organization of the United Nations. doi:92-833-7051-1.

63. Kummu, M., H. de Moel, M. Porkka, S. Siebert, O. Varis, and P. J. Ward. 2012. "Lost Food, Wasted Resources: Global Food Supply Chain Losses and Their Impacts on Freshwater, Cropland, and Fertiliser Use." *Science of the Total Environment* 438:477-89. doi:10.1016/j.scitotenv.2012.08.092.

64. Fanzo, J. 2014. "Strengthening the engagement of food and health systems to improve nutrition security: Synthesis and overview of approaches to address malnutrition. *Global Food Security* 3(3-4): 183-92. doi:10.1016/j.gfs.2014.09.001.

65. Fanzo, J. 2016. "Non-Communicable Diseases, Food Systems and the Sustainable Development Goals." *Sight Life* 30 (1).

66. Tappenden, K. A., B. Quatrara, M. L. Parkhurst, A. M. Malone, G. Fanjiang, and T. R. Ziegler. 2013. "Critical Role of Nutrition in Improving Quality of Care: An Interdisciplinary Call to Action to Address Adult Hospital Malnutrition." *Journal of the Academy of Nutrition and Dietetics* 113 (9): 1219-37. doi:10.1016/j.jand.2013.05.015.

67. Nugent, R. A., and A. B. Feigl. 2010. "Where Have All the Donors Gone? Scarce Donor Funding for Non-Communicable Diseases." Center for Global Development Working Paper 228, November 2010. doi:10.2139/ssrn.1824392.

68. Jan, S., S. W. Lee, J. P. Sawhney, et al. 2016. "Catastrophic Health Expenditure on Acute Coronary Events in Asia: A Prospective Study." *Bulletin of the World Health Organization* 94 (3): 193-200. doi:10.2471/BLT.15.158303.

69. Zoghbi, W. A., T. Duncan, E. Antman, et al. 2014. "Sustainable Development Goals and the Future of Cardiovascular Health: A Statement From the Global Cardiovascular Disease Taskforce." *Journal of the American Heart Association* 3 (5):e000504. doi:10.1161/JAHA.114.000504.

70. Engle, P. L., P. Menon, and L. Haddad. 1999. "Care and Nutrition: Concepts and Measurement." *World Development* 27 (8): 1309-37.

71. Carlson, G. J., K. Kordas, and L. E. Murray-Kolb. 2015. "Associations between Women's Autonomy and Child Nutritional Status: A Review of the Literature. *Maternal & Child Nutrition* 11 (4): 452-82. doi:10.1111/mcn.12113.

72. Agarwala, R., and S. Lynch. 2016. "Refining the Measurement of Women's Autonomy: An International Application of a Multi-Dimensional Construct." *Social Forces* 84 (4): 2077-98.

73. Narayan, Deepa, ed. 2002. "A Framework for Empowerment: Summary." In *Empowerment and Poverty Reduction: A Sourcebook*. Washington, DC: World Bank.

74. O'Reilly A., and D. L. O'Brien Hallstein. 2012. "Maternal Agency." In *Encyclopedia of Motherhood*. doi:10.4135/9781412979276.n366.

75. Ibrahim, S., and S. Alkire. 2007. "Agency & Empowerment: A Proposal for Internationally Comparable Indicators." *Oxford Development Studies* 35 (4): 379-403.

76. Matare, C. R., M. N. N. Mbuya, G. Pelto, K. L. Dickin, and R. J. Stoltzfus. 2015. "Assessing Maternal Capabilities in the SHINE Trial: Highlighting a Hidden Link in the Causal Pathway to Child Health." *Clinical Infectious Disease* 61 (Suppl 7): S745-51. doi:10.1093/cid/civ851.

77. Ickes, S. B., G. A. Heymsfield, T. W. Wright, and C. Baguma. 2017. "Generally the Young Mom Suffers Much: Socio-cultural influences of maternal capabili-

ties and nutrition care in Uganda." *Maternal & Child Nutrition* 13 (3): e12365. doi:10.1111/mcn.12365.

78. Wachs, T. D., H. Creed-Kanashiro, S. Cueto, and E. Jacoby. 2005. "Maternal Education and Intelligence Predict Offspring Diet and Nutritional Status." *Journal of Nutrition* 135 (9): 2179-86. doi:10.1093/jn/135.9.2179.

79. Boyle, M. H., Y. Racine, K. Georgiades, et al. 2006. "The Influence of Economic Development Level, Household Wealth and Maternal Education on Child Health in the Developing World." *Social Science and Medicine* 63 (8): 2242-54. doi:10.1016/j.socscimed.2006.04.034.

80. Abuya, B. A., J. Ciera, and E. Kimani-Murage. 2012. "Effect of Mother's Education on Child's Nutritional Status in the Slums of Nairobi." *BMC Pediatrics* 12 (1): 626. doi:10.1186/1471-2431-12-80.

81. Makoka, D., and P. K. Masibo. 2015. "Is There a Threshold Level of Maternal Education Sufficient to Reduce Child Undernutrition? Evidence from Malawi, Tanzania and Zimbabwe." *BMC Pediatrics* 15 (1): 96. doi:10.1186/s12887-015-0406-8.

82. Ickes, S. B., T. E. Hurst, and V. L. Flax. 2015. "Maternal Literacy, Facility Birth, and Education Are Positively Associated with Better Infant and Young Child Feeding Practices and Nutritional Status among Ugandan Children." *Journal of Nutrition* 145 (11): 2578-86. doi:10.3945/jn.115.214346.

83. Christian, P., R. Abbi, S. Gujral, and T. Gopaldas. 1988. "The Role of Maternal Literacy and Nutrition Knowledge in Determining Children's Nutritional Status." *Food and Nutrition Bulletin* 10 (4): 35-40.

84. Ruel, M. T., J.-P. Habicht, P. Pinstrup-Andersen, and Y. Gröhn. 1992. "The Mediating Effect of Maternal Nutrition Knowledge on the Association between Maternal Schooling and Child Nutritional Status in Lesotho." *American Journal of Epidemiology* 135 (8): 904-14. doi:10.1093/oxfordjournals.aje.a116386.

85. Engle, P. L., L. C. Fernald, H. Alderman, et al. 2011. "Strategies for Reducing Inequalities and Improving Developmental Outcomes for Young Children in Low-income and Middle-income Countries." *The Lancet* 378 (9799): 1339-53. doi:10.1016/S0140-6736(11)60889-1.

86. Fernald, L. C., P. J. Gertler, and L. M. Neufeld. 2008. "Role of Cash in Conditional Cash Transfer Programmes for Child Health, Growth, and Development: An Analysis of Mexico's Oportunidades." *The Lancet* 371 (9615): 828-37. doi:10.1016/S0140-6736(08)60382-7.

87. Food Security Information Network. 2017. *Global Report on Food Crises 2017: Executive Summary.* March.

88. Mates, E., J. Shoham, T. Khara, and C. Dolan. 2017. "Stunting in Humanitarian and Protracted Crises." ENN Discussion Paper, November.

PART FOUR

Key Nutrition-Related Programs and Policies

14

Nutrition-Related Programs and Policies in High-Income Countries

Sara N. Bleich, Johannah M. Frelier, Scott A. Richardson, and Kelsey A. Vercammen

LEARNING OBJECTIVES

- Understand the major federal nutrition assistance programs in the United States
- Discuss efforts at the state and local levels to improve population nutrition status in the United States
- Describe current nutrition-related programs and policies common across high-income countries

Case Study: A Vignette from the Bronx, New York

Hannah is a 6-year-old girl who lives with her mother and father in a small apartment building in the Bronx, New York. Hannah's father works full time at the corner store down the street, and her mother works part time at the neighborhood laundromat. Since the family's gross monthly income is ≤130% of the federal poverty line (i.e., less than $2,311/month for a family of three), they qualify for the Supplemental Nutrition Assistance Program (SNAP), formerly known as "Food Stamps." Each month, the family's Electronic Benefit Transfer (EBT) card is loaded with a maximum of $509 to spend on groceries for the household. They are able to redeem these monetary benefits at any of the approximately 250,000 SNAP-authorized retailers across the United States. Hannah and her family have been receiving SNAP benefits for 2.5 years. Hannah's mother expects to no longer need the program in about six months' time when she will begin working full-time at the laundromat. Hannah attends a local elementary school where she receives free breakfast and lunch as part of the National School Lunch Program (NSLP) and School Breakfast Program (SBP). Because Hannah lives in a high-poverty neighborhood, all of her classmates (regardless of household income) also receive free breakfast and lunch as part of the Community Eligibility Provision (CEP). The CEP was implemented in 2014 to increase NSLP and SBP participation and reduce the administrative burden of schools in determining eligibility.

Hannah's neighbor is a new mother with a 4-month-old baby named Alex. On the weekend, Hannah's neighbor babysits her to earn some extra cash. In addition to receiving SNAP benefits, the mother and infant also receive food packages from the Special Supplemental Nutrition Program for Women, Infants, and Children (WIC). In contrast to SNAP, the food packages for WIC are prescriptive and include an allowance for quantities of certain healthful foods, including infant formula, milk, and whole-wheat bread. For example, each month Hannah's neighbor can use her WIC benefits to redeem one dozen eggs and 18 ounces of peanut butter from WIC-authorized retailers.

Hannah's grandmother lives a few blocks away from her family. She used to work at the laundromat with Hannah's mother, but she has been retired for a few years. She attends an adult day care center during the day, where she receives free, nutritious meals provided by the Child and Adult Care Food Program (CACFP). The CACFP is the same program that provides subsidized meals for the neighborhood day care center where baby Alex will soon attend.

Role and Contributions of Nutrition-Related Programs and Policies in High-Income Countries

Food insecurity refers to inadequate access to sufficient food needed to lead an active, healthy life.[1] Food insecurity, which often coexists with hunger and is associated with poor dietary quality, is a serious concern, particularly among households living at or below the federal poverty line. Food insecure households do not always know where their next meal will come from or are forced to buy less-healthy foods because they lack resources to purchase better options. In the United States, 11.1% of households were food insecure for at least some point in 2018, with 4.3% of households reporting very low food security.[2] In addition to food insecurity, many high-income countries also have high levels of obesity. For example, from 1980 to 2008, the age-standardized prevalence of obesity increased from 11.3% to 31.1% in North America, from 11.1% to 20.0% in Western Europe, and from 2.2% to 5.4% in the Asia Pacific region.[3] Figure 14.1 illustrates how many high-income countries concurrently experience high levels of food insecurity and obesity. Alongside these two major issues are a suite of other diet-related health conditions, including low dietary quality and chronic diseases such as heart disease and type 2 diabetes.

Comprehensive programs and policies are often necessary to adequately address nutrition-related issues.[4] In general, policy approaches have high potential for impact because they are intended to reach large segments of the population and often alter environmental and social drivers of nutrition-related issues.[5] This chapter begins by examining key nutrition-related public sector efforts at the federal, state, and local levels in the United States. The second half of the chapter discusses nutrition-related programs and policies across high-income countries and examines common strategies for improving nutrition through nutrition information (spotlight on dietary guidelines),

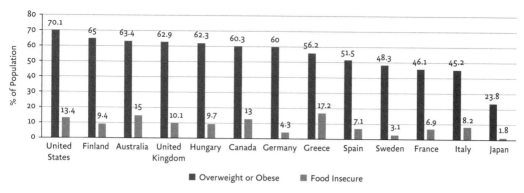

Figure 14.1. Overweight/obesity and food insecurity across high-income countries (2011-2017). *Source:* Data on population with overweight or obesity aged 15+ was obtained from OECD Health Statistics Database. Food insecure data from the following sources: *Foodbank Hunger Report 2017*; Loopstra, R. L., et al. *Financial Insecurity, Food Insecurity, and Disability: The Profile of People Receiving Emergency Food Assistance from The Trussell Trust Foodbank Network in Britain.* Salisbury, England: The Trussell Trust, 2017; *Hunger Count 2016*; *Map the Meal Gap 2017*; Carter, K. N., T. Lanumata, K. Kruse, and D. Gorton. 2010. "What Are the Determinants of Food Insecurity in New Zealand and Does This Differ for Males and Females?" *Australian and New Zealand Journal of Public Health* 34 (6): 602-608. *Note:* Population with overweight or obesity was defined by the OECD according to WHO classifications of BMI: adult BMI of 25-30 and above are classified as having obesity, adult BMI of 30 and above are classified as obese. Definition of food security varies for each country.

hunger relief (spotlight on food banks), and regulatory approaches (spotlight on food marketing to children).

US Federal Nutrition Assistance Programs

To address nutrition-related issues, the US Department of Agriculture (USDA) administers a suite of federal nutrition assistance programs that forms a nationwide safety net to promote the nutrition, health, and well-being of Americans.[6] These programs, administered by the Food and Nutrition Service, are diverse in size, target and scope (table 14.1). This intentional variation helps to address the variety of food needs facing low-income Americans at different stages throughout the life course and responds to different nutrition needs (e.g., acute emergencies vs. long-term challenges).

The USDA funds 15 nutrition assistance programs, with the largest five accounting for 96% of the $104 billion annual budget (73% of the total USDA budget).[7] Those five include the Supplemental Nutrition Assistance Program (SNAP), the National School Lunch Program (NSLP), the Special Supplemental Nutrition Program for Women, Infants, and Children (WIC), the School Breakfast Program (SBP), and the Child and Adult Care Food Program (CACFP). By increasing access to healthy food and nutrition education, these programs promote positive health and nutrition outcomes, consistent

Table 14.1. Overview of the Largest US Department of Agriculture Nutrition Assistance Programs

Program	Focus	Spending in billions, FY2015 (%)	Participation, FY 2015
SNAP	Reduce food insecurity (primary focus) and improve access to a healthy diet (secondary focus)	$74 (71%)	An average of 45.8 million people served monthly (equivalent to 1 in 7 Americans)
NSLP	Provide low-cost or free meals in public and nonprofit private schools to low-income children	$13 (12%)	An average of 30.5 million students served daily in over 100,000 schools
WIC	Provide supplemental food, nutrition education (including breastfeeding promotion and support), and referrals to health care and other social services to low-income, nutritionally at-risk women, infants, and children up to 5 years of age	$6.1 (6%)	An average of 8 million women, infants, and children served monthly[7]
SBP	Provides breakfast programs in schools and residential child care institutions	$3.9 (4%)	An average of 14 million students served monthly
CACFP	Provides aid to child and adult care institutions and family or group day care homes for the provision of nutritious foods as well as emergency at-risk meals	$3.3 (3%)	An average of 4.1 million children and adults served daily

Note: SNAP = Supplemental Nutrition Assistance Program; NSLP = National School Lunch Program; WIC = Special Supplemental Nutrition Program for Women, Infants, and Children; SBP = School Breakfast Program; CACFP = Child and Adult Care Food Program.

with the programs' goals to raise the level of nutrition among low-income households and safeguard the health and well-being of the nation's children.[8]

Supplemental Nutrition Assistance Program (SNAP)

SNAP, formerly known as the "Food Stamp Program," has been a central component of Food and Nutrition Service programming since the authorizing legislation of the Food Stamp Act of 1964.[9,10] Since its inception, it has grown rapidly and is now estimated to serve one in seven Americans (figure 14.2). Compared to other Food and Nutrition Service programs, SNAP has fewer eligibility restrictions (e.g., no age, family structure, or disability status restrictions) and is available to nearly anyone in the United States with low income and few resources. Undocumented immigrants are not eligible for SNAP benefits. Documented immigrants can receive SNAP benefits if they have lived in the United States for at least five years; some noncitizens (e.g., refugees, children, and individuals receiving asylum) are eligible for

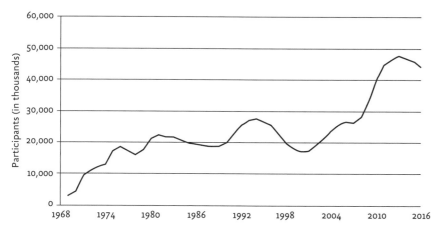

Figure 14.2. Trends in SNAP participation, 1969-2016. *Source:* USDA/FNS SNAP Program Participation and Cost Data.

SNAP with no five-year waiting period.[11] To be eligible for SNAP, households must have a monthly gross income of ≤130% of the federal poverty guideline, monthly net income ≤100% of the federal poverty guideline, and assets of less than $2,250.[12,13] Additionally, households may be considered categorically eligible for SNAP if they participate in other federal programs, including Temporary Assistance for Needy Families (TANF) or Supplemental Security Income (SSI).[13] In fact, most households (76%) receiving SNAP benefits also participate in other safety net programs, excluding Medicaid.[9] Almost half of SNAP participants are children, and many are elderly or disabled.[13]

SNAP participants receive monetary benefits through the Electronic Benefit Transfer (EBT) system, and these benefits can be used to purchase food from nearly 250,000 authorized SNAP retailers across the country.[13] Few restrictions are placed on the type of foods that can be purchased with SNAP benefits, with exceptions including alcohol, hot prepared foods, vitamins and medicines, and nonfood grocery items (e.g., toilet paper).[14] The benefit allotment each household receives is determined based on household size and net monthly income (e.g., $646 is maximum monthly allotment for a family of four).[15]

At its core, SNAP aims to reduce poverty and food insecurity (see box 14.1 for more information about SNAP and the US economy). It is challenging to assess if SNAP reduces poverty because benefits are not counted toward income in official poverty statistics.[9] If SNAP benefits were included as an official measure of income, it is estimated that 13% of households would move above the poverty guidelines.[13] This is likely an underestimate since SNAP may still be reducing extreme poverty even if it does not shift a household above the poverty line.[9] With respect to food insecurity, although estimates differ across sources, one study found that SNAP reduces the likelihood of being food insecure by 30% and of being very food insecure by 20%.[16]

Box 14.1. SNAP, the US Economy and the American Recovery and Reinvestment Act of 2009

SNAP is intrinsically linked to the US economy in two main ways: (1) Participation in SNAP rises and falls depending on economic conditions, and (2) SNAP expenditures stimulate economic activity during economic recessions.[20] First, SNAP participation rises during periods of economic recession and declines during periods of economic growth.[9] In particular, SNAP participation is tightly linked to unemployment rates, with one analysis suggesting that each 1% increase in the unemployment rate increases the per capita participant count by 3.7%.[21] Second, SNAP is an important economy stimulator during times of economic downturn.[20] For example, one extensive analysis found that every $1 billion in SNAP expenditures increased economic activity (GDP) by $1.79 billion.[22] The same study additionally found that $1 billion in SNAP expenditures resulted in 8,900 to 17,900 full-time-equivalent jobs or self-employment.[22] Substantial economic

benefits were also found for nonfood purchases, agricultural GDP, and agricultural jobs.[22]

In 2009, the American Recovery and Reinvestment Act temporarily increased the maximum monthly SNAP benefits by 13.6%, as a way of delivering high "bang-for-the-buck" economic stimulus and easing hardship for the lowest-income Americans.[23] Most eligible four-person households received an $80 increase in their monthly SNAP allotment to spend on groceries.[23] The American Recovery and Reinvestment Act also provided nearly $300 million to states for SNAP administrative expenses in FY 2009 and 2010, and temporarily suspended the three-month time limit for SNAP benefits for Able Bodied Adults Without Dependents until October 2010.[23] Assessments suggest that this successfully decreased food insecurity in low-income households by 2.2 percentage points and increased food spending in these same households by 5.4%.[24]

Improvement in diet quality was not a primary goal of SNAP at its inception. In recent years, there has been a shift in the USDA from using nutrition assistance programs to solely alleviate hunger to also improve diet quality by increasing exposure to healthy foods based on current nutrition science and improving nutrition education. For example, SNAP also includes an education component (SNAP-Ed), which builds partnerships with community organizations to hold nutrition education classes, implement healthy marketing campaigns, and improve policies and environment of the community. Additionally, there is increasing interest at the state level to exclude certain food/beverages (e.g., sugar-sweetened beverages) from the list of eligible SNAP foods, given their poor nutritional quality.[17,18] While there is some evidence that SNAP participants have lower dietary quality than nonparticipants,[19] these types of comparisons are complicated by selection bias and do not imply that receiving SNAP benefits results in lower diet quality (i.e., finding an appropriate comparison group is difficult—people who are income eligible for SNAP but who do not enroll are likely different on key unobserved factors that may also influence diet quality).

National School Lunch Program (NSLP)

The NSLP was signed into law in 1946 with the primary goal of promoting the health and well-being of children.[25] Participation in the NSLP has grown

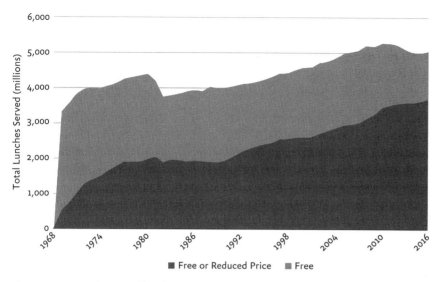

Figure 14.3. Trends in total lunches served through NSLP, 1969–2016. *Source:* USDA/ FNS NSLP Program Participation and Meals Served Data.

substantially over the past 40 years (figure 14.3). Today, the NSLP is the second-largest nutrition assistance program administered by the USDA, providing low-cost or free lunches to nearly 30 million students daily in more than 100,000 public or nonprofit private schools.[26]

Students from households with incomes ≤130% of the federal poverty level are eligible to receive fully subsidized meals, while students from households with incomes between 130% and 185% of the federal poverty level qualify to receive reduced-price lunches.[25] All school-aged children in income-eligible households can receive school meal benefits regardless of the immigration status of household members. In 2014, access to the NSLP was increased through the CEP, a component of the Healthy Hunger-Free Kids Act (HHFKA), which allowed schools to provide meals to all enrolled students based on a formula assessing the proportion of students in the school participating in SNAP and TANF.[27] The Community Eligibility Provision eliminated the school's burden of collecting household income and applications and has been associated with an average 5.2% higher lunch participation than in comparison schools.[28] Also included in the HHFKA were funds to increase the use of direct certification (the process of using income data already verified through applications for means-tested programs such as SNAP to certify children in those households for free meals without requiring a second application).

Schools receive monthly reimbursements based on the number of lunches served, level of economic need (percentage of students eligible for free and reduced-price lunch), and their state geography (to account for higher food costs in Alaska and Hawaii). Federal reimbursements for qualifying meals in the contiguous United States range from $0.31 for a full-price meal in higher-income schools to $3.40 for a free meal in schools serving predominantly low-income students. In 2012, also as part of the Healthy Hunger-Free Kids Act, the USDA ruled that, in order for schools to be reimbursed, their lunches must meet more stringent nutrition requirements aligned with the DGAs.[29] In particular, schools were required to increase the variety and quantity of fruits and vegetables, increase whole grains, decrease sodium and saturated fat levels, and eliminate *trans* fats.[29] The aim of these nutrition standards was to improve the diet quality and health of children while also reducing the risk of childhood obesity.

Relatively few studies have evaluated the association between NSLP participation and nutrition and health outcomes. A USDA review conducted in 2008 (i.e., before new standards)[30] found that NSLP participants generally consume more milk, vegetables, fruit, and 100% fruit juice along with fewer sweets, sugar-sweetened beverages, and snack foods compared to nonparticipants.[31,32] The review also suggested that NSLP participants have higher vitamin and mineral intakes but are also more likely to exceed sodium limits compared to nonparticipants.[32] A more recent analysis found that fruit selection increased by 23.0% and vegetable consumption increased by 16.2% among NSLP participants following the implementation of the new nutrition standards.[33]

School Breakfast Program (SBP)

The SBP is the breakfast equivalent of the NSLP, providing cash assistance to states to operate nonprofit breakfast programs in schools.[34] The SBP started as a pilot project in 1966 and permanent funding for the program was secured

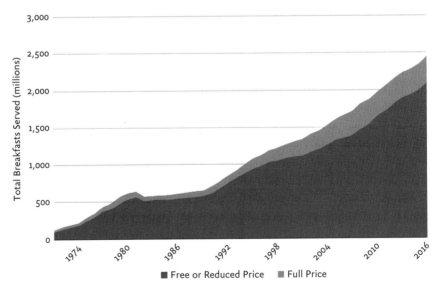

Figure 14.4. Trends in total breakfasts served through the SBP, 1969–2016. *Source:* USDA/FNS SBP Program Participation and Meals Served Data.

by Congress in 1975.[35] Since then, participation in the program has grown consistently (figure 14.4). As with the NSLP, students reliant on free and reduced-price meals comprise the vast majority of total meals served each year. Student household income eligibility thresholds for free or reduced-price breakfasts are the same as the NSLP, as is the ability to receive school meal benefits regardless of the immigration status of household members. The Community Eligibility Provision also applies to the SBP, and its implementation has been associated with a 9.4% increase in breakfast participation.[28]

Similar to the NSLP, very few studies have evaluated whether the SBP is associated with improved health, nutrition, or cognitive outcomes. A recent study reported that, among children who participate in both the SBP and the NSLP, almost half of the day's energy intake was provided by these meals, highlighting the important role these nutrition programs have in influencing low-income children's daily dietary intake.[36]

Special Supplemental Nutrition Program for Women, Infants, and Children (WIC)

WIC is a core USDA Food and Nutrition Service program that serves pregnant, postpartum (up to six months after the birth) and breastfeeding women (up to their infant's first birthday), infants, and children up to age 5.[37] While each state has the autonomy to set income-eligibility standards, almost all states and territories (except Hawaii and Alaska) have determined that eligible participants must have household incomes ≤185% of the federal poverty guideline.[38] Households may also be considered income eligible for WIC if they are currently participating in other federal programs including SNAP, TANF, and Medicaid.[38] Undocumented immigrants may participate in WIC, and WIC does not ask about or track its participants' immigration status. In addition to income requirements, individuals must be considered at nutrition risk, meaning that they have medical-based (e.g., underweight, anemia) or dietary-based (e.g., a poor diet) conditions.[38]

The mission of WIC is to improve the health and nutrition status of participants.[38] To accomplish this, WIC participants receive benefits in the form of a prescriptive supplemental food package.[38] While called a "food package," women actually receive coupons or an Electronic Benefit Transfer redeemable at any WIC-authorized store for the foods included in the food package. The food packages allow participants to redeem a maximum monthly quantity of WIC-approved foods, where the quantity and type of prescribed foods varies by pregnancy/breastfeeding status and child age.[39] There are currently seven food packages: two for infants (0–5 months or 6–11 months), one for individuals with medical needs, one for children, and three for women (depending on if woman is pregnant, postpartum and partially/not breastfeeding, or postpartum and fully breastfeeding). Unlike SNAP, each participant receives the same amount of food in a given food package, irrespective of income. Foods included in the package include infant formula, juice, milk, breakfast cereal, cheese, eggs, whole-wheat bread, fish, and legumes/peanut butter. Participants also receive a cash value voucher that can be used to purchase fruits and vegetables ($8 for children and $11 for women).[39] In addition to food packages, WIC participants also receive nutrition education/counseling, breastfeeding support, and referrals to health and social services.[38]

The current food packages reflect revisions made by the USDA in 2009 in order to more closely align the packages with recommendations from the Dietary Guidelines for Americans. These were the first changes in over 30 years and included the addition of fruits and vegetables, whole-grain options, and cultural food options (e.g., tofu). Unlike SNAP, the WIC program has specific aims to improve the dietary quality and health status of participants. Consistent evidence demonstrates that participation in WIC leads to better pregnancy outcomes—fewer infant deaths, less premature births, and increased birth weights.[40-42] Studies examining breastfeeding among WIC participants compared to nonparticipants are generally inconclusive, with some studies suggesting lower rates of breastfeeding among WIC participants.[41] Studies examining the impact of the new WIC nutrition standards shows that the revisions had a positive impact on food purchases and consumption among WIC households (e.g., more fruits, vegetables, whole grains, and low-fat or non-fat milk), improved the retail food environment in low-income areas, and may have reduced obesity among children.[41,43,44] Studies examining the association between WIC participation and infant growth outcomes are mixed,[41] although the evidence base may strengthen considerably as infants who were fed under the revised WIC food packages are more closely studied. Finally, studies suggest that children who participate in WIC or whose mothers are on WIC have an increased engagement with preventative services and are more connected with the health care system.[41]

Child and Adult Care Food Program (CACFP)

CACFP is a wide-scoping nutrition assistance program that subsidizes nutritious meals and snacks for infants and children attending child care centers, family day care homes, afterschool care programs, and emergency shelters, as well as functionally impaired or older adults (aged 60+) attending adult day care centers (figure 14.5).[45]

Eligible child care centers include public or private nonprofit child care centers, Head Start programs, and before/afterschool care centers. During day care, the center provides enrolled children with eligible healthy foods for which CACFP will reimburse the center at free, reduced-price, or paid rates depending on participant income eligibility.[35] Family day care homes (i.e., day cares in private homes) can also participate in CACFP, with reimbursements rates depending on whether the home is located in a low-income

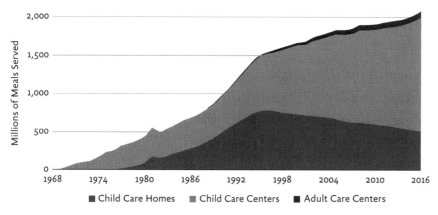

Figure 14.5. Trends in total meals served through CACFP, 1969–2016. *Source:* USDA/FNS CACFP Participation, Meals and Cost Data.

area or higher-income area.[45,46] Eligible afterschool care programs include community-based programs which offer constructive activities during after-school hours and where at least 50% of enrolled children are eligible for free or reduced-price meals.[45,47] These programs are eligible to provide free meals and snacks to all attending children for which the program is fully reimbursed.[45,47] Emergency shelters are also eligible for CACFP reimbursement and can provide up to three free and reimbursable meals a day to children and youth experiencing homelessness.[45,48] In addition to programming aimed at children, CACFP also subsidizes nutritious meals served to adults in public or private nonprofit adult day care centers. Adults must be aged 60 or older or experience significant physical or mental impairment. Similar to child day care centers, adult day care centers provide reimbursements based on participant's eligibility for free, reduced-price or paid meals.[45,49] Given that CACFP is an entitlement program, all eligible homes and centers must be allowed to participate, and all eligible children being cared for in the homes and centers must be served. Immigrant status does not affect eligibility.

As part of the Healthy Hunger-Free Kids Act, nutrition standards for meals and snacks reimbursable for CACFP were also updated to be aligned with the Dietary Guidelines for Americans.[50] In particular, foods served now require a greater variety of vegetables and fruits, more whole grains and protein options, and less added sugar.[12]

Few evaluations of the effectiveness of CACFP in reducing food insecurity and improving dietary quality among participants exist. One reason is that the wide-scoping and decentralized nature of CACFP makes comprehensive evaluations challenging. Existing studies generally focus on assessing the nutrient composition of CACFP meals and snacks,[51,52] although much of this research may be less relevant in light of the recent improvements to CACFP-eligible foods. Several older studies have suggested that preschoolers in CACFP-participating centers have improved dietary intake compared to

In addition to the five main programs, the USDA also administers a number of programs with smaller reach. The remaining 10 USDA nutrition assistance programs account for only 4% of the total budget: the Emergency Food Assistance Program, Summer Food Service Program, Commodity Supplemental Food Program, Fresh Fruit and Vegetable Program, Nutrition Assistance for Puerto Rico, Food Distribution Program on Indian Reservations, Senior Farmers' Market Nutrition Program, WIC Farmers' Market Nutrition Program, Special Milk Program, and the Disaster Food Assistance Program.[55] Two of those are described below:

The *Summer Food Service Program (SFSP)* is designed to continue nutrition support for children in low-income communities during summer months when school is not in session.[17] Attention to nutrition during the summer is particularly important in light of evidence suggesting accelerated summer weight gain for children, particularly among racial/ethnic minorities and those who already have overweight or obesity.[56] While the administration of the SFSP shares administrative similarities with other child nutrition programs at the federal and state levels, local operation of the program differs.[37] At the local level, sponsoring agencies (such as schools, local government agencies, camps, and other nonprofit community organizations) enter into agreements with their state agencies to administer the program at sites located in their community.[37] A variety of settings, including schools, parks, community centers, health clinics, hospitals, apartment complexes, churches, and migrant centers can serve as appropriate meal distribution sites in the SFSP. Participation levels in the SFSP are quite small in comparison to the NSLP or SBP but have risen consistently over the last 15 years as sponsored sites and community outreach has grown. In 2017, the SFSP provided more than 150 million meals and snacks to children during the summer when school was not in session.[17]

The *Fresh Fruit and Vegetable Program (FFVP)* is a small program that provides free fruits and vegetables to elementary students in participating schools during school hours.[57] The program is particularly directed toward low-income schools with high free and reduced-price meal enrollment. As part of the program, participating schools receive a yearly budget per student (e.g., $50 to $75) to purchase fresh fruits and vegetables. These fruits and vegetables must be offered free of cost to students and outside of the normal time frames for the National School Lunch Program and School Breakfast Program; the provision of fruits and vegetables is often accompanied by nutrition education.[17] A recent USDA report summarized the impact of the FFVP, finding that children in FFVP schools consumed one-third of a cup more fruits and vegetables per day compared to children in non-FFVP schools.[57] Additionally, children in FFVP schools had improved knowledge, attitudes, and perception toward fruits and vegetables and were more likely to consume fruits and vegetables outside the school environment.[57]

children in non-CACFP-participating centers, including consuming more milk and vegetables;[53,54] higher daily intakes of vitamin A, riboflavin and calcium;[54] and fewer fats and sweets.[54]

US Federal Nutrition Policies
The Farm Bill

The Farm Bill is a comprehensive piece of legislation that is typically renewed every five years and governs an array of federal programs and policies related to food and agriculture.[58] The Farm Bill consists of a number of components including crop insurance, conservation, farm commodity support, and domestic nutrition assistance programs.[58] At enactment, the 2018 Farm Bill estimated that $326 billion, or 76% of the budget, would be allocated for federal nutrition assistance programs during fiscal year 2019-2023.[58]

One of the key impacts of the 2014 Farm Bill was that it preserved the fundamental structure of USDA nutrition assistance programs (box 14.2)—including, notably, the largest nutrition assistance program, SNAP. Despite strong efforts from opponents, SNAP was not converted to a block grant program (i.e., it is still able to respond automatically to economic change), eligibility was not fundamentally restricted or reduced, participation was not further limited if an individual was unable to secure a job, and categorical eligibility (which greatly simplifies program operations by allowing states to align SNAP financial eligibility rules with other means-tested programs) was not compromised or eliminated. However, allocations to federal nutrition assistance programs have been decreasing slowly since 2012; the 2018 Farm Bill decreased the budget by 4% compared to the 2014 Farm Bill.[58]

Healthy Hunger-Free Kids Act (HHFKA)

In 2010, the HHFKA authorized funding and established policy for USDA's core child nutrition programs to be in alignment with the most current dietary science: the NSLP, the SBP, WIC, Child and Adult Care Food Program, and the Summer Food Service Program.[59] Children spend much of their day in school, and many consume a majority of their daily calories there. However, until passage of the bipartisan Healthy Hunger-Free Kids Act (HHFKA), the federal policies governing the nutrient content of school meals went largely unchanged for 15 years and there had not been a noninflationary reimbursement rate increase in over 30 years.[59]

HHFKA implemented evidence-based reforms to existing nutrition standards for all meals and snacks served in participating schools, and it established additional new guidelines for food sold à la carte through school cafeterias, vending machines, and student stores.[60] HHFKA invested $4.5 billion to improve school nutrition, including a 6-cents-per-lunch increase in reimbursement for school lunches meeting updated school meal standards.[61] The USDA began phasing in these improvements over a three-year period starting with the 2012-2013 school year. This represented the first time in the history of these programs that there was an intentional focus on not only feeding hungry children but on nourishing them as well.

US State- and Local-Level Programs and Policies

In addition to the far-reaching federal programs and policies in the United States, state legislation and local programs also aim to create healthier environments for Americans. The nutrition-related policies and programs covered in this section are not meant to be exhaustive but instead to highlight examples of existing efforts. Also, not included in this section are activities to improve nutrition that are occurring outside of government by private companies or nongovernment organizations.

School-Focused Programs and Policies

Given that students spend half their waking hours and consume at least one-third of their daily calories at school, schools are a natural setting to improve child nutrition, address food insecurity, and prevent childhood obesity.[62] School-focused efforts include school nutrition policies (e.g., "Breakfast After the Bell"), nutrition education, farm-to-school programs, and school wellness policies.[63]

In 2013, 28 states enacted school nutrition policies complementing the federal HHFKA.[63] School breakfast policies like "Breakfast After the Bell"—which provide grab-and-go breakfast, second-chance breakfast between morning classes, or breakfast in the classroom—and other innovative breakfast program models were passed in Arkansas, Colorado, Delaware, the District of Columbia, Illinois, Maryland, Nevada, New Jersey, New Mexico, Texas, Virginia, and West Virginia as of 2016.[64] These new breakfast programs are an improvement on previous models as they do not require students to arrive at school before the start of the school day and therefore may reduce stigma.[64] The Food Research & Action Center surveyed secondary school principals (n = 105) during the 2014-2015 school year to evaluate the effectiveness of "Breakfast After the Bell," with principals reporting fewer occurrences of student hunger, improved student attentiveness, fewer tardy students, and an improved classroom environment.[65] These results are also supported by a more recent No Kid Hungry report that found similar gains in academic achievement and school environment associated with "Breakfast After the Bell" implementation.[64]

Nutrition education is not a federally required component of the standard health education curriculum. Despite its demonstrated benefits,[66] it is estimated that only 71% of primary school districts require nutrition and dietary behavior topics to be taught as part of health education, and 48% require the inclusion of chronic disease prevention (e.g., diabetes or obesity prevention) topics.[67] To address these gaps, Massachusetts enacted a state-level policy mandating the inclusion of nutrition education in schools, and Louisiana and Oregon passed legislation to encourage parent involvement in nutrition education and the inclusion of agriculture-based nutrition education, respectively.[63]

Farm-to-school legislation aims to introduce fresh food into schools, while also increasing students' awareness of food procurement and strengthening local agricultural economies.[63] For example, Mississippi, one of the nine states that enacted farm-to-school policies in 2013, created an innovative Interagency Farm-to-School Council to cultivate farm-to-school programming, encourage local food sourcing for school meals, and facilitate purchasing between local businesses and farms.[63] The implementation of farm-to-school legislation and programming is associated with higher fruit and vegetable availability in schools.[68] Additionally, there is evidence that students participating in farm-to-school programming have increased willingness to try fruits and vegetables, nutrition and agriculture knowledge, and fruit and vegetable consumption (among those with low intakes at baseline).[69]

As part of the Child Nutrition and WIC Reauthorization Act of 2004, schools with child nutrition programs (e.g., NSLP) were required to enact a school wellness policy.[63,70] The HHFKA continued this requirement, while also specifying five elements that must be included in the wellness policies: nutrition education, school meals, physical activity, implementation and evaluation, and competitive foods.[70] While almost all schools nationwide now have a wellness policy, the policies vary in comprehensiveness and strength.[63,70] More recently, state legislation has been implemented to support and expand the implementation of school wellness policies.[63] For example, coordinated school health and wellness pilot programs were funded in Connecticut, Louisiana, and Mississippi, while Massachusetts enacted legislation to include obesity prevention programs with nutrition and wellness components into school curriculum.[63]

Community-Focused Programs and Policies

At the state level, community-focused nutrition programs and policies include increasing healthy food access, initiatives to expand local sustainable food systems (e.g., farmers markets), and implementing fiscal taxes or incentives.[63]

Access to healthy foods is a particular barrier in underserved communities lacking grocery stores that are within walking distance for neighborhood residents and sell fresh, nutritious foods. In 2012, the Illinois Fresh Food Fund, a $10 million program, was enacted to address low access to healthy foods in food-insecure Illinois communities by financing grocery store development to increase the availability of healthy foods.[63] The Pennsylvania Fresh Food Financing Initiative, a similar program funded from 2004–2010, helped build 78 supermarkets and fresh-food outlets in underserved communities that increased access to healthy food for almost 500,000 residents.[71] Other impacts included local job creation and economic revitalization.[71]

In 2013, at least 17 states established initiatives to increase access to local food through farmers markets and other community programs.[63] The 2014 Farm Bill expanded federal funding for USDA's Farmers Market and Local Food Promotion Program to $30 million per fiscal year, which supports farmers markets and other local food suppliers across the country.[63,72] For example, the Appalachian Sustainable Development's Appalachian Harvest program is a regional program that addresses economic and health disparities by increasing food access between local farmers and communities, donating produce to area food banks and pantries, providing agriculture education to schoolchildren, and supporting farmers markets.[63] In 2015, Appalachian Harvest donated almost 130,000 pounds of produce (over 516,000 servings) to families in need, led food tastings for over 1,500 children, and provided nutrition and garden education in 12 school gardens for over 1,000 students.[73] Urban agriculture and community gardens are also on the rise in states. For example, California enacted policy giving power to cities and counties to zone urban areas for local food production, and Tennessee removed a restriction on selling produce from community gardens.[63]

Fiscally, states also enact tax credits/exemptions to encourage healthy choices or levy taxes to deter unhealthy behaviors.[63] For example, Kentucky, Louisiana, Missouri, Oregon, and South Dakota incentivize donations to food banks and pantries.[63] Alternatively, many states continue to consider taxes on sugar-sweetened beverages (SSB) and foods of minimal nutritional value, but, to date, none have been enacted at the state level. Instead, these taxes have been implemented at the local level, with Berkeley, California, placing the first penny-per-ounce excise tax on SSB in 2015.[74] Initial evaluations demonstrate that city-level SSB taxes can be effective in reducing consumption while also raising substantial revenue that can be earmarked for nutrition-related programming.[75]

Comparison of Nutrition-Related Programs and Policies across High-Income Countries
Nutrition Information: Spotlight on Dietary Guidelines

Dietary guidelines provide key recommendations for caloric and food-group intake with the goal of improving population health. Guidelines are primarily developed for professional audiences and are often used to inform programs, policies, and food labeling that target the broader population. For example, the Dietary Guidelines for Americans serve as a foundation for federal nutrition policies and programs across the United States, with several programs recently incorporating the Dietary Guidelines for Americans into their food offerings and nutrition education components, including WIC in 2009, school food programs (e.g., NSLP and SBP) in 2012, and Child and Adult Care Feeding Program in 2015. Additionally, front-of-package food labels are a common translation of dietary guidelines to inform consumer purchasing. For example, the Choices Programme, developed in the Netherlands, adds a check mark to healthy products and has been disseminated worldwide. Similarly, the United Kingdom uses a Traffic Light approach, developed by the Food Standards Agency, to highlight energy, fat, saturated fat, sugar, and salt, which has since been adapted in the United States as Nutrition Keys (figure 14.6).[76]

A recent review reported that 83 out of 215 countries had dietary guidelines, with a clear association between a country's income level and the presa

Each grilled burger (94g) contains

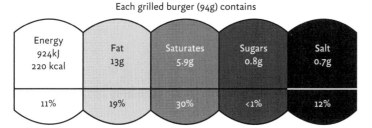

of an adult's reference intake
Typical values (as sold) per 100g: Energy 966kJ/230kcal

b

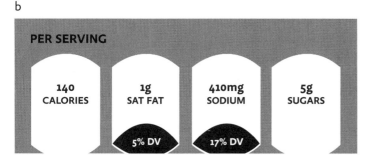

Figure 14.6. Front-of-package food labeling: (a) Traffic Light (UK) and
(b) Nutrition Keys (US). *Source:* Traffic Light, https://www.nutrition.org
.uk/healthyliving/helpingyoueatwell/324-labels.html?start=3. Contains
UK public sector information licensed under the Open Government
License v3.0.

ence of dietary guidelines.[77] Fifty-three percent of high-income countries
have dietary guidelines, 45% of upper-middle-income countries, 24% of low-
middle-income countries, and 6% of low-income countries.[77] The most common messages included in dietary guidelines are reducing sodium, sugar, and
saturated fat intake while increasing fruit and vegetable consumption.[77] Additionally, physical activity recommendations are often included in dietary
guidelines.[77]

Table 14.2 summarizes key recommendations for adults from current dietary guidelines in the United States, Canada, the United Kingdom, Germany,
Sweden, Japan, Australia, and Qatar.[78] The table is not meant to be exhaustive; it provides a sampling of dietary guidelines from a selection of high-
income countries. Food-group categories, serving-specific recommendations, and energy intake recommendations are generally consistent across
the dietary guidelines summarized in table 14.2. For example, the "5 per
Day" minimum recommendation for fruit and vegetables is consistent, although some countries emphasize consuming a variety of fresh, seasonal,
local produce while limiting servings from fruit juice. Additionally, choosing lower-fat foods and beverages, whole grains, and increasing fish consumption is a consistent theme. Discretionary choices, especially products

Table 14.2. Comparison of Dietary Guidelines across High-Income Countries, Adults

Country, dietary guidelines	Recommendations		Additional nutrition and lifestyle advice	Energy intake (kcal/day)
	Food groups	Nutrients		
United States 2015–2020 Dietary Guidelines for Americans (2015) Updated: Every 5 years, since 1980	**Vegetables:** 2.5 cups/day **Fruit:** 2 cups/day **Grain:** 6 oz/day **Dairy:** 3 cups/day **Protein:** 5.5 oz/day **Oils:** 27 g/day	**Carbohydrates** ■ Choose a variety of vegetables from all subgroups ■ At least half of grains should be whole grains **Protein** ■ Choose a variety of protein foods (seafood, lean meats/poultry, eggs, legumes, nuts/seeds, soy products) **Fat** ■ Fat-free or low-fat dairy ■ Limit saturated (<10% of total kcal/day) & *trans* fats	■ Follow a healthy eating pattern across the life span ■ Limit calories from added sugars (<10% of total kcal/day) & reduce sodium intake (<2,300 mg/day) ■ Alcohol consumed in moderation (1 drink/day for women, 2 drinks/day for men) ■ Moderate-intensity exercise ≥150 mins/week or vigorous-intensity aerobic activity 75 mins/week (or a combination)	**Men** *Sedentary:* 2,200–2,400 *Moderately active:* 2,400–2,800 *Active:* 2,800–3,000 **Women** *Sedentary:* 1,600–2,000 *Moderately active:* 1,800–2,200 *Active:* 2,200–2,400
Canada Eating Well with Canada's Food Guide (2007) Updated: Varies, since 1942	Servings/day: **FV:** 7–8 (women), 8–10 (men) **Grain:** 6–7 (women), 8 (men) **Milk:** 2 **Meat:** 2 (women), 3 (men) **Oils & Fats:** 2–3 Tbsp	**Carbohydrates** ■ Choose 1 dark-green & 1 orange vegetable/day ■ Half of your grains should be whole **Protein** ■ Have meat alternatives often ■ 2 servings of fish/week **Fat** ■ Select lower-fat milk alternatives & lean meat ■ Choose unsaturated, limit saturated & *trans* fat	■ Choose prepared foods with little or no added fat, sugar, salt ■ Have breakfast daily ■ Read the nutrition label ■ Eat FV at all meals/snacks ■ Be active, ≥2.5 hours/week of MVPA	**Men** *Sedentary:* 2,350–2,500 *Low active:* 2,600–2,700 *Active:* 2,900–3,000 **Women** *Sedentary:* 1,800–1,900 *Low active:* 2,000–2,100 *Active:* 2,250–2,350

Country / Guideline	Recommended amounts	Food group guidance	Other tips	Energy
United Kingdom Eatwell Guide (2016) Updated: Every ~10 years, since 1994	**FV:** 5 servings/day **Starchy carbohydrates:** ~1/3 of daily intake **Dairy, protein, oils & spreads:** no quantity provided	**Carbohydrates** ■ Base meals on potatoes, bread, rice, pasta, or other starchy carbohydrates ■ Choose whole grains where possible **Protein** ■ 2 servings of fish/week (1 should be an oily fish) **Fat** ■ Choose lower fat & sugar dairy ■ Choose unsaturated oils & spreads	■ Limit fruit juice & smoothies to 150ml/day ■ Drink 6–8 cups of fluid/day ■ Cut down added sugar intake (<30g or 7 sugar cubes per day) ■ Cut down on salt (adults <6g/day) ■ Focus on more sustainable food ■ Read the food labels ■ Don't skip breakfast	**Men:** 2,500 kcal/day **Women:** 2,000 kcal/day
Germany 10 Guidelines of the German Nutrition Society (DGE) for a Wholesome Diet (Vollwertig essen und trinken nach den 10 Regeln der DGE) (2013) Updated: Every 7 years, since 1956	Per day **Whole grain:** 200–300g bread/cereal & 1 serving potatoes/pasta/rice **Vegetables:** 3 servings (400g) **Fruit:** 2 servings (250g) **Dairy:** 200–250g low-fat milk/dairy & 2 slices (50–60g) low-fat cheese **Oils & fats:** 10–15g oil & 15–30g butter/margarine Per week **Meat & eggs:** 300–600g low-fat meat/sausage, 1 serving (80–150g) low-fat seafood, 1 serving (70g) rich fish, up to 3 eggs	**Carbohydrates** ■ 30g/day of fiber especially from whole-grain products ■ Favor seasonal, fresh FV **Protein** ■ White meat is more favorable than red meat **Fat** ■ Choose low-fat products, especially with meat and dairy ■ Favor vegetable fats/oils	■ Focus on a sustainable diet & food diversity ■ Choose mainly plant-based foods ■ Daily fluid intake of 1.5 liters ■ Rarely drink sugar-sweetened beverages & alcohol ■ Exercise 30–60 mins/day	None listed

(continued)

Table 14.2 (continued)

Country, dietary guidelines	Recommendations			Energy intake (kcal/day)
	Food groups	Nutrients	Additional nutrition and lifestyle advice	
Sweden (Nordic) Find your way to eat greener, not too much and to be active! (2015) Updated: Based on 2012 Nordic Nutrition Guidelines	<u>More</u> **FV:** 500g/day **Seafood:** 2–3x/week <u>Switch To</u> **Whole grains:** 70g/day (women), 90g/day (men) **Healthy fats:** unspecified limits **Low-fat dairy:** 2–5 dL/day <u>Less</u> **Red & processed meat:** 500g/week **Salt & sugar:** unspecified limits	**Carbohydrates** ■ Choose high-fiber vegetables, colorful & seasonal FV ■ Choose whole-grain varieties **Protein** ■ Focus on fish/shellfish ■ Vary seafood intake by low-fat and fatty varieties ■ Switch red & processed meat with legumes, fish, eggs, poultry **Fat** ■ Choose unsaturated fats, nuts & seeds ■ Choose dairy products that are low-fat, unsweetened, enriched with vitamin D	■ Holistic, sustainable approach ■ Minimize environmental impact ■ Cut back on sweet drinks & alcohol ■ More exercise (≥30 mins/day)	None listed
Japan Dietary Guidelines for Japanese (食生活指針)[18] (2010) Updated: Every 5 years, since 2000	Servings/day **Grains:** 5–7 **Vegetables:** 5–6 **Fish & meat:** 3–5 **Milk:** 2 (200 ml/day) **Fruits:** 2	**Carbohydrates** ■ Include grain dishes with each meal **Protein** ■ Moderate fish & meat dishes **Fat** ■ Limit greasy dishes	■ Importance of physical activity and water/teas ■ Reduce leftovers & waste through proper cooking and storage ■ Eat well-balanced meals during regular hours ■ Limit consumption of processed snacks, confection, and sugar-sweetened beverages to <200 kcal/day	**Men:** 2,200–2,600 **Women:** 1,800–2,200

	Servings/day	Food group recommendations	Additional recommendations	Energy
Australia Australian Dietary Guidelines (2013) Updated: Every 10 years, since 1982	Servings/day **Vegetables & legumes/beans:** 5 (women), 6 (men) **Fruit:** 2 **Grain:** 6 **Meat, poultry, fish, eggs:** 2.5 (women), 3 (men) **Dairy:** 2.5 **Unsaturated spreads/oils or nuts/seeds:** 14–20g/day (women), 28–40g/day (men)	**Carbohydrates** ■ Variety of vegetables (types & colors) & legumes/beans ■ Mostly whole- & high-fiber grains **Protein** ■ Lean meats ■ Maximum 455g of red meat/week **Fat** ■ Reduced fat dairy ■ Limit saturated fat intake ■ Replace saturated fats with polysaturated/monounsaturated fats	■ Provides serving size examples ■ Limit discretionary choices (e.g., sweets, processed meats, fried foods, salty snacks, sugar-sweetened drinks, alcohol) ■ Drink plenty of water ■ Eat at home more often & try new ways of cooking ■ Use fruit for snacks & desserts ■ Include 1 or 2 meat-free meals/week ■ ≥30 mins/day of moderate-intensity exercise	**Men:** 9,900 kJ/day (~2,350 kcal) **Women:** 8,000 kj/day (~1,900 kcal)
Qatar Qatar Dietary Guidelines (الدلائل الإرشادية الغذائية لدولة قطر) (2015) Updated: Launched in 2015	Servings/day **Vegetables:** 3–5 **Fruit:** 2–4 **Cereals/starchy vegetables:** no quantity provided **Legumes:** Daily (not specific) **Dairy:** Daily (not specific) **Meat:** no quantity specified	**Carbohydrates** ■ Aim for a variety of seasonal, fresh FV & eat with most meals/snacks ■ Favor whole fruit over juices (no more than ½ cup/day) ■ Eat more greens & leafy vegetables ■ Substitute refined products with high-fiber whole grains with little/no added fat, sugar, salt **Protein** ■ Variety of fish 2x/week ■ Choose skinless poultry & low-fat meat ■ Avoid processed meats ■ Choose legumes, nuts, seeds as alternative protein sources **Fat** ■ Choose low-fat, unsweetened, vitamin D-fortified dairy products ■ Avoid saturated, hydrogenated, *trans* fat ■ Use healthy vegetable oils	■ Provides serving size examples ■ Limit sugar, salt (<5g/day), fat ■ Avoid sweetened beverages ■ Eat less fast foods & processed foods ■ Read nutrition labels ■ Eat homemade food more often ■ Emphasize plant-based diet, choose local foods, reduce waste ■ Drink 2–3 liters of fluid/day, choosing water often ■ Adopt safe & clean food preparation methods ■ Be physically active (moderate intensity 5 days/week for at least 30 minutes; vigorous intensity 3 days/week & include muscle-strengthening activities	None listed

Note: FV = fruits and vegetables; MVPA = moderate to vigorous physical activity.

with added sugar (e.g., sugar-sweetened beverages), high levels of sodium (e.g., salty snacks and processed meats), and excessive alcohol consumption are discouraged in most of the guidelines. Finally, many countries also provide specific dietary recommendations for important subgroups in the population (e.g., children, women of childbearing age, and older adults), versions for vulnerable peoples (e.g., First Nations, Inuit, and Métis[79] in Canada and Aboriginal and Torres Strait Islanders[80] in Australia), and highlight alternative eating patterns (e.g., Mediterranean and Vegetarian in the United States[81]).

In addition to use by professional audiences, simplified dietary guidelines are often distributed to consumers through visual representations. Figure 14.7 depicts the various styles of food guides corresponding to the dietary guidelines listed in table 14.2. At the time of writing, the United States and Canada both use a plate illustration to highlight recommended relative consumption of fruits, vegetables, grains, and protein. Sweden's dietary guidelines, based on the 2012 Nordic Guidelines, suggest consumers consume "more," "less," and "switch to" certain food groups, with the color scheme reflecting the green, red, and yellow traffic light visual.[82] Notably, Japan's culturally relevant spinning top contradicts the consensus that fruit and vegetables should represent the largest part of the diet, placing grains as the highest proportion of the diet in the model.[78]

There is a global shift toward the promotion of sustainable diets in current dietary guidelines. A sustainable diet is characterized by shifting to a plant-based diet, selecting seasonal and locally grown produce, limiting meat consumption, and avoiding processed foods.[77] This sustainability theme is a strong focus in the dietary guidelines for the high-income countries of Sweden, Qatar, and Germany, along with the upper-middle-income country of Brazil. High-income countries of the United States and Australia have attempted to include sustainable considerations but have yet to gain government approval.[77] The FAO review also highlights the emerging transition of the United Kingdom, France, Netherlands, and Estonia (all high-income countries) toward sustainable-minded dietary recommendations.[77]

Adherence to Dietary Guidelines

Overall, dietary recommendations are not being met across most high-income countries. Most adults in high-income countries fail to meet the recommendations for fruit and vegetables, with only 30% of adults in the United Kingdom and 26% of Canadians meeting their country's recommended intakes for fruits and vegetables.[83,84] Similarly, 87% of Americans fall below the US recommendation for vegetables and 75% fall below the recommendation for fruit.[81] Most adults in high-income countries exceed the guidelines for saturated fat, sodium, and added sugar. For example, among Nordic populations in Denmark, Finland, Iceland, and Sweden, the majority of adults consume excess saturated fat and sodium.[85] Likewise, 70% of Americans exceed the

US recommendation for added sugars, 71% exceed the recommendation for saturated fat, and 89% exceed the recommendation for sodium.[81]

Hunger Relief: Spotlight on Food Banks and Pantries

Food insecurity and hunger in high-income countries are often addressed through food banks and food pantries. A **food bank** is defined as a "charitable organization that solicits, receives, inventories, and distributes donated food and grocery products . . . to charitable human service agencies (e.g., food pantries), which provide the products directly to clients through various programs."[86] Feeding America in the United States, Foodbank in Australia, and The Trussell Trust Foodbank Network in the United Kingdom are examples of large hunger relief organizations. Food banks were originally created as emergency food assistance, but with changing economic conditions, such as substantial wage stagnation over the last 40 years in the United States, they often serve as ongoing food assistance. Feeding America reports that 36% of clients use their pantries regularly each month.[86]

In the United States, many food-insecure households often combine both public (e.g., SNAP and WIC) and private (e.g., food banks and pantries) resources to alleviate food insecurity and hunger. The most recent Hunger in America Report by Feeding America found that at least 55% of households using food banks are also receiving SNAP benefits.[87] Food banks are also an important resource for food-insecure households who are not eligible for federal nutrition assistance programs. For example, SNAP limits eligibility by income, excludes all undocumented immigrants as well as many documented immigrants who have lived in the United States for less than five years, and some states have a time limit to apply for SNAP benefits.[87,88] Based on a Feeding America's 2014 Client Survey, 39% of households that use food banks were not eligible for SNAP benefits based on income eligibility requirements (above 130% of the federal poverty line).[87] Frequent food bank usage and inadequate support from federal safety net programs is not unique to the United States, with Food Banks Canada reporting a 28% increase in food bank recipients from 2008 to 2016, with a large proportion of households using food banks also receiving government assistance (e.g., pension, disability, welfare).[88] In the United Kingdom, a 2017 report found similar drivers of recurrent food bank usage, including welfare benefit delays, income shocks, and poverty.[89]

Regulatory Approaches: Spotlight on Restrictions on Marketing to Children

There is considerable global debate around the ethical concerns of marketing unhealthy foods and beverages to vulnerable populations (e.g., children) given the implications that this may contribute to obesogenic environments.[90] US food and beverage companies spend nearly $2 billion annually marketing to children, with 84% of advertisements viewed by children promoting

Plate

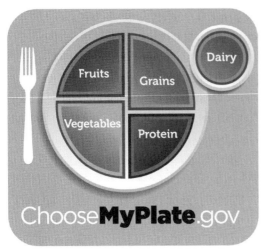

United States (2015)

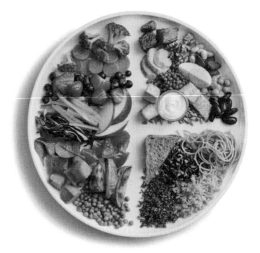

Canada (2019)

Traffic Light

Find *your* way

to eat **greener**, **not too much**, and **be active**

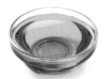

MORE	SWITCH	TO	LESS
vegetables, fruit and berries	white flour	whole grain	red and processed meat
fish and shellfish	butter-based fats	vegetable fats and oils	salt
nuts and seeds	high-fat dairy products	low-fat dairy products	sugar
exercise			alcohol

Sweden (2015)

Figure 14.7. Visual representation of food guides across high-income countries.

foods and beverages high in fat, sugar, and salt, as no regulations for broadcasting advertisements for foods high in fat, sugar, and salt currently exist.[91] Cross-promotion is a common marketing method where industries use channels such as popular movies, TV shows, and cartoon characters to advertise food and beverage products.[92] For example, it is common practice for companies to display characters from popular children's movies like *Frozen* or *Ice Age* on fruit snacks, cereal, and candy to incentivize purchases.[92] The

Pie Chart

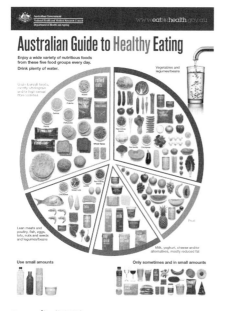

Australia (2013)

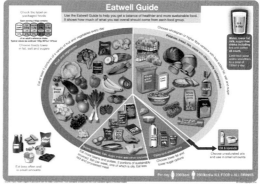

United Kingdom (2016)

Spinning Top

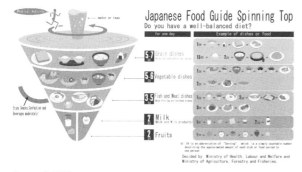

Japan (2010)

strength of the food and beverage industries have made it very challenging to pass national legislation on marketing restrictions to children.[90]

A 2016 UNICEF report found that while most countries have national legislation regulating *general* marketing and advertising to consumers, only 10 countries *explicitly* address marketing and advertising to children: Argentina, Austria, Belgium, Denmark, Ecuador, France, Germany, India, the United Arab Emirates, and the United Kingdom.[93] For example, the United Kingdom has general statutes and codes regulating marketing to consumers but additionally restricts marketing products that are harmful to children (e.g., foods high in fat, sugar, and salt), timing and placement of marketing to children, and the use of certain marketing techniques to children (e.g., cross-promotion).[93] China, France, Poland, Russia, Switzerland, and the United Kingdom have restrictions on marketing and advertising in schools or other places children regularly visit, while Australia, Brazil, Ghana, Indonesia, Italy, Spain, Sweden, and the United Kingdom have restrictions on marketing and advertising techniques that target children.[93] The United Kingdom has been a leader in restricting marketing to children as the first country to ban foods high in fat, sugar, and salt advertisements on television channels and programs aimed at children aged 4-15 years.[94] However, there are many loopholes in the current restrictions (i.e., lack of enforcement), and restrictions are absent at the point of purchase, for product packaging, and for foods high in fat, sugar, and salt sponsorship and promotion at sporting events.[95] Similarly, the Marketing Act in Sweden bans any advertisements targeting children under the age of 12 on national radio and television before and during children's programs.[96] Despite the lag in marketing restrictions for American children, the 2010 HHFKA included restrictions on marketing to children in schools by restricting food and beverage advertisements to those that meet the Smart Snacks in School nutrition standards.

There has been some notable industry self-regulation related to marketing to children. For example, in the United States more than a dozen major food and beverage companies launched the Children's Food and Beverage Advertising Initiative (CFBAI) in 2009 and pledged to advertise only healthier products to children. A similar industry self-regulation initiative was launched in 2015 in Canada—the Canadian Children's Food and Beverage Advertising Initiative (CAI)—with commitments from 17 corporations (Campbell Canada, Coca-Cola, Danone, Ferrero, General Mills, Hershey's, Kellogg Canada, Kraft Canada, Mars, McDonald's, Mondelēz, Nestlé, Parmalat, PepsiCo, Post, Unilever, and Weston Bakeries).[97] The core principles of the CAI are directed at children 12 years and under and include advertising only healthy products, integrating healthier products in interactive games, reducing the use of licensed characters in advertising, eliminating product placement in channels specifically directed at children, and stopping all advertising in schools.[97] While the participating companies are following their pledges, the evidence suggests that the pledges may not have a meaningful impact on shifting the food and beverage advertising on television toward healthier products since the standards are not high.[98,99] Also, many companies do not participate, which limits impact.[98]

Conclusion

Government programs and policies are an effective way for high-income countries to address nutrition-related issues including food insecurity and obesity. Within the United States, a comprehensive suite of federal nutrition assistance programs administered by the USDA form a nationwide safety net that works to promote the nutrition, health, and well-being of Americans across the life course. There are additional efforts at the state and local level that aim to improve nutrition by directing efforts at the school and community level. Across high-income countries, the creation of national dietary guidelines, the contribution of food banks, and restriction of marketing to children are three examples of efforts aimed toward improving population health and nutrition.

Review Questions

1. Describe the five major federal nutrition assistance programs in the United States and discuss which populations they target and the aims of each program.
2. Identify ways in which state- and local-level efforts in the United States can tackle nutrition-related issues.
3. How are dietary guidelines used in high-income countries to promote nutrition?
4. What is the role of food banks in addressing food insecurity?

References

1. Campbell, Cathy C. 1991. "Food Insecurity: A Nutritional Outcome or a Predictor Variable?" *Journal of Nutrition* 121 (3): 408-15.

2. Coleman-Jensen, Alisha, Matthew Rabbitt, Christian Gregory, and Anita Singh. 2019. *Household Food Security in the United States in 2018, EER-270*. US Department of Agriculture, Economic Research Service.

3. Stevens, Gretchen A., Gitanjali M. Singh, Yuan Lu, Goodarz Danaei, John K. Lin, Mariel M. Finucane, Adil N. Bahalim, et al. 2012. "National, Regional, and Global Trends in Adult Overweight and Obesity Prevalences." *Population Health Metrics* 10 (1): 22. https://doi.org/10.1186/1478-7954-10-22.

4. Swinburn, Boyd, and Garry Egger. 2002. "Preventive Strategies against Weight Gain and Obesity." *Obesity Reviews* 3 (4): 289-301.

5. Swinburn, Boyd A., Gary Sacks, Kevin D. Hall, Klim McPherson, Diane T. Finegood, Marjory L. Moodie, and Steven L. Gortmaker. 2011. "The Global Obesity Pandemic: Shaped by Global Drivers and Local Environments." *The Lancet* 378 (9793): 804-14. https://doi.org/10.1016/S0140-6736.

6. "Programs and Services." 2016. US Department of Agriculture (USDA), Food and Nutrition Services (FNS). https://www.fns.usda.gov/programs-and-services.

7. *Program Information Report: US Summary, FY 2015-FY 2016*. 2016. US Department of Agriculture (USDA), Food and Nutrition Services (FNS). http://www.fns.usda.gov/sites/default/files/datastatistics/keydata-february-2016.pdf.

8. "Programs and Services." 2018. US Department of Agriculture (USDA), Food and Nutrition Services (FNS). https://www.fns.usda.gov/programs-and-services.

9. Bartfeld, Judith, Craig Gundersen, Timothy Smeeding, and James Ziliak. 2016. *SNAP Matters: How Food Stamps Affect Health and Well-Being*. Redwood City, CA: Stanford University Press.

10. "A Short History of SNAP." 2014. US Department of Agriculture (USDA), Food and Nutrition Services (FNS). https://www.fns.usda.gov/snap/short-history-snap.

11. "SNAP Policy on Non-Citizen Eligibility." 2017. US Department of Agriculture (USDA), Food and Nutrition Services (FNS). https://www.fns.usda.gov/snap/snap-policy-non-citizen-eligibility.

12. "Nutrition Standards for CACFP Meals and Snacks." 2017. US Department of Agriculture (USDA), Food and Nutrition Services (FNS). https://www.fns.usda.gov/cacfp/meals-and-snacks.

13. "Building a Healthy America: A Profile of the Supplemental Nutrition Assistance Program." 2012. US Department of Agriculture (USDA), Food and Nutrition Services (FNS). https://fns-prod.azureedge.net/sites/default/files/BuildingHealthyAmerica.pdf.

14. "SNAP Eligible Food Items." 2017. US Department of Agriculture (USDA), Food and Nutrition Services (FNS). https://www.fns.usda.gov/snap/eligible-food-items.

15. "SNAP Eligibility." 2020. US Department of Agriculture (USDA), Food and Nutrition Services (FNS). https://www.fns.usda.gov/snap/recipient/eligibility.

16. Ratcliffe, Caroline, and Signe-Mary McKernan. 2010. "How Much Does SNAP Reduce Food Insecurity?" *The Urban Institute*. Washington, DC.

17. "Summer Food Service Program." 2017. US Department of Agriculture (USDA), Food and Nutrition Services (FNS). https://www.fns.usda.gov/sfsp/summer-food-service-program.

18. "Full Committee—Public Hearing RE: Pros and Cons of Restricting SNAP Purchases." 2017. *House Committee on Agriculture*. https://agriculture.house.gov/calendar/eventsingle.aspx?EventID=3644.

19. Cole, Nancy, and Mary Kay Fox. 2008. "Diet Quality of Americans by Food Stamp Participation Status: Data from the National Health and Nutrition Examination Survey, 1999-2004." Alexandria, VA. https://fns-prod.azureedge.net/sites/default/files/NHANES-FSP.pdf.

20. "Supplemental Nutrition Assistance Program (SNAP) Linkages with the General Economy." 2017. US Department of Agriculture, Economic Research Service. https://www.ers.usda.gov/topics/food-nutrition-assistance/supplemental-nutrition-assistance-program-snap/economic-linkages/.

21. Mabli, James, Emily Sama Martin, and Laura A. Castner. 2009. *Effects of Economic Conditions and Program Policy on State Food Stamp Program Caseloads, 2000 to 2006*. Washington, DC: US Department of Agriculture, Economic Research Service.

22. Hanson, K. 2010. "The Food Assistance National Input-Output Multiplier (FANIOM) Model and Stimulus Effects of SNAP." Washington, DC: US Department of Agriculture, Economic Research Service.

23. Castner, Laura, and Julieete Henke. 2011. "Benefit Redemption Patterns in the Supplemental Nutrition Assistance Program (SNAP)." Alexandria, VA: US Department of Agriculture, Food and Nutrition Services.

24. Nord, Mark, and Mark A. Prell. 2011. *Food Security Improved Following the 2009 ARRA Increase in SNAP Benefits*. Washington, DC: US Department of Agriculture, Economic Research Service.

25. "National School Lunch Program Fact Sheet." 2017. US Department of Agriculture (USDA), Food and Nutrition Services (FNS). https://fns-prod.azureedge.net/sites/default/files/cn/NSLPFactSheet.pdf.

26. Guthrie, Joanne, and Katherine Ralston. 2018. "National School Lunch Program." Washington, DC: US Department of Agriculture, Economic Research Service. https://www.ers.usda.gov/topics/food-nutrition-assistance/child-nutrition-programs/national-school-lunch-program.

27. "Community Eligibility Provision." 2017. US Department of Agriculture (USDA), Food and Nutrition Services (FNS). https://www.fns.usda.gov/school-meals/community-eligibility-provision.

28. "Community Eligibility Provision Evaluation (Summary)." 2014. US Department of Agriculture (USDA), Food and Nutrition Services (FNS). https://fns-prod.azureedge.net/sites/default/files/CEPEvaluation_Summary.pdf.

29. "Final Rule: Nutrition Standards in the National School Lunch and School Breakfast Programs." 2012. US Department of Agriculture (USDA), Food and Nutrition Services (FNS).

30. Ralston, Katherine, Constance Newman, Annette Clauson, Joanne Guthrie, and Jean Buzby. 2008. "The National School Lunch Program: Background, Trends, and Issues, ERR 61." Washington, DC: US Department of Agriculture.

31. Gordon, Anne, Mary Kay Crepinsek, Renee Nogales, and Elizabeth Condon. 2007. "School Nutrition Dietary Assessment Study III, Volume I: School Food Service, School Food Environment, and Meals Offered and Served." Alexandria, VA: US Department of Agriculture, Food and Nutrition Services.

32. Gordon, Anne, Mary Kay Fox, Melissa Clark, Rénee Nogales, Elizabeth Condon, Philip Gleason, and Ankur Sarin. 2007. "School Nutrition Dietary Assessment Study III, Volume II: Student Participation and Dietary Intakes." Alexandria, VA: US Department of Agriculture, Food and Nutrition Services.

33. Cohen, Juliana F. W., Scott Richardson, Ellen Parker, Paul J. Catalano, and Eric B. Rimm. 2014. "Impact of the New US Department of Agriculture School Meal Standards on Food Selection, Consumption, and Waste." *American Journal of Preventive Medicine* 46 (4): 388–94.

34. "School Breakfast Program." 2017. US Department of Agriculture (USDA), Food and Nutrition Services (FNS). https://www.fns.usda.gov/sbp/school-breakfast-program-sbp.

35. "School Breakfast Program (SBP) Program History." 2017. US Department of Agriculture (USDA), Food and Nutrition Services (FNS). https://www.fns.usda.gov/sbp/program-history.

36. Cullen, Karen Weber, and Tzu-An Chen. 2017. "The Contribution of the USDA School Breakfast and Lunch Program Meals to Student Daily Dietary Intake." *Preventive Medicine Reports* 5: 82–85.

37. "Special Supplemental Program for Women, Infants, and Children (WIC)." n.d. US Department of Agriculture (USDA), Food and Nutrition Services (FNS). https://www.fns.usda.gov/wic.

38. "About WIC: WIC at a Glance." 2015. US Department of Agriculture (USDA), Special Supplemental Nutrition Program for Women, Infants, and Children (WIC). https://www.fns.usda.gov/wic/about-wic-wic-glance.

39. "WIC Food Packages: Maximum Monthly Allowances." 2016. US Department of Agriculture (USDA), Food and Nutrition Services (FNS). https://www.fns.usda.gov/wic/wic-food-packages-maximum-monthly-allowances.

40. Carlson, Steven, and Zoë Neuberger. 2015. "WIC Works: Addressing the Nutrition and Health Needs of Low-Income Families for 40 Years." *Center on Budget and Policy Priorities*.

41. Colman, Silvie, Ira P. Nichols-Barrer, Julie E. Redline, Barbara L. Devaney, Sara V. Ansell, and Ted Joyce. 2012. "Effects of the Special Supplemental Nutrition Program for Women, Infants, and Children (WIC): A Review of Recent Research." Mathematica Policy Research.

42. Fox, Mary Kay, William L. Hamilton, and Biing-Hwan Lin. 2004. "Effects of Food Assistance and Nutrition Programs on Nutrition and Health: Volume 4, Executive Summary of the Literature Review." US Department of Agriculture, Economic Research Service.

43. Kong, Angela, Angela M. Odoms-Young, Linda A. Schiffer, Yoonsang Kim, Michael L. Berbaum, Summer J. Porter, Lara B. Blumstein, Stephanie L. Bess, and Marian L. Fitzgibbon. 2014. "The 18-Month Impact of Special Supplemental Nutrition Program for Women, Infants, and Children Food Package Revisions on Diets of Recipient Families." *American Journal of Preventive Medicine* 46 (6): 543–51.

44. Whaley, Shannon E., Lorrene D. Ritchie, Phil Spector, and Judy Gomez. 2012. "Revised WIC Food Package Improves Diets of WIC Families." *Journal of Nutrition Education and Behavior* 44 (3): 204–9.

45. "Why CACFP Is Important." 2014. US Department of Agriculture (USDA), Food and Nutrition Services (FNS). https://www.fns.usda.gov/cacfp/why-cacfp -important.

46. "Family Day Care Homes." 2015. US Department of Agriculture (USDA), Food and Nutrition Services (FNS). https://www.fns.usda.gov/cacfp/family-day -care-homes.

47. "Afterschool Meals." 2016. US Department of Agriculture (USDA), Food and Nutrition Services (FNS). https://www.fns.usda.gov/cacfp/afterschool-meals.

48. "Meals in Emergency Shelters." 2016. US Department of Agriculture (USDA), Food and Nutrition Services (FNS). https://www.fns.usda.gov/cacfp/meals -emergency-shelters.

49. "Adult Day Care Centers." 2017. US Department of Agriculture (USDA), Food and Nutrition Services (FNS). https://www.fns.usda.gov/cacfp/adult-day-care-centers.

50. "Final Rule: Child and Adult Care Food Program: Meal Pattern Revisions Related to the Healthy, Hunger-Free Kids Act of 2010." 2016. US Department of Agriculture (USDA), Food and Nutrition Services (FNS). https://www.gpo.gov /fdsys/pkg/FR-2016-04-25/pdf/2016-09412.pdf.

51. Crepinsek, Mary Kay, Nancy R. Burstein, Ellen B. Lee, and William L. Hamilton. 2002. "Meals Offered by Tier 2 CACFP Family Child Care Providers: Effects of Lower Meal Reimbursements." USDA Economic Research Service, Electronic Publications from the Food Assistance and Nutrition Research Program, E-FAN.

52. Fox, Mary Kay, Frederic B. Glantz, and Lynn Geitz. 1997. "Early Childhood and Child Care Study: Nutritional Assessment of the CACFP: Volume II, Final Report." US Department of Agriculture.

53. Korenman, Sanders, Kristin S. Abner, Robert Kaestner, and Rachel A. Gordon. 2013. "The Child and Adult Care Food Program and the Nutrition of Preschoolers." *Early Childhood Research Quarterly* 28 (2): 325–36.

54. Bruening, Kay Stearns, Judith A. Gilbride, Marian R. Passannante, and Sandra McClowry. 1999. "Dietary Intake and Health Outcomes among Young

Children Attending 2 Urban Day-Care Centers." *Journal of the American Dietetic Association* 99 (12): 1529–35.

55. Brown, Kay E. 2015. "Domestic Food Assistance: Multiple Programs Benefit Millions of Americans, but Additional Action Is Needed to Address Potential Overlap and Inefficiencies." http://www.gao.gov/assets/680/670313.pdf.

56. Franckle, Rebecca, Rachel Adler, and Kirsten Davison. 2014. "Accelerated Weight Gain Among Children During Summer Versus School Year and Related Racial/Ethnic Disparities: A Systematic Review." *Preventing Chronic Disease* 11 (June): 130355. https://doi.org/10.5888/pcd11.130355.

57. Bartlett, Susan, Lauren Olsho, Jacob Klerman, Kelly Lawrence Patlan, Michelle Blocklin, Patty Connor, Karen Webb, Lorrene Ritchie, and Patricia Wakimoto. 2013. "Evaluation of the Fresh Fruit and Vegetable Program (FFVP): Final Evaluation Report." Alexandria, VA. https://fns-prod.azureedge.net/sites /default/files/FFVP.pdf.

58. Johnson, Renée, and Jim Monke. 2019. "What Is the Farm Bill?" https://fas .org/sgp/crs/misc/RS22131.pdf.

59. "Healthy Hunger-Free Kids Act." 2017. US Department of Agriculture (USDA), Food and Nutrition Services (FNS). https://www.fns.usda.gov/school -meals/healthy-hunger-free-kids-act.

60. "National School Lunch Program and School Breakfast Program: Nutrition Standards for All Foods Sold in School as Required by the Healthy, Hunger-Free Kids Act of 2010." 2013. US Department of Agriculture (USDA), Food and Nutrition Services (FNS). https://www.gpo.gov/fdsys/pkg/FR-2013-06-28/pdf/2013-15249.pdf.

61. "Certification of Compliance with Meal Requirements for the National School Lunch Program Under the Healthy, Hunger-Free Kids Act of 2010." 2012. US Department of Agriculture (USDA), Food and Nutrition Services (FNS).

62. Committee on Accelerating Progress in Obesity Prevention, Food and Nutrition Board, and Institute of Medicine. 2012. *Accelerating Progress in Obesity Prevention: Solving the Weight of the Nation.* Edited by D. Glickman, L. Parker, L. J. Sim, H. Del Valle Cook, and E. A. Miller. Washington, DC: National Academies Press.

63. Winterfeld, A. 2014. "State Actions to Reduce and Prevent Childhood Obesity in Schools and Communities: Summary and Analysis of Trends in Legislation." In *Washington, DC: National Conference of State Legislatures*.

64. "School Breakfast: Changing State Policy to Increase Access to Breakfast." 2018. No Kid Hungry Center for Best Practices. https://bestpractices.nokidhungry .org/school-breakfast/school-breakfast-policy-0.

65. "School Breakfast After the Bell." 2015. Food Research & Action Center. http://frac.org/wp-content/uploads/secondary-principals-bic-report.pdf.

66. Contento, I., George I. Balch, and Yvonne L. Bronner. 1995. "The Effectiveness of Nutrition Education and Implications for Nutrition Education Policy, Programs and Research a Review of Research." *Journal of Nutrition Education* 27:277–418.

67. CDC. 2016. "Results from the School Health Policies and Practices Study." United States Health and Human Services Department, Centers for Disease Control and Prevention.

68. Nicholson, Lisa, Lindsey Turner, Linda Schneider, Jamie Chriqui, and Frank Chaloupka. 2014. "State Farm-to-School Laws Influence the Availability of Fruits

and Vegetables in School Lunches at US Public Elementary Schools." *Journal of School Health* 84 (5): 310–16.

69. Yoder, Andrea B. Bontrager, Janice L. Liebhart, Daniel J. McCarty, Amy Meinen, Dale Schoeller, Camilla Vargas, and Tara LaRowe. 2014. "Farm to Elementary School Programming Increases Access to Fruits and Vegetables and Increases Their Consumption among Those with Low Intake." *Journal of Nutrition Education and Behavior* 46 (5): 341–49.

70. Chriqui, Jamie, Elizabeth Pickarz, and Rebecca Schermbeck. 2016. "School District Wellness Policies: Evaluating Progress and Potential for Improving Children's Health Eight Years after the Federal Mandate." Chicago: Institute for Health Research and Policy, University of Illinois at Chicago. http://www .bridgingthegapresearch.org/_asset/98nbk1/WP_2016_monograph.pdf.

71. Treuhaft, Sarah, and Allison Karpyn. 2010. "The Grocery Gap: Who Has Access to Healthy Food and Why It Matters." PolicyLink & The Food Trust. http://thefoodtrust.org/uploads/media_items/grocerygap.original.pdf.

72. "Farmers Market Promotion Program: 2016 Report." 2016. Washington, DC: USDA Agricultural Marketing Service. https://www.ams.usda.gov/sites/default /files/media/FMPP2016Report.pdf.

73. Appalachian Sustainable Development. 2015. "2015 Annual Report." Abingdon, VA. http://asdevelop.org/wp-content/uploads/2016/05/ASD-2015-annual-report -for-web.pdf.

74. City of Berkeley, CA. 2016. "Frequently Asked Questions (FAQ) for the Sweetened Beverage Tax of Berkeley, CA."

75. Silver, Lynn D., Shu Wen Ng, Suzanne Ryan-Ibarra, Lindsey Smith Taillie, Marta Induni, Donna R. Miles, Jennifer M. Poti, and Barry M. Popkin. 2017. "Changes in Prices, Sales, Consumer Spending, and Beverage Consumption One Year after a Tax on Sugar-Sweetened Beverages in Berkeley, California, US: A before-and-after Study." Edited by Claudia Langenberg. *PLOS Medicine* 14 (4): e1002283. https://doi.org/10.1371/journal.pmed.1002283.

76. Hawley, Kristy L., Christina A. Roberto, Marie A. Bragg, Peggy J. Liu, Marlene B. Schwartz, and Kelly D. Brownell. 2013. "The Science on Front-of-Package Food Labels." *Public Health Nutrition* 16 (3): 430–39.

77. Fischer, C. Gonzalez, and Tara Garnett. 2016. "Plates, Pyramids, Planet: Developments in National Healthy and Sustainable Dietary Guidelines: A State of Play Assessment." *Rome: Food and Agriculture Organization of the United Nations and The Food Climate Research Network at The University of Oxford.*

78. "Japanese Food Guide Spinning Top." 2010. Ministry of Health, Labour and Welfare and Ministry of Agriculture, Forestry and Fisheries. http://www.maff.go .jp/e/data/publish/attach/pdf/index-63.pdf.

79. "Eating Well with First Nations, Inuit, and Métis." 2007. Ottawa, Ontario: Minister of Health Canada. https://www.canada.ca/content/dam/hc-sc/migration /hc-sc/fn-an/alt_formats/fnihb-dgspni/pdf/pubs/fnim-pnim/2007_fnim-pnim _food-guide-aliment-eng.pdf.

80. "Aboriginal and Torres Strait Islander Guide to Healthy Eating." 2015. Australian Government, National Health and Medical Research Council, Department of Health. https://www.nhmrc.gov.au/_files_nhmrc/file/your_health

/healthy/nutrition/final_-_atsi_guide_to_healthy_eating_a4_size_double_sided
_poster_d15-11061411.pdf.

81. "2015–2020 Dietary Guidelines for Americans." 2015. US Department of
Agriculture (USDA), Food and Nutrition Services (FNS). https://health.gov
/dietaryguidelines/2015/guidelines/.

82. "Find Your Way to Eat Greener, Not Too Much and Be Active." 2015.
Livsmedelsverket National Food Agency. http://www.fao.org/3/a-az854e.pdf.

83. Bates, Beverley, Alison Lennox, Ann Prentice, Christopher J. Bates, Polly
Page, Sonja Nicholson, and Gillian Swan. 2014. "National Diet and Nutrition
Survey: Results from Years 1, 2, 3 and 4 (Combined) of the Rolling Programme
(2008/2009–2011/2012): A Survey Carried Out on Behalf of Public Health England
and the Food Standards Agency." London: Public Health England and Food
Standards Agency.

84. Black, Jennifer L., and Jean-Michel Billette. 2013. "Do Canadians Meet
Canada's Food Guide's Recommendations for Fruits and Vegetables?" *Applied
Physiology, Nutrition, and Metabolism* 38 (3): 234–42.

85. Jonsdottir, Svandis Erna, Lea Brader, Ingibjorg Gunnarsdottir, Ola Kally
Magnusdottir, Ursula Schwab, Marjukka Kolehmainen, Ulf Risérus, et al. 2013.
"Adherence to the Nordic Nutrition Recommendations in a Nordic Population
with Metabolic Syndrome: High Salt Consumption and Low Dietary Fibre Intake
(The SYSDIET Study)." *Food and Nutrition Research* 57 (1): 21391.

86. "Food Banks: Hunger's New Staple." 2011. Chicago, IL: Feeding America.
http://www.feedingamerica.org/research/hungers-new-staple/hungers-new-staple
-full-report.pdf.

87. "Hunger in America 2014 National Report." 2014. Feeding America.
http://help.feedingamerica.org/HungerInAmerica/hunger-in-america-2014-full
-report.pdf.

88. "Map the Meal Gap 2017: Highlights of Findings for Overall and Child Food
Insecurity." 2017. Chicago, IL: Feeding America.

89. Loopstra, Rachel, and Doireann Lalor. 2017. "Financial Insecurity, Food
Insecurity, and Disability: The Profile of People Receiving Emergency Food
Assistance from The Trussell Trust Foodbank Network in Britain." Salisbury,
England: The Trussell Trust. https://www.trusselltrust.org/wp-content/uploads
/sites/2/2017/07/OU_Report_final_01_08_online2.pdf.

90. Nill, Alexander. 2015. *Handbook on Ethics and Marketing*. Northhampton, MA:
Edward Elgar Publishing.

91. Powell, Lisa M., Rebecca M. Schermbeck, and Frank J. Chaloupka. 2013.
"Nutritional Content of Food and Beverage Products in Television Advertisements
Seen on Children's Programming." *Childhood Obesity* 9 (6): 524–31.

92. Commission, Federal Trade. 2012. "A Review of Food Marketing to
Children and Adolescents: Follow-up Report." Washington, DC: US Government
Printing Office.

93. UNICEF. 2016. "Advertising & Marketing to Children: Global Report." New
York: United Nations Children's Fund.

94. WHO. 2013. "Nutrition, Physical Activity, and Obesity: United Kingdom of
Great Britain and Northern Ireland." World Health Organization. http://www.euro

.who.int/__data/assets/pdf_file/0020/243335/United-Kingdom-WHO-Country
-Profile.pdf?ua=1.

95. "UK's Restrictions on Junk Food Advertising to Children." 2017. The Food
Foundation. http://foodfoundation.org.uk/wp-content/uploads/2017/07/3-Briefing
-UK-Junk-Food_vF.pdf.

96. WHO. 2013. "Nutrition, Physical Activity and Obesity: Sweden." World
Health Organization. http://www.euro.who.int/__data/assets/pdf_file/0003
/243327/Sweden-WHO-Country-Profile.pdf.

97. "The Canadian Children's Food and Beverage Advertising Initiative: 2016
Compliance Report." 2016. Ad Standards. 2016.

98. Kunkel, Dale L., Jessica S. Castonguay, and Christine R. Filer. 2015. "Evaluating Industry Self-regulation of Food Marketing to Children." *American Journal of Preventive Medicine* 49 (2): 181-87.

99. Kent, Monique Potvin, Lise Dubois, and Alissa Wanless. 2011. "Self-regulation by Industry of Food Marketing Is Having Little Impact during Children's Preferred Television." *Pediatric Obesity* 6 (5-6): 401-8.

15

A Deeper Look: The Special Supplemental Nutrition Program for Women, Infants, and Children (WIC)

Julie A. Reeder

LEARNING OBJECTIVES

- Trace the history of the WIC program from its inception to today
- Describe the core components of a WIC certification visit
- Differentiate WIC from other food assistance programs
- Recognize the interaction between the WIC food packages and the larger community food environment
- Be able to identify allied programs and resources (website, videos, materials) addressing common issues among the WIC population
- Illustrate at least two ways in which WIC is more than a food assistance program
- Propose a course of action for WIC's future challenges and opportunities

Case Study: Vignettes from WIC Participants in Oregon

I wasn't expecting to have babies. All my friends would tell me that there's just not enough room in your heart for all the love that a baby brings. But once my baby was born, I found out that is so true! I like to think I'm a pretty loving person already as is, but I just didn't think I was capable of being that loving. —Oregon WIC participant sharing what she loves about being a mom

I really love to just be there for my children and I try to be a good role model for them. Sometimes you think you need to correct your children, but you actually need to correct yourself. I learned this the hard way. I was really grateful for WIC because I had so much going on—between leaving work and trying to make time for my family—so being able to get food vouchers was a very big help.

And I'm really grateful for this program because it has been a consistent source of support, and that's something I needed. I'm very blessed to have that in WIC, and I've learned that you just have to keep going forward. I think it's really important that we're just not another person in line, that there's a story behind us. —Oregon WIC participant sharing what the program has meant to her during difficult times

The Special Supplemental Nutrition Program for Women, Infants, and Children (WIC) arose from the antipoverty and civil rights movements of

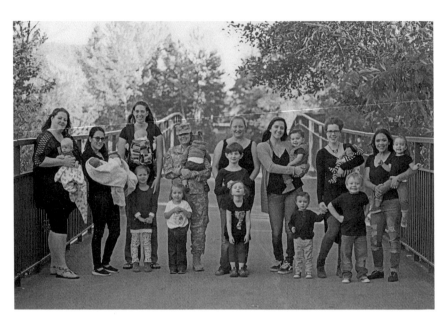

Figure 15.1. WIC families.

the late 1960s (box 15.1). WIC began as a two-year pilot program in 1972 and was initially called the Special Supplemental Food Program. The words *Women, Infants, and Children* were added in 1973. In 1975 legislation was passed making WIC a permanent national health and nutrition program.[1,2] The program's mission is to safeguard the health of low-income women, infants, and children up to age 5 who are at nutrition risk by providing nutritious foods to supplement diets, information on healthy eating, and referrals to health care (figures 15.1-15.6). The name and core components of the program as well as the food items offered by the program have changed in the decades since its inception[3] (table 15.1). A specific emphasis on breastfeeding promotion was added in 1989. The program's name was changed again in 1994 to the Special Supplemental Nutrition Program to better emphasize WIC's nutrition focus. Other additions to the original program include the WIC Farmers' Market Nutrition Program and breastfeeding peer counselors. In 2009, significant changes were made to the items included in the WIC food packages to better align with the Dietary Guidelines for Americans. These changes included a cash-value voucher to purchase fruits and vegetables, whole-grain products, and options for tofu and soy milk.[1-3] The program continues to evolve as new research identifies key nutrients of concerns for the maternal and child population, the expanding diversity of WIC participants brings about a shift in food preferences, and as technology plays an ever-increasing role in accessing health information and services.

WIC is administered by the US Department of Agriculture, Food and Nutrition Service. Federal funding is provided to 50 state, 5 territorial, and 34

Table 15.1. Major Milestones of the Special Supplemental Nutrition Program for Women, Infants, and Children (WIC)

Year	Milestone
1978	Nutrition education becomes a required program component
1987	First infant formula rebate program
1988	Grants awarded to 10 states for farmers market demonstration programs
1989	Child Nutrition Reauthorization Act requires all states to use competitive bidding to procure infant formula. Adjunctive eligibility established. USDA required to promote breastfeeding.
1992	WIC Farmers' Market Nutrition Program established
1992	An enhanced food package was introduced to promote breastfeeding
1994	Legislation changes name to Special Supplemental Nutrition Program for Women, Infants, and Children to emphasize nutrition focus
1997	Loving Support national breastfeeding campaign to encourage WIC participants to initiate and continue breastfeeding
2004	Breastfeeding Peer Counselor Initiative launched
2009	New WIC food packages introduced based on Institute of Medicine recommendations and in alignment with the Dietary Guidelines for Americans. Whole grains added to the food packages as well as infant foods. A cash dollar amount provided for produce.

intertribal organizations to administer the program. There are over 10,000 WIC clinic sites nationwide located in county health departments, community centers, medical clinics, hospitals, mobile sites, and migrant health centers. WIC is the nation's third-largest nutrition assistance program, behind SNAP and the School Meals Program. Over 7 million women, infants, and children participate in the program each year. WIC reaches just over half of all pregnant women in the nation.[1]

WIC Eligibility and Services

To participate in WIC, an individual must meet categorical and income requirements. WIC serves (1) pregnant women, (2) breastfeeding women for up to one-year postpartum, (3) nonbreastfeeding postpartum women up to six months, (4) infants, and (5) children up until their fifth birthday.[1] WIC can also provide services to the children of single fathers, those being raised by grandparents, and children in the foster care system. To be income eligible, household incomes must be ≤185% of the federal poverty level. Individuals can be adjunctively eligible through participation in other programs such as Medicaid. Participants must also have a nutrition risk, as determined by a WIC health professional. This can be a dietary or health risk

For a detailed history of the origins of the WIC Program, view "Saving the Children: The Story of WIC" on YouTube.

Concept Check

WIC services currently end for nonbreastfeeding women at 6 months and breastfeeding women at 12 months postpartum. With an increased interest in improving the health of women before and between pregnancies, suggestions have been made to extend the amount of time women remain on the program.

If you were writing a policy proposal to increase the length of time women could participate in WIC, what would your main arguments be for doing so? How would you address the main barriers to extending the duration of participation?

Did You Know?

WIC is not an entitlement program. Entitlement programs such as Social Security, Medicare, Medicaid, and many veterans' benefits are guaranteed to serve all eligible individuals. WIC, however, receives a yearly amount of funding from Congress that is less than the amount required to serve every eligible individual.

---

such as over- or underweight, low iron levels, tobacco use, or inadequate dietary intake.

WIC participants are typically eligible to receive benefits for a six-month period. Pregnant women are certified for the duration of their pregnancy and up to six weeks postpartum. State WIC agencies can opt to provide certifications lasting up to a one-year period, with the ability for infants and breastfeeding women to be certified up to the infant's first birthday. Once the certification period ends, the participant must be recertified to continue receiving benefits.

A WIC certification visit includes nutrition and health screening, referrals to other health and social service programs, nutrition education, breastfeeding education and support, and issuance of food benefits. In a typical WIC visit, a participant's height or length and weight are measured. Iron levels (hemoglobin or hematocrit) may be assessed. A brief health and dietary screening are conducted, with corresponding nutrition education based on identified risks and the participant's desired focus. Food benefits are distributed via paper voucher or loaded on to an electronic debit card. A second contact in approximately three months is scheduled, which could be for a group class, follow-up visit with a dietitian, an online nutrition education course, or a pre-approved community-based nutrition-related event. WIC services are provided by registered dietitians, nurses, and trained paraprofessional staff. International Board-Certified Lactation Consultants and breastfeeding peer counselors are also available in some clinics.

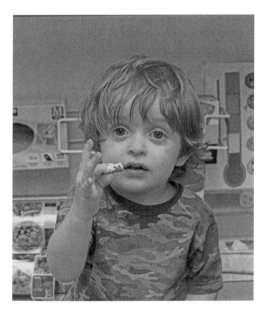

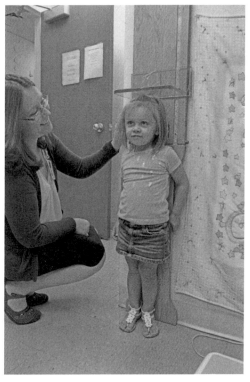

Figure 15.2. Child receiving hemoglobin testing at WIC office.

Figure 15.3. Child having height measured at WIC office.

WIC Food Packages

The WIC food packages are meant to be supplemental and not a source of primary food assistance.[1] WIC food benefits differ from those of other assistance programs in that participants are issued specific quantities of a limited set of WIC-approved food items rather than a dollar amount to spend on any desired food item. For example, women and children are issued 36 ounces of dry breakfast cereal per month and the cereal must meet WIC guidelines for minimum iron and maximum sugar content. The food items and amounts of monthly food benefits are determined by the participant's category and medical needs. Seven different food packages are offered, and all include foods that are high in iron, vitamin C, vitamin A, protein, or calcium. Infants are provided iron-fortified infant formula if they are non-breastfeeding as well as infant cereal, and infant fruits and vegetables starting at 6 months of age. Fully breastfeeding infants are not provided formula and instead receive greater quantities of baby food fruits and vegetables as well as infant food meats at 6 to 12 months of age. Mothers who are fully breastfeeding receive a larger food package than mothers who are not breastfeeding. The core food items in the women's and children's food packages include milk; cheese or yogurt; eggs; dried or canned beans; peanut butter;

whole grains (whole-wheat bread, whole-wheat tortillas, brown rice, corn tortillas, bulgur, barley); low-sugar, iron fortified breakfast cereal; juice; and a voucher to purchase fruits and vegetables.[4] An option to substitute dairy items for soy milk and tofu is available.[4] WIC is transitioning from delivering its food benefits via a paper voucher system to electronic debit cards (EBT), with all programs required to have EBT in place by October 1, 2020. Most WIC participants purchase the WIC-approved foods through the retail food stores, with the majority of WIC transactions occurring in large grocery store chains or supercenters.[5]

WIC's Impact on the Larger Community Food Environment

WIC participants redeem their food benefits at over 47,000 retail food stores nationwide. As WIC is the nation's third-largest nutrition program and serves over 7 million individuals each year, it can have a major impact on the food manufacturing and retail grocery environments (box 15.2).[6] Many companies would like their food products to be on the WIC-approved food list, and some have altered the nutritional content to meet WIC's stringent standards. Not only do these changes assist WIC families in accessing healthier food but the larger community as well. When whole-grain benefits were added to the WIC food package in 2009, the standard 24-ounce loaf of whole-wheat bread did not meet the WIC size requirement of 16 ounces. Although availability of the smaller loaf of bread had limited availability in the first months after roll-out, manufacturers quickly stepped up to make the WIC-approved product.

WIC also impacts the retail food environment by requiring its authorized vendors to carry a minimum stock of WIC-approved foods.[6] WIC-authorized stores are mandated to carry at least one whole-grain cereal, lower-fat milk,

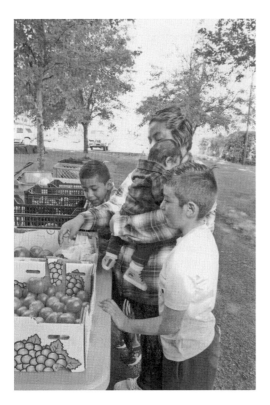

Figure 15.4. Mother and children at farmers market.

and at least two fruits and two vegetables.[7] Some studies have demonstrated a positive impact on the food environment of small stores related to the WIC minimum stock requirements.[8] At the same time, another study suggests that WIC's provision of infant formula without cost to its participants may increase the retail shelf-cost for non-WIC participants.[9]

Finally, WIC supports local agriculture through the WIC Farm Direct Nutrition Program.[10] Each summer, program participants over 4 months of age are issued a set dollar amount per person in vouchers to spend on fruits and vegetables at local farmers markets and farm stands. Having this base of ready consumers can help support new and fledgling markets. At the same time, only 1.7 million of the 7 million WIC participants in the last year reported receiving Farm Direct vouchers[10] due to insufficient federal funding to support voucher issuance to all eligible participants. The federally set minimum Farm Direct benefit dollar value is $10 and the maximum amount $30 per recipient for the summer. Typically, a household is issued only one set of vouchers per participant at the beginning of summer. A state agency can opt to increase the dollar value or number of recipients if they are able to supplement federal funds with local, private, or state funds.[10]

Moving beyond Food Assistance to Address Larger Causes of Health Inequities
Social Determinants of Health

The past decade has seen a growing recognition of the importance of the social determinants of health and their influence on current health inequities. As defined by the World Health Organization, "social determinants of health are the conditions in which people are born, grow, work, live, and age, and the wider set of forces and systems shaping the conditions of daily life."[11] This broader vision of the factors influencing health challenges programs such as WIC to expand their definition of nutrition education as well as moving beyond a focus on individual behavior change as the key mechanism to improving nutrition and health. Food choices and nutrition do not happen in a vacuum. Recognizing the social, emotional, structural, societal, and policy factors that shape these choices is essential. Although referrals are one of the core services of the WIC program, fully addressing the social determinants of health may require WIC to initiate or enhance partnerships with housing, employment and workforce development agencies, environmental health organizations, the criminal justice system, and community mental health programs (box 15.3).

Expanding the Definition of Nutrition Education

A broader focus on the social determinants of health may seem beyond WIC's mission to safeguard the health of low-income women, infants, and children by providing nutritious foods to supplement diets, information on healthy eating, and referrals to health care. However, expanded definitions of nutrition education are increasingly widening the lens of what are viewed as nutrition-related services. The Society for Nutrition Education and Behavior's consensus definition of nutrition education is "any combination of educational strategies, accompanied by environmental supports, designed to facilitate voluntary adoption of food choices and other food and nutrition-related behaviors conducive to health and well-being [*of individuals, community, planet*]. It is delivered through multiple venues and involves activities at the individual, community, and appropriate policy levels."[12] With a new focus on enhancing environmental supports for healthy food and nutrition behaviors and an opportunity to act through multiple venues, WIC has new opportunities to advance it mission of safeguarding the health of low-income women and children.

WIC and Early Learning

Developmental disabilities are common in early childhood, affecting one in six US children. Common developmental conditions include speech/language delays, gross and/or fine motor delays, autism spectrum disorder (ASD), attention-deficit/hyperactivity disorder (ADHD) cerebral palsy, and genetic

Box 15.3. Find Out More

Visit http://www.aylabirth.org/ to learn more about one county's WIC program collaboration with a state women's prison to help mothers provide breastmilk to their infants while separated due to incarceration. The site features a multimedia toolkit as well as videos for parents and foster care providers.

Sesame Street has produced the series "Little Children, Big Challenges." The multimedia toolkit includes caregiver and child resources on topics such as incarceration and divorce. https://www.sesamestreet.org /toolkits/incarceration.

Concept Check

How does the definition of nutrition education in the paragraph above differ from those you have read before?

In your opinion, which of the social determinants of health most closely link to the mission of the WIC program?

Did You Know?

Early Intervention provides services and supports to infants and children with disabilities or developmental delays. As good nutrition and feeding are tied to child development and can be impacted by disabilities, Early Intervention is a critical partner to help safeguard the health and nutrition of WIC participants.

For more information and to find program contact information for your state, visit https://www .cdc.gov/ncbddd/actearly/parents /states.html.

---

conditions such as Down syndrome.[13] For children with these conditions, early access to community-based diagnosis and therapy services is essential. Low-income and racial and ethnic minority children are at risk for under-identification and treatment of developmental disabilities. These children are less likely to participate in early intervention services, which provides free evaluations and services for young children with developmental delays and are more likely to have unmet therapy needs. A recent study found that although it is outside the primary scope of their work, developmental and behavioral concerns are frequently raised and addressed by WIC staff.[13] A majority of staff either noticed concerns or were asked about concerns more than once per week and between once per week and once per month. Although many staff mentioned referring concerns to early intervention services or public health nurses, few WIC staff felt well connected to pediatricians or early intervention staff. Therefore, while WIC staff play an important role in child development, early learning, and identification of delays, further work is needed to improve timely referrals to services and coordination of care.

Referrals are one of the cornerstones of the WIC program, yet communication between WIC and health, early learning, and social service providers relies largely on the WIC participant to follow through with referral information and communicate their referral experience or outcome back to WIC staff. Through policy initiatives, state WIC programs can create standardized workflows for WIC staff when a participant's health, developmental, or social need is identified. Key to the success of these workflows will be the establishment of ongoing, two-way communication between WIC and the referral organizations to ensure continuity of care. The placement of patient navigators—individuals paid by health care systems to help patients with health and social needs to navigate service systems—in WIC would assure a warm hand-off for WIC participants when WIC staff identify an issue that is outside of their scope of practice or requires more intensive case management.

Automated data sharing systems, similar to those in use currently by health systems to track emergency room visits within and outside of their own health networks, could help support continuity of care. Technologies currently exist that could facilitate the automatic extraction and communication of designated information from one organization to another. For example, if WIC staff identify an infant with potential failure to thrive, the system would automatically initiate a data transfer to the WIC participant's primary care provider, thus spurring follow-up by a case manager. Likewise,

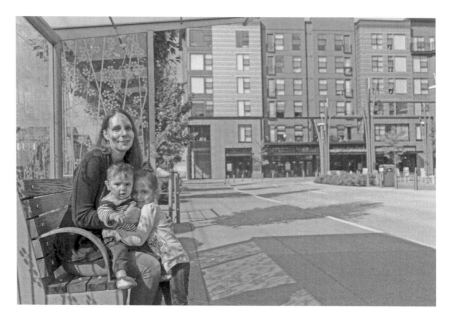

Figure 15.5. WIC family.

automated notification could be sent to WIC staff if a woman is diagnosed with gestational diabetes after her initial WIC visit or has certain complications with labor and delivery, leading to more tailored prenatal or postpartum WIC services.

Transportation is a commonly cited barrier to attending WIC appointments. Non-emergency medical transportation (NEMT) is benefit for Medicaid participants who need to get to and from medical services but have no means of transportation. Federal law requires states to ensure that eligible, qualified Medicaid beneficiaries have NEMT to take them to and from providers. However, states may vary in their implementation of the program. As the vast majority of WIC participants are also Medicaid patients, expanding NEMT to include rides to WIC could lessen the transportation barrier. However, research is needed to determine whether this could be executed in all states and territories given the varied implementation of this program.

Considering Literacy, Numeracy, and Digital Inclusion When Adopting New Technologies

Literacy, numeracy, and more recently health literacy have been identified as important factors in health outcomes. The most recent International Survey of Adult Skills noted, "Literacy skills are linked not only to employment outcomes, but also to personal and social well-being. In the United States the odds of being in poor health are four times greater for low-skilled adults than those with the highest proficiency."[14]

The study also found that adults in the United States had lower literacy and numeracy skills compared to those in other countries. Most US adults had literacy levels corresponding to between the sixth and ninth grades. Numeracy fared worse, with just under two-thirds of US adults scoring at a level 2 or below on a scale of 1 to 5. Problem-solving in technology-rich environments (PSTRE) is defined as the capacity to access, interpret, and analyze information found, transformed, and communicated in digital environments. Two in three US adults scored a level 1 or below, with 3 being the highest level of skill. Online tasks such as completing an unfamiliar form, navigating across pages, and completing multiple steps corresponds with a level 2 score. This means that two-thirds of US adults do not have the skills necessary to complete online application forms, navigate web portals, and go online to connect with their child's school or find and evaluate health information.[14]

At the same time, WIC is rapidly embedding technology throughout every aspect of its services. The program is transitioning from paper vouchers to EBT, has apps, offers online nutrition education and interactive two-way texting, and is seeking to explore online pre-ordering and delivery to ease the shopping experience. Yet for all the technology that has been introduced in WIC, no formal, comprehensive assessment of the digital skill levels of WIC participants has been conducted. Furthermore, the needs of WIC participants with the lowest levels of literacy, numeracy, and those of immigrants and refugees and others who have limited English proficiency have not always been fully incorporated into new technological offerings. Thus, WIC runs the risk of adopting new technologies that may not be a best fit to the digital literacy skills of participants. While technology can produce many efficiencies, it can also unintentionally increase disparities by excluding those with lower skills or access. A digital inclusion framework provides an approach to understanding *both barriers and benefits* to the adoption of technological innovations (box 15.4). Adding such a framework will be critical as WIC moves forward with technology.

Addressing Periconceptual Health and Emphasizing Women's Health

Most women enroll in WIC while pregnant and can continue in the program through six months or one year postpartum, depending on their breastfeeding status. By initiating services in the prenatal period and continuing them into the postpartum phase, WIC has the unique opportunity to interact with women between pregnancies to improve their own health as well as positively influence the outcomes of future births.

There are numerous health issues faced by the women served by WIC. More than half of the women who participate in WIC have a pre-pregnancy body mass index (BMI) that is classified as overweight or obese, half gain

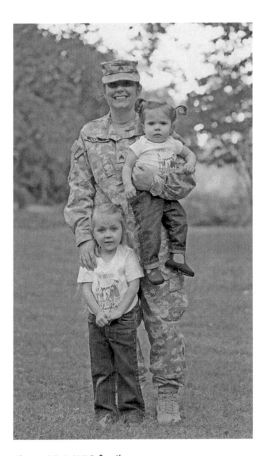

Figure 15.6. WIC family.

more than the recommended amount of weight during their pregnancy, and many retain the weight beyond the early postpartum period. Just over 5% of WIC participants have gestational diabetes and over 6% have gestational hypertension.[15] Depression and other mental and emotional health issues are prevalent with 20% of WIC mothers experiencing postpartum depression.

The need to better understand the underlying causes of these maternal health risk factors in the WIC population as well as how WIC can modify and enhance its current services to better address them is a critical area for study. This would include exploring innovative approaches to addressing postpartum health issues that fall within the appropriate scope of practice for WIC and building partnerships with the medical community to provide services that are beyond that scope.

Few women enroll in WIC during the early weeks of their pregnancy. As such, most have passed the critical time periods for fetal development before they began interacting with WIC. Exploring ways to encourage pregnant women to enroll earlier in WIC is a promising approach to have a greater impact on the critical periods of early fetal development. Designing and testing postpartum health messages or interventions tailored to a woman's health, nutritional, and breastfeeding status as well as her future pregnancy plans would be equally important. Creating and evaluating partnerships between WIC and behavioral or mental health professionals to address maternal depression is another critical area for future initiatives. Improving the health of women during their reproductive years not only holds promise for improving pregnancy outcomes but for reducing the mothers' risk of chronic disease over her lifetime.

Increasing Cultural Diversity

The WIC population is more diverse than the general population, with 58.6% of all WIC participants self-identifying as white only, 20.8% black or African American only, 10.3% American Indian or Alaska Native only, and 4.4% either Asian only or Native Hawaiian or Other Pacific Islander only; 41.8% identified as being of Hispanic ethnicity.[16] Yet, the core components of the WIC food package may not be in keeping with traditional food ways of the diversity of families served by WIC. In its 2017 report, the National Academy of Sciences, Engineering and Medicine recommended that "USDA-FNS should support the cultural food preferences and special dietary needs of WIC participants by requiring states to offer additional options for the WIC food categories."[17] How WIC will balance its traditional nutrient-rich food requirements with changing food trends and increased cultural diversity remains an area for rich exploration.

Instant Access to Nutrition Expertise

Current research demonstrates that people are using social media sites and online searches to find information about topics related to health and nutrition. Results from a study on social media and behavior change showed that of the 74% of American adults who regularly went online, 80% are searching for health information.[18] After checking email and using Internet search engines, searching for health information was the third most popular online activity, among all participants.[19] Social media sites such as Facebook, Tumblr, and Pinterest are all tools currently used for sharing health and nutrition information, including diet, exercise, recipes, and breastfeeding. Women are significantly more likely to use social media to follow topics about health, medicine, and other lifestyle topics than men.[20] Although social media use for the pursuit of information about health may be widespread, what influence it has on perceptions of healthy foods and child feeding approaches, particularly with WIC participants, is limited. However, with open access to an unlimited of amount of advice and information about many of the topics WIC traditionally covers, the program may need to adapt to this changing environment.

Conclusion

The WIC program has been safeguarding the health and well-being of low-income women and children for over four decades and will continue to do so for decades to come. By continually evolving and adapting the core components of its offerings and being a dynamic vs. static program, WIC truly recognizes that each participant is more than just a person standing in line waiting for benefits but is a person with a story. As long as WIC continues to deliver personalized and caring services to some of our most vulnerable citizens, it will remain an essential support for improving maternal and child health.

Review Questions

1. In what year was the WIC program established?
2. Name three significant changes or additions to the WIC program over the decades.
3. WIC food benefits can only be redeemed for a limited set of WIC-approved food items. In contrast, SNAP benefits are a dollar amount that can be spent on a much wider variety of food items. Some have suggested that SNAP should follow WIC's lead and restrict the food items that can be purchased to only "healthy" options. List three pros and three cons to modifying SNAP benefits in this way.
4. You have been charged with writing a policy document to encourage your state legislature to provide supplemental funds to the Farm Direct Nutrition Program. The extra funds could allow you to either give vouchers to more participants or increase the dollar amount with the same number of participants. What key arguments would you put forth to the legislature to justify this use of state funds? If awarded, in which way would you use the extra funds?
5. You receive a phone call from a start-up technology company wanting to expand their product offerings to the WIC program. They have heard that most WIC participants are "young" and therefore they assume that all WIC participants will have the knowledge, skills, and access to use their latest app or online services. What would you share with this company about digital literacy and inclusion?
6. A local organization serving newly arrived immigrant and refugee families reaches out to you to learn more about WIC. One of the first questions they ask is whether the foods offered by WIC will be familiar to the families they serve. How would you respond?
7. You are teaching a childbirth education class at a local hospital. You overhear one mother-to-be telling another mom about a Facebook pregnancy group she is in. When you get to the part of the class where you mention WIC, this mom says that she gets all the information she needs from her Facebook group and isn't sure what else WIC would have to offer. How would you respond?

References

1. Oliveira, Victor, and Frazão Elizabeth. 2015. "The WIC Program: Background, Trends, and Economic Issues, 2015 Edition, EIB-134." United States Department of Agriculture, Economic Research Service.

2. "About WIC: WIC at a Glance." 2015. United States Department of Agriculture (USDA), Women Infants Children (WIC). https://www.fns.usda.gov/wic/about-wic-wic-glance.

3. "WIC Program Overview and History." n.d. National WIC Association. https://www.nwica.org/overview-and-history.

4. "Final Rule: Revisions in the WIC Food Package." 2014. United States Department of Agriculture, Food and Nutrition Services. www.fns.usda.gov/wic/fr-030414.

5. Ploeg, Michele Ver, Lisa Mancino, Jessica E. Todd, Dawn Marie Clay, and Benjamin Scharadin. 2015. "Where Do Americans Usually Shop for Food and How Do They Travel to Get There? Initial Findings from the National Household Food Acquisition and Purchase Survey, EIB-138." USDA United States Department of Agriculture, Economic Research Service.

6. Ploeg, Michele Ver. 2009. "Do Benefits of US Food Assistance Programs for Children Spillover to Older Children in the Same Household?" *Journal of Family and Economic Issues* 30 (4): 412-27. https://doi.org/10.1007/s10834-009-9164-9.

7. Oliveria, Victor, and Elizabeth Frazão. 2015. "Painting a More Complete Picture of WIC: How WIC Impacts Nonparticipants." United States Department of Agriculture, Economic Research Service.

8. Andreyeva, Tatiana, Joerg Luedicke, Ann E. Middleton, Michael W. Long, and Marlene B. Schwartz. 2012. "Positive Influence of the Revised Special Supplemental Nutrition Program for Women, Infants, and Children Food Packages on Access to Healthy Foods." *Journal of the Academy of Nutrition and Dietetics* 112 (6): 850–58. https://doi.org/10.1016/j.jand.2012.02.019.

9. Oliveira, Victor, Elizabeth Frazão, and David Smallwood. n.d. "The Infant Formula Market: Consequences of a Change in the WIC Contract Brand." United States Department of Agriculture, Economic Research Service.

10. "WIC Farmers' Market Nutrition Program." 2016. USDA United States Department of Agriculture. https://fns-prod.azureedge.net/sites/default/files/fmnp/WICFMNPFactSheet.pdf.

11. "Social Determinants of Health." n.d. Geneva, Switzerland: World Health Organization. https://www.who.int/social_determinants/en/.

12. "Nutrition Education." 2018. Society for Nutrition Education and Behavior. https://www.sneb.org/.

13. Zuckerman, Katharine E., Alison E. Chavez, and Julie A. Reeder. 2017. "Decreasing Disparities in Child Development Assessment." *Journal of Developmental & Behavioral Pediatrics* 38 (5): 301-9. https://doi.org/10.1097/DBP.0000000000000446.

14. "United States Country Note: Survey of Adult Skills First Results." 2013. Organisation for Economic Cooperation and Development (OECD). https://www.oecd.org/skills/piaac/Country note - United States.pdf.

15. "Pediatric Nutrition Surveillance Survey." 2011. https://www.health.ny.gov/statistics/prevention/nutrition/pednss/2011/.

16. Thorn, Betsy, Nicole Kline, Chrystine Tadler, Eric Budge, Elaine Wilcox-Cook, Jason Michaels, Michele Mendelson, et al. 2018. "WIC Participant and Program Characteristics 2016." Arlington, VA: United States Department of Agriculture (USDA), Food and Nutrition Services (FNS), Office of Policy Support.

17. *Review of WIC Food Packages*. 2017. Washington, DC: National Academies Press. https://doi.org/10.17226/23655.

18. Korda, Holly, and Zena Itani. 2013. "Harnessing Social Media for Health Promotion and Behavior Change." *Health Promotion Practice* 14 (1): 15–23. https://doi.org/10.1177/1524839911405850.

19. American Press Institute, and Associated Press-NORC Center for Public Affairs Research. 2014. "The Media Insight Project: The Personal News Cycle Report." The Media Insight Project. http://www.mediainsight.org/Pages/the -personal-news-cycle.aspx.

20. Greenwood, Shannon, Andrew Perrin, and Maeve Duggan. 2016. "Social Media Update 2016." Pew Research Center, Internet and Technology.

16

A Deeper Look: Cash Transfer Programs

Garrison J. Spencer, Melissa Hidrobo, Damien de Walque, Paul Gertler, and Lia C. Haskin Fernald

LEARNING OBJECTIVES

- Define types of cash transfer (CT) programs, including CCT (conditional cash transfer) and UCT (unconditional cash transfer) programs and describe the variations among different programs

- Identify the pathways by which participation in CT programs could lead to improved health, nutrition, development, or education outcomes

- Analyze and review results from CT programs worldwide on a range of health, nutrition, development, and education indicators

- Using Mexico's *Prospera* CCT program as a case study, explain the components of the program and the results of the program on infant, child, and adult outcomes

- Compare the costs and benefits of different types of CCT and UCT programs

- Evaluate criticisms of CT programs and how various program types have addressed previous criticisms

Case Study: *Prospera*—Mexico's CCT

In 1994-1995, Mexico experienced a period of political upheaval and economic crisis that resulted in a 6% decline in GDP.[1] This loss of economic activity was expected to have an enormous impact on the nation's poor, and motivated policy makers to adopt a new approach to social programs.[1] The result was a new type of program that combined transferring cash to poor households with the promotion of positive health, education, and nutrition behaviors.[2] This program, initially called *PROGRESA,* subsequently rebranded as *Oportunidades,* and now known as *Prospera,* was rolled out in 1997 and was one of the first of what has become known as a conditional cash transfer (CCT) program. *Prospera* was financed primarily by the elimination of general food subsidies and represented a shift toward a more narrowly targeted and rural antipoverty program.[3] Within three years *Prospera* had expanded to cover 2.6 million families living in 50,000 rural villages, accounting for 40% of rural families and 10% of Mexican families overall.[2] Today, the program reaches over 6 million, or approximately 20%, of all Mexican households.[4]

Conditional and Unconditional Cash Transfer Programs

Cash transfer (CT) programs are a type of noncontributory social assistance designed to support the poor and vulnerable through regular transfers of money in order to protect against shocks, promote human capital accumulation, and disrupt cycles of poverty.[5] Since the earliest CT programs began in the mid-1990s (*Prospera* in Mexico and *Bolsa Familia* in Brazil[6]), CT programs have spread rapidly in low- and middle-income countries (LMICs) as a central part of poverty alleviation and social protection strategies.[7] Today, 130 LMICs have at least one unconditional cash transfer (UCT) program and 63 countries have at least one conditional cash transfer (CCT) program.[7]

There are two types of CT programs: unconditional cash transfers (UCTs) and conditional cash transfers (CCTs). In UCT programs, the recipient must belong to the broadly defined eligibility category but no other conditions are required to receive the transfer.[8] Eligibility categories can be income based (living below an established poverty line), geographically based (living in a defined region), or demographically based (belonging to a defined group such as indigenous peoples or being an orphan). Unlike UCT programs, in CCT programs the provision of the cash transfer is tied to compliance with a set of predetermined actions or behaviors, the "conditions" of the transfer. The conditions of CCTs are intended to induce positive behaviors and activities, such as mandatory school attendance or preventative health care appointments, that are expected to reduce the conditions of poverty for the beneficiaries.[9] CCTs are operationally more complex and costly for governments to implement than UCTs because they require monitoring compliance with the conditions of the transfer. Additionally, health and education conditions require functioning health care and school systems.

Despite common features of many of CT programs, there is a great deal of heterogeneity across countries and programs regarding program benefits, the conditions of transfers, and targeted outcomes. Examples of the different types of UCT and CCT programs that exist around the world today include the following:

- The Uganda Social Assistance Grants for Empowerment (SAGE) program is a UCT that disperses approximately US$9 every other month to two groups of beneficiaries: vulnerable families who are eligible based on a composite index of demographic indicators and the elderly whose eligibility is based on age.[10]
- The *Bono de Desarrollo Humano* (BDH) in Ecuador is an example of a CCT with "soft conditionalities," meaning that compliance with the conditions is weakly monitored or enforced. *Bono de Desarrollo Humano* transfers a flat rate of US$50 each month to eligible families with school-aged children.[11]

Box 16.1. *Prospera's* Conditions and Transfers

Prospera is a CCT with both health and education conditions and transfers. Qualifying households receive a monthly health-related transfer of approximately US$15 per household per month.[12] The characteristics and conditionalities of the health transfer are as follows:

- The transfer amount is fixed and does not depend on the size of the household or age of children.
- Each member of the family must attend regular preventive medical care appointments.
- Family members must attend *pláticas*, health education sessions on various topics.
- The primary beneficiary, usually the mother, must also attend monthly program meetings.[1,12]

The education transfer varies with the number of children in the household and with their year in school. The amount of the transfer increases with each additional year of schooling and varies from approximately US$9 per month for first and second graders in rural areas to US$57 per month for

women age 14 to 21 in their third year of high school.[4] Characteristics and conditionalities of the education transfer include the following:

- Students must not have more than four unjustified absences per month, or more than 12 in an academic year in order to receive the monthly transfer.
- Students who graduate from high school receive an additional one-time transfer.
- Subsidies are provided for school supplies.
- The maximum amount of monthly benefits per household is approximately $92 for families with no high school students and $150 for families with high school students.[4,12]

Prospera also includes an in-kind component that provides nutritional supplements of approximately 20% of kilocalories and 100% of micronutrients for pregnant or nursing women, infants between 4 months and 2 years of age, and undernourished children up to the age of 5.[1]

- Cash Transfer for Orphans and Vulnerable Children (CT-OVC) is Kenya's primary antipoverty program that provides a fixed amount of approximately US$20 each month to households with one deceased parent or who are caring for an orphan, and to all households with children in the lowest expenditure quintile.[13] The transfer is unconditional, though recipients are instructed to use the transfer for the care of the orphaned or vulnerable children.[13]

Conceptual Framework

Despite the heterogeneity in program design across countries, cultures, and contexts, CT programs hinge on the same conceptual framework. CT programs assume that households are fundamentally income constrained and do not have sufficient money to pay for pressing requirements, such as nutritious food and medical care. Furthermore, children born into poor households are much more likely to become poor adults than their nonpoor peers because they are likely to receive poorer education and health care, both of which are powerful determinants of future earnings.[14] CCT programs in particular aim to reduce poverty in the short term through cash transfers while also reducing the intergenerational transmission of poverty in the long term through conditionalities that promote investments in health and education (box 16.1).[9]

There are many policy options available to governments to address poverty, so why choose CTs over interventions such as investing in infrastructure, using subsidies to reduce costs, or providing in-kind transfers in the form of food or other commodities? One compelling reason is that while improving infrastructure and public services can lead to efficiency and productivity gains, the benefits often fail to reach the poorest communities, especially in LMICs.[15] For example, in the late 1990s in Nicaragua only 10% of the poorest quintile had access to electricity while 90% of the top quintile was tapped in to the electricity infrastructure.[16] Additionally, subsidies, which artificially lower the cost of commodities, can disproportionately benefit the nonpoor over the poor and the urban poor over the rural poor.[1] For example, although subsidies on fuel are frequently justified as a policy to alleviate poverty, in reality they are regressive with much of the benefit going to the middle and upper class, who use more fuel in the form of motorized transportation or air conditioning.[17]

Unlike in-kind transfers, cash allows individuals to use the transfer however they see fit and thereby maximize welfare gains (the utility achieved by individuals resulting from an increased consumption of goods and services).[18] Not only do beneficiaries choose how to spend their money, they also transfer benefits to the community as they spend that money on locally produced goods and services.[19] In contrast, the benefits of in-kind food transfers stop when the recipient consumes the transferred food. Last, because of the infrastructure required to distribute in-kind transfers, cash transfers are considered less expensive, especially after the requisite administrative structures are established.[18] Therefore, because cash transfers can be given directly to the poorest households, they can contribute to poverty alleviation more effectively and efficiently than other forms of public investment.[15]

In addition to directly targeting the poor, CT programs can create positive externalities, especially when the transfers are conditioned on health and education requirements. The pathways by which CT programs create these positive outcomes all begin with the transfer of cash to poor families. According to the conceptual framework developed by Bastagli et al.,[7] the immediate outcomes of a CT program are what families choose to do with the cash they receive. First, a family can spend the money on goods and services, such as school tuition, transportation costs, food, or health care. Second, a family can save the money for emergencies or to increase their access to credit. Third, they may choose to invest the money in assets or services, such as purchasing farm equipment. For CCTs, the conditions themselves can be an immediate outcome as well when the transfer is at a point of service, for example, when the cash is dispersed at a local health clinic after a family has attended a preventive health care appointment.

The intermediate outcomes of CT programs are the results of spending, saving, or investing cash transfers.[7] For example, a child may be able to attend school more consistently if the transfer is used on tuition or school supplies. The nutritional diversity of a family may improve due to the ability to purchase higher-quality and/or more nutritious foods. And, feelings of pride and self-acceptance could result from expenditures on new clothes or hygiene products. If the transfer was saved by the family, they may be able to better cope with a shock, such as a poor harvest, without withdrawing a child from school. Or, if the money was invested in farm equipment or fertilizers, the family may be able to improve their agricultural productivity. For CCTs, the intermediate outcomes of conditions are the results of meeting those conditions, such as a student graduating who might not have otherwise due to a school attendance conditionality.

Lastly, the cumulative effects of intermediate outcomes result in the longer-term impacts of the program.[7] For example, consider a young adult who was able to stay in school due to reduced absenteeism from not paying school fees or from illness. They then were able to graduate with good grades as a result of improved cognitive abilities from better nutrition and were therefore able to find a higher-paying job to better support their family. Investment in productive assets, such as agricultural machinery, could also increase long-term consumption of goods and services. For example, evidence from Zambia[20] and Mexico[21] shows that household consumption is substantially higher following program participation, demonstrating the effect of investment in productive assets that allows for improved standards of living even after the cash transfers are stopped.

Through these various pathways, CT programs promote the accumulation of human capital—the set of productive skills, abilities, health, education, and expertise of the labor force that are produced through investment decisions that weigh the opportunity costs of an individual's time and money.[22] By reducing income constraints and providing incentives, CT programs reduce the opportunity cost of accumulating human capital.

The extent to which these intended pathways actually lead to improved long-term outcomes is dependent on numerous interacting variables and underlying assumptions, such as that

- the poor underutilize health and education services and cash transfers will increase utilization;
- increased utilization will improve health and education outcomes;
- for CCTs, the imposition, monitoring, and enforcement of conditions is necessary to increase utilization; and
- there are sufficient and adequate services available for the poor to utilize.[23]

Improved nutrition may not lead to increased growth if poor sanitation prevents nutrient absorption, or higher school attendance may not lead to higher test scores if the quality of instruction is poor. Health and education

The opportunity cost of pursuing education is the money that otherwise could be made by working in either the informal or formal economy, which could be in or outside the home. The opportunity cost of education is low for young children who do not have great earning potential. However, for children in secondary school who have more opportunities for employment, the opportunity cost of education, and thus the risk of dropping out, is much higher. This is reflected in the design of *Prospera*, which significantly increases the amount of transfer when students transition from primary to secondary school, lowering the opportunity cost of secondary school.[14]

conditions may not be effective if the quality of care or instruction is inadequate or simply unavailable. Additionally, for the poorest households, the cash transfer may not be enough to compensate for the costs of the conditionalities or to substantially improve consumption (box 16.2). Therefore, it is important to carefully evaluate CT programs to effectively allocate funding and design programs to maximize the intended outcomes.

Evaluating CT Programs

CCT and UCTs have been extensively studied to determine if they are producing results, to improve program design, and to help policy makers allocate resources effectively. Many impact evaluations have been done on CT program to establish causality between an intervention and outcomes. There are multiple impact evaluation methodologies, and the ones most commonly used to study CT programs are briefly described below.

Randomized control trials (RCTs), in which randomly assigned treatment groups receive the intervention and are compared to control groups that did not receive the intervention, is an experimental design considered to be the gold standard of impact evaluations (box 16.3).[14] Random assignment helps to ensure that the only difference between the groups is that one receives the intervention and the other does not. If receiving the intervention is the only difference between two groups, then differences in observed outcomes can be attributed to the intervention.[14]

When RCTs are not feasible or realistic, there are several quasi-experimental methods that can be used to construct treatment and control groups. Propensity score matching (PSM) constructs a control group by matching nonparticipants to those who have received the treatment based on a number of observable characteristics.[14] PSM relies on the assumption that individuals

---

Box 16.3. The Impact of *Prospera*

An important component of *Prospera* is that it was carefully studied from its inception through randomized control trials that allowed for rigorous evaluations of its impact. A 2017 review[3] of *Prospera* impact evaluations found that the program has largely had significant positive effects on nutrition, health, and education indicators. For example, participation in *Prospera* has been shown to increase the number of children who continue on to secondary school by 4% to 10%;[24] decrease the number of newborns reported as sick in the previous month by 25% in the first year of the program;[2] and to increase the average birth weight by 127 grams in treatment groups from 1997 to 2003.[25]

---

with similar observable characteristics also have similar unobservable characteristics. PSM is helpful when designing an evaluation after an intervention has been implemented and randomization is not possible. The difference-in-differences method can also be used after an intervention has already been implemented by comparing the change in an outcome for a group that did not receive treatment to the change in that outcome for a group that did receive treatment.[14] Then, subtracting the change in the control group from the change in the treatment group leaves the impact, or the difference in differences, of the intervention. Last, regression discontinuity designs (RDD) can be used when participation in an intervention is determined by a given threshold, such as a poverty line.[14] RDDs assume that individuals who fall just above the threshold are essentially the same as those that fall just below the threshold, so that any difference in outcomes can be attributed to enrollment in an intervention.

Impact of CT Programs on Health Outcomes

Having explored the theoretical underpinnings of how CT programs are intended to work, we now turn to existing empirical evidence on the effects of UCT and CCT programs on health, nutrition, development, and education outcomes.

Birth Weight

Low birth weight, defined as under 2,500 grams, is a significant determinant of health outcomes later in childhood and as an adult. In several Latin American countries, both UCT and CCT programs have been shown to increase birth weight (box 16.4).[12,26,27] Studies in other countries have also found improvements in birth weights but with slightly different conclusions. A study

Box 16.4. *Prospera* and Birth Weights

The results from a study by Barber and Gertler[10] showed that babies born to *Prospera* program participants were 127.3 grams heavier and were 44.5% less likely to have a low birth weight compared to births to nonpartici-pants. When considering pathways, the study found that the average number of prenatal consultations for nonparticipants was 6.4, higher than the required five visits under *Prospera*. Therefore, the condition that women attend five prenatal visits did not likely impact birth weight through increased prenatal care utilization. To measure improved nutrition, time enrolled in the program was used as a proxy since the longer a person has been enrolled, the more food they have been able to buy and

the longer they could have benefitted from receiving supplements. This was not found to have any effect on birth weight outcomes. Lastly, quality of care was measured by the types of services and procedures patients received throughout the pregnancy and was found to be correlated with increased birth weight and decreased likelihood of low birth weight. The study concluded that these improve-ments were primarily attributable to *Prospera* empowering women to demand their rights to quality care by informing them of what quality prenatal care should include, the importance of this care, their rights to this care, and by providing social support and encouragement to be active and informed patients.

in Colombia found the effect to only be significant in urban areas.[26] In Uru-guay, improvements were attributed to improved maternal nutrition and decreased levels of mothers working and smoking.[27]

Hypothesized mechanisms by which a CCT, such as *Prospera*, could im-pact birth weight include (1) improved nutrition due to nutritional supple-ments distributed to pregnant women as a part of the program and from us-ing the cash transfer to purchase more or higher-quality foods; (2) prenatal care utilization due to the five prenatal care visits that are one of the condi-tions of the program; and (3) increased quality of health care by promoting more informed and active patients through the required *pláticas* sessions.[12]

Perinatal, Neonatal, and Infant Mortality

The effects of CT programs on perinatal mortality (having a stillbirth after 28 weeks of pregnancy or death within one week of birth), neonatal mortal-ity (death within one month of birth), and infant mortality (death within one year of birth) have also been examined by several evaluations (box 16.5). Stud-ies of Brazil's *Bolsa Família* CCT program[28,29] and India's *Janani Suraksha Yojana* (JSY) CCT program[30] have found significant decreases in mortality rates. However, not all studies have found positive effects. Nepal's Safe Delivery

Incentive Programme (SDIP) provides a cash transfer to mothers conditioned on giving birth in a facility and to health care providers attending births either in a facility or in the home.[32] Powell-Jackson et al.[32] found that while Nepal's SDIP increased skilled birth attendance in communities with women's groups that shared information about the program, it had no impact on neonatal mortality. This demonstrates how a CT program may change health care utilization behavior but have no impact on health outcomes if the care sought is suboptimal.

Self-Reported Child Health and Morbidity

A particular challenge of assessing morbidity with CCT programs is that some indicators may underestimate benefits because of more frequent visits to clinics, resulting in more regular or accurate diagnoses.[23] Therefore, incidence of a disease could appear to increase as a result of a CCT when really it is just being documented more frequently. Studies have shown that most programs have had beneficial effects on indicators of morbidity, such as reported diarrhea, reported respiratory problems, or sick days (box 16.6). Studies of CT programs in Brazil,[33] Malawi,[34] Burkina Faso,[35] and Tanzania[36] all found a significant decrease in the number of reported sick days and illnesses. In Jamaica, program participation was found to have no effect on reported illness.[37] In contrast, an evaluation in Ghana found that program participation was associated with an increase in reported illness in children aged 0 to 5.[38]

Anthropometric Measures

Anthropometric indicators are commonly used to assess the nutritional status of children. Severe or persistent malnutrition directly affects linear growth and a child's ability to accumulate fat and muscle mass.[43] The three main measurements of anthropometry are height-for-age (stunting), weight-for-height (wasting), and weight-for-age (underweight). These measurements use z-scores, or the number of standard deviations the measurement is from

Box 16.6. *Prospera* and Morbidity

Studies of *Prospera*'s effect on morbidity have shown mixed results. While three studies did find significant reductions in morbidity rates in the treatment group,[2,39,40] a fourth study found that the decrease was only significant in rural areas but not in urban areas.[41] Last, a study by Fernald et al.[42] found that increasing the size of the cash transfer had no effect on the number of children sick days reported by *Prospera* beneficiaries.

the median measurement for a reference group of the same age and gender.[7] A child is considered to be stunted, wasted, or underweight if their height-for-age z-scores (HAZ), weight-for-height z-scores (WHZ), or weight-for-age z-scores (WAZ) are more than 2 standard deviations away from the median in the reference population, respectively.[7]

Stunting is a measurement of chronic malnutrition, since a child with poor nutrition over long periods of time does not grow to be as tall as a healthy child of the same age. Wasting represents a deficit in muscle and fat mass, which can be lost over shorter periods of time and is thus a measurement of acute malnutrition. Underweight is a composite indicator that can be caused by either chronic malnutrition, causing shortness for age, or acute undernutrition, causing thinness for height.[44]

Stunting

Though the evidence for positive effects of both CCT and UCT programs is stronger for stunting than the other two anthropometric indicators, the findings are mixed both within and across countries (box 16.7). For example, in Tanzania[36] and Brazil,[45] evaluations found no effect of CCTs on children's height. A CCT program in Burkina Faso led to improvements in HAZ after one year; however, after two years these gains could no longer be detected.[46] An evaluation of Colombia's *Familias en Acción* CCT program found significant improvements in HAZ but only for those age 24 months or younger.[26]

There are similarly inconclusive results for evaluations of UCT programs as well. In Sri Lanka, a UCT program was found to have significant improvements on children's HAZ, while in Zambia and Ecuador no effect was found.[53,54] Variations in program design and implementation increase the difficulty in identifying trends. For example, the UCT program in Ecuador transfers the lowest amount of cash of all CT programs in Latin America, which could help explain why there was no impact on children's HAZ.[53] Additionally, due to study design limitations, it is not possible to identify potential causes of these null findings. Characteristics such as small sample size, delays or errors in program implementation, transfers failing to improve nutritional intake, or children being older and less responsive to improved nutrition could help explain a lack of significant findings.

Wasting

Both UCT and CCT programs have no consistent effect on WHZ or wasting (box 16.8). Impact evaluations of CT programs in Bangladesh,[55] Indonesia,[56] Tanzania,[36] and Nicaragua[57] found no impact on WHZ or wasting. In their study on Nicaragua's CCT program, Maluccio and Flores[57] note that the null findings are not surprising because in the program areas wasting was not of much concern to begin with, as only 0.2% of children under 5 were wasted in both control and intervention areas prior to the program. There have also been some partially positive findings as well. An evaluation of a UCT program in Sri Lanka[58] found a statistically significant increase in WHZ, but only in children ages 36-60 months.

Underweight

CCTs and UCTs have no statistically significant improvements for WAZ or underweight;[7] the majority of results show either no effect or only effects for subgroups. Evaluations of CCT programs in Bangladesh[55] and Tanzania[36] found no effect on WAZ or underweight. Results from CCTs in Nicaragua have been mixed, with one study finding a significant reduction in underweight[57] and a more recent study finding no effect.[59] UCT programs have also had inconclusive results; an evaluation in Malawi[34] did not find any impact on prevalence of underweight while in Zambia a UCT was found to increase WAZ but did not have an impact on the prevalence of underweight.[54]

Counterintuitively, results from Brazil[45] actually find a decrease in weight among treatment groups. In their study on the effect of Brazil's *Bolsa Família* CCT program, Morris et al.[45] hypothesize that this could be the result of an adverse incentive where mothers believe that their participation in the CCT program was due to their child being underweight and that they would stop receiving benefits if the child's growth improved. Though this was not the case, a previous program in Brazil did halt transfers of milk powder to mothers of underweight children if they were no longer underweight. Many of the recipients of transfers under *Bolsa Família* were likely beneficiaries of the previous program and there have been anecdotal, but unverifiable, reports of deliberately keeping children underweight in order to qualify for benefits.[45]

Impact of CT Programs on Child Development and Education

Early childhood development and education are important components of human capital accumulation and are of great interest to CT programs. A 2016 systematic review[7] of CCT and UCT evaluations that measured school attendance, test scores, and cognitive development (as indicated by language acquisition, memory, information processing ability, intelligence, and reasoning) found that while cash transfers are effective at improving access to education and attendance, there is mixed evidence for the impact on cognitive development and learning outcomes (box 16.9).

Both UCTs and CCTs are effective at improving enrollment and attendance, however, the effects of CCTs are always larger, especially for CCTs that strictly monitor compliance and penalize noncompliance.[60] Childhood development studies are less clear. A study in Uganda[61] found that cash transfers increased cognitive scores, while a UCT in Zambia had no impact on language and cognition assessments.[54] A CCT program in Peru showed no effect on language outcomes,[62] while studies from Nicaragua showed cognitive benefits from participating in two separate CT programs.[59,63]

The mixed results of CCTs on childhood development demonstrate the dynamic interaction between the social, biological, and environmental determinants of childhood development.[7] Additionally, there are multiple intermediate pathways by which CT programs can affect children's development, such as improved food consumption, increased health care utilization, higher immunization coverage, or improved physical and pyschological well-being of the family. A systematic review of the effects of CCTs on child

Box 16.9. *Prospera*'s Effect on Cognitive Development and Education Outcomes

Results from *Prospera* show small but significant positive results on several indicators of cognition, development, and education. A 10-year follow-up study[51] found children that were enrolled early on and received an additional 18 months of inclusion in the program had improved socio-emotional development. While the study found no effect of early enrollment on cognitive or language development, it did identify a statistically significant positive association between the cumulative amount of cash received, determined by the interaction of time of enrollment and baseline household demographic structure, and cognition and vocabulary scores, as well as decreased behavioral problems. This is supported by another study[42] that found that a doubling of the cumulative amount of cash received was associated with improvements in memory, language development, and motor skills. Additionally, *Prospera* has been found to decrease aggressive and oppositional problems by 10% in beneficiary children.[64]

health[65] found that while they are largely effective in improving health by addressing multiple determinants of health, such as nutrition, morbidity risk, income poverty, and increased access to care, it is not possible to identify which pathway is most important. More research will need to be done to determine which pathways are the most responsible for improved child health outcomes.

Role of Design and Implementation Features

There are several characteristics of program design and implementation that can impact outcomes. For example, the study of *Educación Inicial* and *Prospera*[66] demonstrates how complementary interventions can improve the outcomes of CT programs (box 16.10). Other characteristics include the duration of exposure, payment mechanisms, the types of conditionalities, and the timing and frequency of transfers. The role of three other features—conditionality, primary recipients, and targeting methods—are described in more detail below.

To Condition or Not to Condition Cash Transfers

One of the first steps in designing a CT program is deciding whether or not the cash transfer should be conditioned or unconditioned. CCT programs are more expensive and complex to administer than UCT programs due to the costs of monitoring compliance and ensuring availability of the health care and education services required of the program.

Box 16.10. Integration of Early Childhood Development Promotion with CCTs

In Mexico, there is a parental support program called *Educación Inicial* (EI) that provides training and support to parents in poor rural communities where access to preschool is limited.[66] The content of the program includes promoting motor skills development, early childhood stimulation for cognitive and language development, and supporting psycho-social development.[66] A cluster randomized control trial[66] compared a control group that only received benefits from the *Prospera* CCT program with two treatment groups in which the EI program was also implemented. In one treatment group the EI program was implemented in its usual method, with no links or coordination between EI and *Prospera*. In the second group, *Prospera* was responsible for promoting EI and encouraging participation by disseminating information, bringing attention to weekly meetings, and emphasizing the benefits of participation in the program on child development. The two programs also coordinated with each other so that there were no conflicts between meetings, allowing families to fully participate in both programs. The results of the experiment showed that children in the second treatment group (coordinated implementation of *Prospera* and EI) performed better on child development tests, while there was no difference in cognitive outcomes for children in communities where EI was not offered and in communities where EI was offered but not coordinated with *Prospera*.

CCT programs are an example of top-down development strategies in which the implementing organization makes decisions about what is best for poor children and incentivizes their parents to achieve these objectives with cash transfers. UCTs, on the other hand, are bottom-up initiatives that rely on the assumption that when a family's income is raised, the parents will make appropriate decisions regarding investing in their children's human capital.

While it may seem that social programs should maximize freedom of choice and thus favor UCTs, there are three main arguments in favor of imposing conditions on cash transfers. First, people may have incomplete or incorrect information about the benefits of investments in health or education.[15] Second, research shows that individuals can also suffer from myopia, problems with self-control, and procrastination that result in short-term behavior that is incompatible with their own long-term goals for the future.[15] Last, there can be intrahousehold conflicts of interest between parents and children that may result in parents making decisions that are rational to them but may be inconsistent with what the child would choose for themselves.[15]

A systematic review[60] of effects of UCTs compared to CCTs found that CCTs with strict monitoring and enforcement increase the likelihood of enrolment in school by 60%, programs with minimal monitoring and enforcement increase the likelihood by 25%, and UCTs with no conditions increase the likelihood of enrollment by 18%. There have been few studies comparing CCTs and UCTs in the same context, and within the same trial (e.g., Baird et al.[67] and Akresh et al.[46]). One study took place in Malawi[67] and compared the effects of a UCT and a CCT (conditional on school attendance) on dropout rates, test scores, and teenage pregnancy and marriage among girls from different schools. While the UCT caused a small reduction in dropout rates, it was not as large as the decline in dropouts caused by the CCT. The UCT, however, was found to cause a 27% reduction in the teenage pregnancy rate and a 44% reduction in the marriage rate, whereas the CCT had no impact on either of these indicators. The effect of the UCT on these indicators is accounted for by girls who dropped out of school and were able to delay marriage and pregnancy with the cash transfer. This result shows the tradeoffs that can be made in choosing whether or not to condition a transfer based on the goal of the program. The success of the CCT arm of the study in reducing the dropout rate was achieved at the expense of those who did dropout, who are at risk for early marriage and pregnancy, and who are no longer eligible for the cash transfer that helped delay marriage and pregnancy in the UCT arm of the study.[14] A follow-up study,[68] however, found that there was a spike in marriage and pregnancy among UCT beneficiaries immediately following the end of the program and that the improvements in teen pregnancy and marriage had disappeared within two years. The CCT arm of the study, on the other hand, had lasting effects on school attainment and teen pregnancy and marriage, but only for those who had previously dropped out and returned to school with the CCT.

An alternative to conditionality is using social marketing, finding ways to induce beneficiaries to use transfers for the intended purpose of the program without enforcing conditions, such as by labeling the money dispersed.[14] The *Bono de Desarrollo Humano* (BDH) program in Ecuador, which does not monitor or enforce the conditions of the transfer, used radio and television announcements to imply transfers were linked to school enrollment and found that households that believed the transfer condition was monitored and enforced had higher enrollment rates than those that did not.[69] Additionally, there was a significant improvement in height-for-age scores for children of mothers who believed that *Bono de Desarrollo Humano* was a CCT rather than a UCT.[53]

Main Recipient

The main recipient of cash transfers is an important feature of CCT and UCT programs. Most CT programs where education and health are the goal target transfers at women because women are perceived to be more likely to use the transfer for children's welfare than men.[14] This assumption is supported by numerous studies on intra-household bargaining, showing that resources controlled by the mother have a stronger positive impact than resources controlled by the father on a child's health and schooling[70-72] because women are more likely to spend the money on things such as nutritious food or preventive health care.

Because the vast majority of CT programs target transfers at mothers, it is difficult to determine to what extent the gender of the recipient influences outcomes. One of the few studies doing a direct comparison of CT recipients, based in Burkina Faso, found that CCTs given to women were marginally more effective than transfers given to men at increasing child health visits,[35] while giving transfers to fathers was associated with improved anthropometric outcomes.[46] A study of the Give Directly UCT program in Kenya showed that while transferring to women resulted in improved psychological well-being and female empowerment, there was no statistically significant difference between male and female recipients on child health, education, and food security indices.[73]

Another interesting consideration is that while women may be more likely to use transfers for health and education, transfers to men could be more effective for investing in productive assets that increase the household's income and consumption in the long run.[14] A study of the PROCAMPO cash transfer program in Mexico (designed to compensate farmers for expected losses due to NAFTA) found that for every dollar transferred to men, a second dollar was generated due to investments in fertilizers and other agricultural inputs that increased production capacity.[74] Investing cash transfers in order to increase a household's productive capacity, rather than spending it directly on education or health care, could also lead to increased access to education and health care in the long run. However, more research is needed to determine what, if any, effect the gender of the recipient has on intended outcomes.

Targeting

Because the demand for cash transfers will always be higher than available resources, implementing organizations or agencies must decide on how to select or target the beneficiaries of the CT program (box 16.11). The benefit of effective targeting is that it reduces errors in excluding poor people who should benefit from the program or in including the nonpoor who should not benefit.[14] There are also several costs of targeting, such as the administrative costs of accurately identifying who is poor and who is not; private costs incurred by households, such as waiting in line to receive transfers or the stigma of participation; the indirect costs that can be caused by negative incentives, such as a household reducing their labor supply to meet the

Box 16.11. Targeting in Practice

Prospera targets specific households with a method called proxy means testing, which uses a set of correlates of poverty to calculate a score that determines eligibility. Typical variables include characteristics of the home (cement or dirt floor), ownership of certain goods (refrigerator), demographic characteristics, and type of employment. The seven variables used by *Prospera* are kept secret to help prevent cheating.[14] The CCT program in Honduras, on the other hand, uses group targeting. Using census data, the program identifies the poorest municipalities in the country and then makes the CCT program available to all residents of those municipalities.[75] While this type of targeting is cheaper and easier to implement, it results in larger inclusion errors (providing benefits to the nonpoor), due to intra-municipality heterogeneity of incomes.

qualifying income threshold; and the political costs of excluding those who do not meet the criteria.[76]

Effective targeting is especially difficult because of hidden or asymmetrical information about the income or assets of potential beneficiaries and because nonbeneficiaries will try to mimic the characteristics of beneficiaries in order to receive benefits.[14] According to Coady et al.,[76] there are three approaches to targeting: targeting individuals or households, targeting groups of individuals or households, and self-targeting.

Critiques, Unintended Consequences, and Ethical Considerations of CT Programs

Though there have been many documented successes of CT programs and they have spread rapidly in LMICs, the programs have also been criticized. What follows is not an exhaustive list of critiques but a sampling of some of the common concerns with CT programs. Many of the concerns are specifically about CCTs and have to do with the conditions placed on recipients. For example, enforcing conditions may have the unintended consequence of excluding the poorest households if the transfer is not enough to cover the costs of compliance. These could include transportation costs to health clinics, enrollment fees, or school uniforms. If the poorest families do not have enough resources to meet the conditions, are kicked out of the program, and stop receiving transfers, the program can fail to help those who need it most. By imposing additional burdens on already vulnerable and marginalized populations, conditions can result in exacerbating existing injustices.[77] Another critique of education conditions is that it disqualifies poor families without children or with older children, which can be a substantial number of individuals who may also need assistance.[78]

CCT programs aim to increase the demand for education and health services. However, stimulating demand by requiring recipients to enroll in school or attend health care appointments may be an inefficient use of funds if there is not an adequate supply of those services. If the quality of health and education systems is poor or even nonexistent, then scarce program resources may be better spent strengthening the health and education sectors.

Another line of critique of CT programs is the necessary targeting and exclusion that it requires, which may cause feelings of injustice, resentment, or envy.[79] This is supported by a study that found that households that were deemed ineligible for transfers based on a needs assessment have much stronger negative reactions to their exclusion than those excluded due to randomized assignment to treatment and control groups.[79] There may be physical negative externalities resulting from exclusion as well. Introducing a large amount of cash into communities can cause prices of food and services to increase, especially when there is a high concentration of beneficiaries.[79] A study from a large CCT program in the Philippines[80] found that, in addition to increased food prices, the program increased stunting in nonbeneficiaries and that this impact was higher in areas with more program recipients.

There are also feminist critiques of CCT programs. First, intra-household power relations may mean that making women the main beneficiary of the program does not automatically mean she has control over the use of funds or increased economic autonomy.[81] Second, the conditionalities of programs draw on traditional notions of womanhood and a mother's participation is as an intermediary for improving children's human capital without regard for women's education, employment, or empowerment.[82] Last, the conditions imposed on primary beneficiaries, who are predominantly women, such as attending weekly meetings, can lead to a "feminization of responsibility and obligation" when dealing with poverty.[83]

Distributing cash may worsen health if it is used to purchase unhealthy food, alcohol, or tobacco products. Evidence from Mexico shows that higher cumulative cash transfers is associated with increased BMI and incidence of overweight, obesity, and hypertension.[84] In Colombia, women's participation in the *Familias en Acción* CCT was associated with increased BMIs and an elevated risk for obesity.[85] While there is anecdotal evidence of some recipients using cash transfers for alcohol and tobacco, a systematic review of program evaluations found that on the whole transfers are not used to purchase alcohol and tobacco and may even lead to a decrease in consumption of these products.[86]

Last, the conditions and cash transfers of CCT programs can have very real implications for millions of people's lives and therefore merit careful ethical consideration. Krubiner et al.[87] identifies the following moral questions that policy makers should take into account when designing CCT programs:

Box 16.12. Summary of Arguments in Favor of and Against CCTs

In favor of	Against
■ Ensures that recipients engage in the intended positive behaviors of the program	■ May exclude households who are for some reason unable to meet conditions but are still in need of assistance
■ Helps families make long-term investments in human capital accumulation	■ Expensive to monitor and enforce compliance
■ People may have incomplete or incorrect information regarding health and education	■ Not effective if education or health care systems are inadequate or inaccessible
■ Parents and children may have conflicting interests	■ Parents will choose what is best for their children when income constraints are relieved
■ People suffer from short-sightedness, self-control, and procrastination	■ Conditions are paternalistic and represent a top-down approach to development
■ Conditions improve effectiveness of cash transfers in achieving improved health and education outcomes	■ Complying with conditions imposes additional burdens and costs on poor families
■ Increases women's empowerment and autonomy	■ Enforces traditional gender roles and adds additional burdens to women
■ Increases demand for health and education services	■ Conditions on education can exclude poor households without school-aged children
■ Can increase poor individuals' feelings of dignity and social inclusion	■ Can cause feelings of jealousy and lead to social exclusion
	■ Transfers can be used for unhealthy food, alcohol, and tobacco

- Is there sufficient evidence linking the conditionality to the desired outcome? To what extent can the conditionality be expected to benefit participants? And, are the benefits of compliance sustainable and will they lead to lasting positive changes?
- Does compliance with conditionalities expose participants to physical, social, or psychological risks or impose unnecessary burdens?
- How do beneficiary communities perceive conditionalities and intended outcomes? Does the program respect individual and collective rights to self-determination?
- Is compliance with a conditionality realistically attainable, and what barriers may participants face? Are ancillary services needed to help participants meet conditions?
- Could there be negative externalities or indirect harm for individuals or communities resulting from participation in the program?

Many of the concerns and ethical considerations regarding CCT and UCT programs can be either avoided or mitigated with careful planning, extensive research, diligence, and respect (box 16.12).

Conclusion

This chapter reviews the conceptual framework for CCT and UCT programs; explores the evidence for how these programs affect health, nutrition, development, and education; describes variations in design and implementation; and reviews some of the concerns these programs have raised. Comparisons across programs, countries, and regions are difficult because of the variance in objectives, conditions, targeting, and other differences in design. These programs also differ due to varying levels of quality of education and health care systems. For example, if households comply with a condition to seek health care then utilization of health services will increase. However, this may not lead to improved health outcomes if the health system has inadequate infrastructure, insufficient supplies, or high levels of staff absenteeism.

CT programs generally show positive effects on birth weight, infant mortality, morbidity, cognitive development, and access to education. There have been mixed results for CT effects on stunting, and generally few results for wasting and underweight. CCTs generally result in greater effects than UCTs, however, there are far fewer UCT studies than CCTs, and UCTs are more common in sub-Saharan Africa while CCTs are more common in Latin America. This makes it difficult to differentiate the effects of conditionalities from regional differences. When considering whether to impose conditions, or what type of conditions to impose, programs need to carefully consider the desired outcomes, administrative capacity, and available resources.

CT programs are an innovative form of social protection that aim to break the intergenerational transfer of poverty through reducing income restraints in the short run and promoting the accumulation of human capital in the long run. They have caused clear and significant impacts on multiple health and education indicators; however, many questions still remain. Additional research is needed to better understand how UCTs and CCTs differ in effectiveness, to adapt CT programs to focus on obesity and prevention of noncommunicable diseases, to map the pathways linking program participation to outcomes, and to identify what changes or complimentary programs can be added to make CT programs more effective. By advancing our comprehension of how and why cash transfer programs function, their effectiveness on improving health, nutrition, development, and education can be improved for vulnerable populations across the globe.

Review Questions

1. To what extent is it appropriate for the government to instruct poor families how they should raise their children?
2. How do CT programs differ from other social programs designed to reduce poverty?

3. What types of programs are best designed with UCTs, and what are best designed with CCTs? Why?
4. What are some of the reasons that CT programs may not lead to improved nutrition?
5. Could CT programs be used to address obesity and chronic disease? If so, what types of alterations would you make to the design and implementation of a CT intervention?
6. What changes could be made to CT programs to address some of the common criticisms they face?

References

1. Levy, Santiago. 2007. *Progress against Poverty Sustaining Mexicos Progresa-Oportunidades Program.* Washington, DC: Brookings Institution Press.

2. Gertler, Paul. 2004. "Do Conditional Cash Transfers Improve Child Health? Evidence from PROGRESA's Control Randomized Experiment." *The American Economic Review,* Papers and Proceedings of the One Hundred Sixteenth Annual Meeting of the American Economic Association, 94 (2): 336-41.

3. Parker, Susan W., and Petra E. Todd. 2017. "Conditional Cash Transfers: The Case of Progresa/Oportunidades." *Journal of Economic Literature* 55 (3): 866-915. https://doi.org/10.1257/jel.20151233.

4. Dávila Lárraga, Laura G. 2016. "How Does Prospera Work? Best Practices in the Implementation of Conditional Cash Transfer Programs in Latin America and the Caribbean." Technical Note IDB-TN-971. Inter-American Development Bank.

5. *The State of Social Safety Nets 2015.* 2015. Washington, DC: World Bank.

6. Tepperman, Jonathan. 2016. "Brazil's Antipoverty Breakthrough." *Foreign Affairs* 95 (1): 34-44.

7. Bastagli, Francesca, Jessica Hagen-Zanker, Luke Harman, Georgina Sturge, Valentina Barca, Tanja Schmidt, and Luca Pellerano. 2016. "Cash Transfers: What Does the Evidence Say? A Rigorous Review of Impacts and the Role of Design and Implementation Features." London: Overseas Development Institute.

8. Pega, Frank, Stefan Walter, Sze Yan Liu, Roman Pabayo, Stefan K. Lhachimi, and Ruhi Saith. 2014. "Unconditional Cash Transfers for Reducing Poverty and Vulnerabilities: Effect on Use of Health Services and Health Outcomes in Low- and Middle-Income Countries." *Cochrane Database of Systematic Reviews,* no. 11 (June). https://doi.org/10.1002/14651858.CD011135.

9. Morais de Sá e Silva, Michelle. 2017. *Poverty Reduction, Education, and the Global Diffusion of Conditional Cash Transfers.* Cham, Switzerland: Springer International Publishing.

10. Merttens, Fred, Esméralda Sindou, Ramlatu Attah, and Chris Hearle. 2016. "Evaluation of the Uganda Social Assistance Grants for Empowerment (SAGE) Programme." Final Evaluation. Oxford Policy Management.

11. Mideros Mora, Andres, and Franziska Gassmann. 2017. "Fostering Social Mobility: The Case of the 'Bono de Desarrollo Humano' in Ecuador." Working Paper 2017-002. Maastricht, The Netherlands: United Nations University—Maastricht Economic and Social Research Institute on Innovation and Technology (MERIT).

12. Barber, Sarah L., and Paul J. Gertler. 2010. "Empowering Women: How Mexico's Conditional Cash Transfer Programme Raised Prenatal Care Quality and Birth Weight." *Journal of Development Effectiveness* 2 (1): 51-73. https://doi.org/10.1080/19439341003592630.

13. Handa, Sudhanshu, Amber Peterman, Carolyn Huang, Carolyn Halpern, Audrey Pettifor, and Harsha Thirumurthy. 2015. "Impact of the Kenya Cash Transfer for Orphans and Vulnerable Children on Early Pregnancy and Marriage of Adolescent Girls." *Social Science & Medicine* 141 (September): 36-45. https://doi.org/10.1016/j.socscimed.2015.07.024.

14. Janvry, Alain De, and Elisabeth Sadoulet. 2016. *Development Economics: Theory and Practice*. London; New York: Routledge, Taylor & Francis Group.

15. Fiszbein, Ariel, Norbert Rüdiger Schady, Francisco H. G. Ferreira, Margaret Ellen Grosh, Nial Kelleher, and Weltbank, eds. 2009. *Conditional Cash Transfers: Reducing Present and Future Poverty*. A World Bank Policy Research Report. Washington, DC: World Bank.

16. Ferranti, David M. De, ed. 2004. *Inequality in Latin America: Breaking with History?* World Bank Latin American and Caribbean Studies. Washington, DC: World Bank.

17. Smith, Joel E., and Johannes Urpelainen. 2017. "Removing Fuel Subsidies: How Can International Organizations Support National Policy Reforms?" *International Environmental Agreements: Politics, Law and Economics* 17 (3): 327-40. https://doi.org/10.1007/s10784-017-9358-9.

18. Hidrobo, Melissa, John Hoddinott, Amber Peterman, Amy Margolies, and Vanessa Moreira. 2014. "Cash, Food, or Vouchers? Evidence from a Randomized Experiment in Northern Ecuador." *Journal of Development Economics* 107 (March): 144-56. https://doi.org/10.1016/j.jdeveco.2013.11.009.

19. Davies, Simon, and James Davey. 2008. "A Regional Multiplier Approach to Estimating the Impact of Cash Transfers on the Market: The Case of Cash Transfers in Rural Malawi." *Development Policy Review* 26 (1): 91-111. https://doi.org/10.1111/j.1467-7679.2008.00400.x.

20. Handa, Sudhanshu, Luisa Natali, David Seidenfeld, Gelson Tembo, and Benjamin Davis. 2018. "Can Unconditional Cash Transfers Raise Long-Term Living Standards? Evidence from Zambia." *Journal of Development Economics* 133 (July): 42-65. https://doi.org/10.1016/j.jdeveco.2018.01.008.

21. Gertler, Paul J, Sebastian W Martinez, and Marta Rubio-Codina. 2012. "Investing Cash Transfers to Raise Long-Term Living Standards." *American Economic Journal: Applied Economics* 4 (1): 164-92. https://doi.org/10.1257/app.4.1.164.

22. Goldin, Claudia. 2016. "Human Capital." In *Handbook of Cliometrics.*, edited by Claude Diebolt and Michael J. Haupert. Heidelberg: Springer Reference.

23. Gaarder, Marie M., Amanda Glassman, and Jessica E. Todd. 2010. "Conditional Cash Transfers and Health: Unpacking the Causal Chain." *Journal of Development Effectiveness* 2 (1): 6-50. https://doi.org/10.1080/19439341003646188.

24. Paul Schultz, T. 2004. "School Subsidies for the Poor: Evaluating the Mexican Progresa Poverty Program." *Journal of Development Economics* 74 (1): 199-250. https://doi.org/10.1016/j.jdeveco.2003.12.009.

25. Barber, Sarah, and Paul Gertler. 2008. "The Impact of Mexico's Conditional Cash Transfer Programme, Oportunidades, on Birth weight." *Tropical Medicine & International Health* 13 (11): 1405-14.

26. Attanasio, Orazio, Erich Battistin, Emla Fitzsimons, Alice Mesnard, and Marcos Vera-Hernandez. 2005. "How Effective Are Conditional Cash Transfers? Evidence from Colombia." Briefing Note 54. London: The Institute for Fiscal Studies.

27. Amarante, Verónica, Marco Manacorda, Edward Miguel, and Andrea Vigorito. 2011. "Do Cash Transfers Improve Birth Outcomes? Evidence from Matched Vital Statistics, Social Security and Program Data." Working Paper 17690. Cambridge, MA: National Bureau of Economic Research.

28. Rasella, Davide, Rosana Aquino, Carlos AT Santos, Rômulo Paes-Sousa, and Mauricio L Barreto. 2013. "Effect of a Conditional Cash Transfer Programme on Childhood Mortality: A Nationwide Analysis of Brazilian Municipalities." *The Lancet* 382 (9886): 57-64. https://doi.org/10.1016/S0140-6736(13)60715-1.

29. Shei, Amie. 2013. "Brazil's Conditional Cash Transfer Program Associated With Declines In Infant Mortality Rates." *Health Affairs* 32 (7): 1274-81. https://doi.org/10.1377/hlthaff.2012.0827.

30. Lim, Stephen S., Lalit Dandona, Joseph A. Hoisington, Spencer L. James, Margaret C. Hogan, and Emmanuela Gakidou. 2010. "India's Janani Suraksha Yojana, a Conditional Cash Transfer Programme to Increase Births in Health Facilities: An Impact Evaluation." *The Lancet* 375 (9730): 2009-23. https://doi.org/10.1016/S0140-6736(10)60744-1.

31. Barham, Tania. 2011. "A Healthier Start: The Effect of Conditional Cash Transfers on Neonatal and Infant Mortality in Rural Mexico." *Journal of Development Economics* 94 (1): 74-85. https://doi.org/10.1016/j.jdeveco.2010.01.003.

32. Powell-Jackson, T., B. D. Neupane, S. Tiwari, K. Tumbahangphe, D. Manandhar, and A. M. Costello, eds. 2009. "The Impact of Nepal's National Incentive Programme to Promote Safe Delivery in the District of Makwanpur." *Advances in Health Economics and Health Services Research* 21:221-49.

33. Reis, Mauricio. 2010. "Cash Transfer Programs and Child Health in Brazil." *Economics Letters* 108 (1): 22-25. https://doi.org/10.1016/j.econlet.2010.04.009.

34. Miller, Candace M., Maxton Tsoka, and Kathryn Reichert. 2010. "Targeting Cash to Malawi's Ultra-Poor: A Mixed Methods Evaluation." *Development Policy Review* 28 (4): 481-502. https://doi.org/10.1111/j.1467-7679.2010.00493.x.

35. Akresh, Richard, Damien de Walque, and Harounan Kazianga. 2012. "Alternative Cash Transfer Delivery Mechanisms: Impacts on Routine Preventative Health Clinic Visits in Burkina Faso." Working Paper 17785. Cambridge, MA: National Bureau of Economic Research.

36. Evans, David, Brian Holtemeyer, and Katrina L. Kosec. 2016. "Cash Transfers and Health: Evidence from Tanzania." Policy Research Working Paper WPS 7882. Washington, DC: World Bank Group.

37. Levy, Dan, and Jim Ohls. 2007. "Evaluation of Jamaica's PATH Program: Final Report." Princeton, NJ: Mathematica Policy Research.

38. Handa, Sudhanshu, Michael Park, Robert Osei Darko, Isaac Osei-Akoto, Benjamin Davis, and Silvio Diadone. 2013. "Livelihood Empowerment Against

Poverty Program Impact Evaluation." Chapel Hill: The University of North Carolina, Carolina Population Center.

39. Gertler, Paul. 2000. "The Impact of Progresa on Health." Washington, DC: International Food Policy Research Institute.

40. Gutiérrez, J. P., S. Bautista, P. J. Gertler, M. Hernandez Avila, and S. M. Bertozzi. 2006. "Impacto de Oportunidades En El Estado de Salud, Morbilidad y Utilización de Servicios de Salud de La Población Beneficiaria En Zonas Urbanas." In *Evaluación Externa de Impacto Del Programa Oportunidades 2006*, edited by M. H. Ávila, B. H. Prado, and J. E. U. Salomón. Mexico, DF: Instituto Nacional de Salud Pública.

41. Gutiérrez, J. P., S. Bautista, P. J. Gertler, M. Hernandez Avila, and S. M. Bertozzi. 2004. "Impacto de Oportunidades En La Morbilidad y El Estado de Salud de La Población Beneficiana y En La Utilización de Los Servicios de Salud: Resultados de Corto Plazo En Zonas Urbanas y de Mediano Plazo En Zonas Rurales." In *Evaluación Externa de Impacto Del Programa Oportunidades 2004*, edited by B. H. Prado and M. H. Avila. Mexico, DF: Instituto Nacional de Salud Pública.

42. Fernald, Lia C. H., Paul J. Gertler, and Lynnette M. Neufeld. 2008. "Role of Cash in Conditional Cash Transfer Programmes for Child Health, Growth, and Development: An Analysis of Mexico's Oportunidades." *The Lancet* 371 (9615): 828-37. https://doi.org/10.1016/S0140-6736(08)60382-7.

43. Hoddinott, John, and Lucy Bassett. 2009. "Conditional Cash Transfer Programs and Nutrition in Latin America: Assessment of Impacts and Strategies for Improvement." Working Paper 9. United Nations Food and Agriculture Organization (FAO) Hunger-Free Latin America and the Caribbean Initiative.

44. "Nutrition Landscape Information System (NLIS) Country Profile Indicators Interpretation Guide." 2010. Geneva, Switzerland: World Health Organization.

45. Morris, Saul S., Pedro Olinto, Rafael Flores, Eduardo A. F. Nilson, and Ana C. Figueiró. 2004. "Conditional Cash Transfers Are Associated with a Small Reduction in the Rate of Weight Gain of Preschool Children in Northeast Brazil." *The Journal of Nutrition* 134 (9): 2336-41. https://doi.org/10.1093/jn/134.9.2336.

46. Akresh, Richard, Damien de Walque, and Harounan Kazianga. 2016. "Evidence from a Randomized Evaluation of the Household Welfare Impacts of Conditional and Unconditional Cash Transfers Given to Mothers or Fathers." Policy Research Working Paper 7730. Washington, DC: World Bank.

47. Behrman, Jere R., and John Hoddinott. 2005. "Programme Evaluation with Unobserved Heterogeneity and Selective Implementation: The Mexican PRO-GRESA Impact on Child Nutrition." *Oxford Bulletin of Economics and Statistics* 67 (4): 547-69. https://doi.org/10.1111/j.1468-0084.2005.00131.x.

48. Neufeld, Lynnette M., D. Sotres Alvarex, P. J. Gertler, L. Tolention Mayo, J. Jimenez Ruiz, et al. 2005. "Impacto de Oportunidades En El Crecimiento y Estado Nutricional de Niños En Zonas Rurales." In *Evaluación Externa de Impacto Del Programa Oportunidades 2004*, edited by M. Hernandez Avila, III: Aliment-ación:17-52. Mexico, DF: Instituto Nacional de Salud Pública.

49. Leroy, Jef L., Armando García-Guerra, Raquel García, Clara Dominguez, Juan Rivera, and Lynnette M. Neufeld. 2008. "The Oportunidades Program Increases the Linear Growth of Children Enrolled at Young Ages in Urban Mexico." *The Journal of Nutrition* 138 (4): 793-98. https://doi.org/10.1093/jn/138.4.793.

50. Rivera, Juan A., Daniela Sotres-Alvarez, Jean-Pierre Habicht, Teresa Shamah, and Salvador Villalpando. 2004. "Impact of the Mexican Program for Education, Health, and Nutrition (Progresa) on Rates of Growth and Anemia in Infants and Young Children: A Randomized Effectiveness Study." *JAMA* 291 (21): 2563. https://doi.org/10.1001/jama.291.21.2563.

51. Fernald, Lia C. H., Paul J. Gertler, and Lynnette M. Neufeld. 2009. "10-Year Effect of Oportunidades, Mexico's Conditional Cash Transfer Programme, on Child Growth, Cognition, Language, and Behaviour: A Longitudinal Follow-up Study." *The Lancet* 374 (9706): 1997-2005. https://doi.org/10.1016/S0140-6736(09)61676-7.

52. Neufeld, L. 2005. "Estudio Comparative Sobre El Estado Nutricional y La Adquisición de Lenguage Entre Niños de Localidades Urbana Con y Sin Oportunidades." In *Evaluación Externa de Impacto Del Programa Oportunidades 2004*, edited by M. Hernandez Avila. Vol. III: Salud. Mexico, DF: Instituto Nacional de Salud Pública.

53. Fernald, Lia C. H., and Melissa Hidrobo. 2011. "Effect of Ecuador's Cash Transfer Program (Bono de Desarrollo Humano) on Child Development in Infants and Toddlers: A Randomized Effectiveness Trial." *Social Science & Medicine* 72 (9): 1437-46. https://doi.org/10.1016/j.socscimed.2011.03.005.

54. Seidenfeld, David, Leah Prencipe, Sudhanshu Handa, and Laura Hawkinson. 2015. "The Impact of an Unconditional Cash Transfer on Early Child Development: The Zambia Child Grant Program." ED562535. Society for Research on Educational Effectiveness.

55. Ahmed, Akhter U., Agnes R. Quisumbing, Mahbuba Nasreen, John F. Hoddinott, and Elizabeth Bryan. 2009. "Comparing Food and Cash Transfers to the Ultra-Poor in Bangladesh." Research Reports 163. Washington, DC: International Food Policy Research Institute.

56. Alatas, Vivi. 2011. "Program Keluarga Harapan: Impact Evaluation of Indonesia's Pilot Household Conditional Cash Transfer Program (English)." Working Paper 72506. Washington, DC: World Bank.

57. Maluccio, John A., and Rafael Flores. 2004. "Impact Evaluation of a Conditional Cash Transfer Program: The Nicaraguan Red de Protección Social." FCND Discussion Paper 184. Washington, DC: International Food Policy Research Institute.

58. Himaz, Rozana. 2008. "Welfare Grants and Their Impact on Child Health: The Case of Sri Lanka." *World Development* 36 (10): 1843-57. https://doi.org/10.1016/j.worlddev.2008.02.003.

59. Macours, Karen, and Norbert Schady. 2012. "Cash Transfers, Behavioral Changes, and Cognitive Development in Early Childhood: Evidence from a Randomized Experiment." *American Economic Journal: Applied Economics* 4 (2): 247-73.

60. Baird, Sarah, Francisco H.G. Ferreira, Berk Özler, and Michael Woolcock. 2014. "Conditional, Unconditional and Everything in between: A Systematic Review of the Effects of Cash Transfer Programmes on Schooling Outcomes." *Journal of Development Effectiveness* 6 (1): 1-43. https://doi.org/10.1080/19439342.2014.890362.

61. Gilligan, Daniel O., and Shalini Roy. 2013. "Resources, Stimulation, and Cognition: How Transfer Programs and Preschool Shape Cognitive Development in Uganda," 2013 Annual Meeting, Agricultural and Applied Economics Association, August 4-6. Washington, DC.

62. Andersen, Christopher T., Sarah A. Reynolds, Jere R. Behrman, Benjamin T. Crookston, Kirk A. Dearden, Javier Escobal, Subha Mani, et al. 2015. "Participation in the Juntos Conditional Cash Transfer Program in Peru Is Associated with Changes in Child Anthropometric Status but Not Language Development or School Achievement." *The Journal of Nutrition* 145 (10): 2396–2405. https://doi.org/10.3945/jn.115.213546.

63. Barham, Tania, Karen Macours, and John A. Maluccio. 2013. "Boys' Cognitive Skill Formation and Physical Growth: Long-Term Experimental Evidence on Critical Ages for Early Childhood Interventions." *The American Economic Review* 103 (3): 467–71. https://doi.org/10.1257/aer.103.3.467.

64. Ozer, E. J., L. C. H. Fernald, J. G. Manley, and P. J. Gertler. 2009. "Effects of a Conditional Cash Transfer Program on Children's Behavior Problems." *Pediatrics* 123 (4): e630–37. https://doi.org/10.1542/peds.2008-2882.

65. Owusu-Addo, Ebenezer, and Ruth Cross. 2014. "The Impact of Conditional Cash Transfers on Child Health in Low- and Middle-Income Countries: A Systematic Review." *International Journal of Public Health* 59 (4): 609–18. https://doi.org/10.1007/s00038-014-0570-x.

66. Fernald, Lia C. H., Rose M. C. Kagawa, Heather A. Knauer, Lourdes Schnaas, Armando Garcia Guerra, and Lynnette M. Neufeld. 2017. "Promoting Child Development through Group-Based Parent Support within a Cash Transfer Program: Experimental Effects on Children's Outcomes." *Developmental Psychology* 53 (2): 222–36. https://doi.org/10.1037/dev0000185.

67. Baird, S., C. McIntosh, and B. Ozler. 2011. "Cash or Condition? Evidence from a Cash Transfer Experiment." *The Quarterly Journal of Economics* 126 (4): 1709–53. https://doi.org/10.1093/qje/qjr032.

68. Baird, Sarah, Craig T. McIntosh, and Berk Özler. 2017. "When the Money Runs Out: Do Cash Transfers Have Sustained Effects on Human Capital Accumulation?" Policy Research Working Paper 7901. Washington, DC: World Bank.

69. Schady, Norbert, and Maria Caridad Araujo. 2008. "Cash Transfers, Conditions, and School Enrollment in Ecuador." *Economia* 8 (2): 43–77.

70. Lundberg, Shelly J., Robert A. Pollak, and Terence J. Wales. 1997. "Do Husbands and Wives Pool Their Resources? Evidence from the United Kingdom Child Benefit." *Journal of Human Resources* 32 (3): 463–80.

71. Schultz, T. Paul. 1990. "Testing the Neoclassical Model of Family Labor Supply and Fertility." *Journal of Human Resources* 25 (4): 599–634.

72. Thomas, Duncan. 1990. "Intra-Household Resource Allocation An Inferential Approach." *Journal of Human Resources* 25 (4): 635–64.

73. Haushofer, Johannes, and Jeremy Shapiro. 2016. "The Short-Term Impact of Unconditional Cash Transfers to the Poor: Experimental Evidence from Kenya." *The Quarterly Journal of Economics* 131 (4): 1973–2042. https://doi.org/10.1093/qje/qjw025.

74. Sadoulet, Elisabeth, Alain de Janvry, and Benjamin Davis. 2001. "Cash Transfer Programs with Income Multipliers: PROCAMPO in Mexico." *World Development* 29 (6): 1043–56. https://doi.org/10.1016/S0305-750X(01)00018-3.

75. Moore, Charity. 2008. "Assessing Honduras? CCT Programme PRAF, Programa de Asignación Familiar: Expected and Unexpected Realities." Country

Study 15. Brasilia: United Nations Development Programme International Poverty Centre.

76. Coady, David, Margaret E. Grosh, and John Hoddinott. 2004. *Targeting of Transfers in Developing Countries.* [Electronic Resource]: *Review of Lessons and Experience.* World Bank Regional and Sectoral Studies. Washington, DC: World Bank.

77. Pérez-Muñoz, Cristian. 2017. "What Is Wrong with Conditional Cash Transfer Programs?" *Journal of Social Philosophy* 48 (4): 440-60. https://doi.org/10 .1111/josp.12215.

78. Cecchini, Simone, and Aldo Madariaga. 2011. *Conditional Cash Transfer Programmes: The Recent Experience in Latin America and the Caribbean.* Cuadernos de La CEPAL. Santiago, Chile: United Nations, ECLAC.

79. Stecklov, Guy, Alexander Weinreb, and Paul Winters. 2016. "The Exclusion from Welfare Benefits: Resentment and Survey Attrition in a Randomized Controlled Trial in Mexico." *Social Science Research* 60 (November): 100-109. https://doi.org/10.1016/j.ssresearch.2016.06.002.

80. Filmer, Deon, Jed Friedman, Eeshani Kandpal, and Junko Onishi. 2018. "General Equilibrium Effects of Targeted Cash Transfers: Nutrition Impacts on Non-Beneficiary Children." Policy Research Working Paper 8377. Washington, DC: World Bank.

81. Tabbush, Constanza. 2010. "Latin American Women's Protection after Adjustment: A Feminist Critique of Conditional Cash Transfers in Chile and Argentina." *Oxford Development Studies* 38 (4): 437-59. https://doi.org/10.1080 /13600818.2010.525327.

82. Molyneux, Maxine. 2007. "Change and Continuity in Social Protection in Latin America: Mothers at the Service of the State?" Gender and Development Programme Paper 1. Geneva, Switzerland: United Nations Research Institute for Social Development.

83. Chant, Sylvia. 2008. "The 'Feminisation of Poverty' and the 'Feminisation' of Anti-Poverty Programmes: Room for Revision?" *The Journal of Development Studies* 44 (2): 165-97. https://doi.org/10.1080/00220380701789810.

84. Fernald, Lia C. H., Paul J. Gertler, and Xiaohui Hou. 2008. "Cash Component of Conditional Cash Transfer Program Is Associated with Higher Body Mass Index and Blood Pressure in Adults." *The Journal of Nutrition* 138 (11): 2250-57. https://doi.org/10.3945/jn.108.090506.

85. Forde, I., T. Chandola, S. Garcia, M. G. Marmot, and O. Attanasio. 2012. "The Impact of Cash Transfers to Poor Women in Colombia on BMI and Obesity: Prospective Cohort Study." *International Journal of Obesity* 36 (9): 1209-14. https: //doi.org/10.1038/ijo.2011.234.

86. Evans, David, and Anna Popova. 2017. "Cash Transfers and Temptation Goods." *Economic Development & Cultural Change* 65 (2): 189-221.

87. Krubiner, Carleigh B., and Maria W. Merritt. 2017. "Which Strings Attached: Ethical Considerations for Selecting Appropriate Conditionalities in Conditional Cash Transfer Programmes." *Journal of Medical Ethics* 43 (3): 167-76. https://doi.org /10.1136/medethics-2016-103386.

Glossary

absenteeism: The time absent from work because of a condition or illness, with costs accrued in the form of lost productivity or increased pay-outs for sick leave.

adequacy assessment: Assessment of whether expected changes occurred in indicators of interest as compared to previously established adequacy criteria.

anthropometry: The measurement of physical dimensions that helps to assess body composition and growth, such as height, weight, skinfold assessment, and waist circumference.

assessment: The collection, assembly, analysis, and communication of information on the health of the community, including statistics on health status, community health needs, and epidemiologic and other studies of health problems.

assets: Individuals, organizations, material resources, and existing policies that support and positively influence the health of communities.

biomarker: Any substance, structure, or process in the body or its products that influences and predicts the incidence of disease or other outcome, such as biological specimens of blood and urine.

body mass index (BMI): A person's weight in kilograms divided by the square of height in meters.

catabolism: The degradation and breakdown of molecules to produce energy.

climate change: Shifts in global climate patterns linked to solar output or altered atmospheric composition. Climate change is characterized by increased levels of greenhouse gases, which contribute to atmospheric warming; affect ocean temperatures, sea level, and precipitation patterns; and cause extreme weather events.

climate-smart agriculture: An agricultural practice that aims to increase productivity in ways that reduce or remove greenhouse gas emissions and build resilience to climate change.

communicable disease (infectious disease): A disease caused by microorganisms such as bacteria, viruses, parasites, and fungi that can be spread, directly or indirectly, from one person to another.

community: A group of people with common characteristics or interests, not necessarily restricted by geographical location, in which membership occurs mutually through self-identification and group consensus.

community health assessment: A systematic process for summarizing the needs and assets in a community, undertaken specifically for the purpose of taking action to improve health.

complementary feeding: The process starting when breast milk alone is no longer sufficient to meet the nutritional requirements of infants and therefore other foods and liquids are needed, along with breast milk.

complex system: A system that may contain several elements whose relationships may be unknown, be unpredictable, or may adapt over time.

concepts: The overarching vision or big idea that the theory postulates.

constructs: The road map or the guiding force directing the overarching concept.

descriptive statistics: Measurements of central tendency (mean, median, mode), frequencies, trends over time, and relationships (correlation).

dietary guidelines: Key recommendations for caloric and food-group intake developed for professional audiences and used to inform programs, policies, and food labeling with the goal of improving population health.

dietary intake assessment: The collection of methods for studying individual dietary intake such as food records, 24-hour dietary recalls, and food frequency questionnaires.

dietary screener: A short dietary assessment instrument that often focuses on one aspect of diet (e.g., fruit and vegetable intake, beverage intake, dietary screen questionnaire).

disability: The short- and long-term absence from the workplace because a condition or illness precludes one's ability to meet occupational demands.

disability-adjusted life year (DALY): A combined metric that includes data on both fatal events and nonfatal disease states in an effort to provide a single measure that strives to measure population health.

disability weight (DW): Assigned ranges to various health states, ranging from 0 to less than 1; a disability weight of 1 is equivalent to death.

disease burden: The impact of a cause or risk factor on the combined concepts of morbidity and mortality.

ecological model (EM): A model that recognizes that there are multiple layers of influence on individuals' behaviors.

energy expenditure: The amount of energy used to carry out a physical function.

energy imbalance: Longer-term, cumulative effect of energy intake greater than energy expenditure (positive) or energy expenditure greater than intake (negative).

energy intake: The amount of energy (calories) consumed from foods and beverages.

environmental enteropathy: A condition in which the microvilli of the small intestine are flattened and permeable through repeated bouts of infection, leading to poor absorption of nutrition and malnutrition.

epidemiologic transition: The gradual shift in disease burden from communicable disease, undernutrition, and injuries (resulting in high infant, under 5, and maternal mortality, and low life expectancy) to noncommunicable disease.

exosystem: The social settings an individual is indirectly affected by (i.e., loss of a job carries over into a parent's interactions with a child at home).

exposure-disease relationship: The degree to which exposure to a risk factor increases risk of disease.

first 1,000 days: The period from conception to approximately 2 years of life, a highly vulnerable stage of the life cycle when nutrition insults may have irreparable consequences.

focus group: A small-group discussion guided by a trained leader. It is used to learn about opinions on a designated topic and to guide future action.

food bank: A charitable organization that solicits, receives, inventories, and distributes donated packaged food and grocery produce to charitable human service agencies (e.g., food pantries), which provide the products directly to clients through various programs.

food frequency questionnaire (FFQ): A structured questionnaire that contains a written list of usually 60 to 150 commonly consumed foods.

food insecurity: Inadequate access to sufficient food to lead an active, healthy life, which often coexists with hunger and is associated with poor dietary quality.

food loss and waste: The decrease of food throughout the food supply chain intended for human consumption. Food is lost or wasted somewhere from initial production to final household consumption, due to problems in harvesting, storage, packing, transport, and infrastructure as well as institutional and legal frameworks.

formative evaluation: Assessment of the feasibility, acceptability, and appropriateness of a new program. Formative evaluation aims to improve program design prior to its development and implementation through a needs assessment and preprogram research.

Gini index: A measure of the extent to which the distribution of income within an economy deviates from a perfectly equal distribution. A Gini index of 0 represents perfect equality, while an index of 100 implies perfect inequality.

globalization: The increased interconnectedness and interdependence of peoples and countries. Globalization is characterized by the movement of goods, services, and ideas across international borders.

gross domestic product (GDP): The monetary value of all goods and services produced within a country over a specified period of time.

gross national income (GNI): The gross domestic product plus the value from resident wages, property income, taxes, and subsidies received from abroad.

gross national product (GNP): The market value of all goods and services produced by citizens of a country (either within the country itself or abroad) over a specified period of time.

health belief model: A model in which the accumulation of knowledge is used to perceive risks or benefits of a health behavior change. This assessment is used to change beliefs and attitudes and leads to change in behavior.

Health Impact Pyramid: A public health–specific model that considers the societal factors that are in most urgent need of intervention and illustrates how program planners can have the greatest impact on large numbers of the population. It is an ecologically focused model that identifies socioeconomic factors as the foundation of nutrition-related health, followed by environmental context, protective interventions, clinical interventions, and finally, counseling and educational interventions.

high-income countries: Countries with a gross national income ≥$12,236 per capita.

homestead food production: A program where participants are given resources and training to create or improve existing systems of household crop production, animal husbandry, or aquaculture.

Human Development Index (HDI): Developed by the United Nations Development Program, the HDI combines data on life expectancy, education, and GNI to create a summary measure not driven entirely by income.

impact evaluation: The assessment of a program's effectiveness in achieving its ultimate goal.

implementation: Putting an intervention into action.

implementation theory: The details of how a program is implemented to achieve desired interactions with the target population and provide the planned services.

inputs: Resources or assets within the organization or agency to complete the program such as materials, resources, and human capital.

interpersonal theories: Health theories such as the social cognitive theory that encourage healthy eating and enhanced nutrition through the provision of social support.

intrapersonal theories: Individual-level health theories, including the health belief model, theory of reasoned action, and transtheoretical model, that focus on the behaviors manifested within people based on knowledge, beliefs, cognitions, motivations, and perceptions.

Knowledge-Attitude-Behavior Model (KBAM): A model that postulates that behavior change stems from an accumulation of knowledge, leading to shifting of attitudes and resulting in changes in behavior.

logic model: Visual representations and descriptions of the steps in the program planning process, including program inputs, process, outputs, outcomes, and impact, in the form of a flow chart, map, or table. It guides program planning and management.

macrosystem: The cultural setting and constructs such as beliefs, values, and traditions that one lives in.

mesosystem: The interrelationships between microsystems, such as issues in one microsystem affecting how an individual functions in another microsystem (i.e., family conflict impacts behavioral or academic difficulties at school).

meta-analysis: A study design that combines the results of numerous observational studies (or randomized controlled trials) to come up with a single combined estimate of the association between a dietary factor and a health outcome based on the weight of the published science.

microsystem: The immediate physical and social environment in which the individual interacts and functions and includes the most proximal level of influence on an individual.

morbidity: Any departure, subjective or objective, from a state of physiological or psychological well-being, including disease, injury, and disability.

mortality: The rate of deaths by place, time, and cause.

need: The gap between what is and what should be.

nominal group technique (NGT): Structured method for group brainstorming that encourages contributions from everyone.

noncommunicable disease (chronic disease): A disease caused by a combination of genetic, physiological, environmental, and behavioral factors that tends to be of long duration.

nutrition assessment: The collection and interpretation of data such as anthropometry, dietary intake assessment, and biomarker data that examines dietary behaviors and intake and nutrition-related health status of individuals or groups of individuals.

nutrition epidemiology: The science of identifying the relationship between diet and disease.

nutrition monitoring: Assessment of the diet and nutrition of a population or population subgroup for the purposes of detecting changes but not necessarily for initiating public health action.

nutrition-sensitive approaches: Research that studies underlying determinants of undernutrition, such as agriculture and food systems, water, sanitation and hygiene, social protection, women's empowerment, and early childhood development.

nutrition-sensitive interventions: Interventions that address some of the underlying and basic causes of malnutrition by incorporating nutrition goals and actions from a wide range of sectors.

nutrition-specific interventions: Interventions that address the immediate causes of undernutrition, such as inadequate dietary intake due to feeding practices and access to food.

nutrition surveillance: A form of surveillance that involves the repeated collection or collation of nutrition-related data for a population or a selected population subgroup for the purpose of detecting trends that may trigger action to improve nutrition.

nutrition transition: A shift away from a traditional plant- and cereal-based diet high in fiber to a more "Western" diet characterized by increasing consumption of foods high in sugar, salt, animal protein, and fat.

obesity: A body mass index ≥ 30 kg/m^2 in adults and >2 standard deviations in children aged >5 to 18 years and >3 standard deviations in children from birth to 5 years

obesogenic environment: The sum of influences that the surroundings, opportunities, or conditions of life have on promoting obesity in individuals or populations.

objectives: Building blocks leading toward the overall goal.

outcomes: Changes in knowledge, intention, motivation, attitude or behavior (impact), or health status, quality of life, or disease risk (outcome).

output: A direct result of a program activity or activities.

overweight: A body mass index of ≥ 25 to <30 kg/m^2 in adults and >1 to 2 standard deviations in children aged >5 to 18 years and >2 to 3 standard deviations in children from birth to 5 years.

plausibility assessment: Assessment of whether impact observed is due to the program as opposed to other external influences.

premature mortality: Death that occurs before the average age of death in a specific population.

presenteeism: The costs accrued when an employee is present at work but not able to function at full capacity or productivity due to a health condition.

primary data: Data that are directly obtained from an individual by the investigator, including interviews, surveys, questionnaires, focus groups, or environmental assessments.

probability assessment: Assessment of whether the changes observed in a target population are causal.

process evaluation: The evaluation of whether program activities have been implemented as intended. Process evaluation uses mixed methods of data collection to understand implementation components (i.e., program recruitment, maintenance, context, and barriers to implementation).

program effectiveness: Whether the intervention or set of interventions have an effect under "real-life" conditions or circumstances, such as in the context of an ongoing government-led nutrition program.

program efficacy: Whether an intervention or set of interventions have an effect under ideal or strict conditions or circumstances of implementation.

program evaluation: The systematic and rigorous assessment of the results achieved by a program and its interventions. Program evaluation broadly encompasses monitoring and evaluation activities that ultimately promote systematic improvement and accountability in a program and informs public health policy.

program monitoring: The continuous process of setting and tracking goals, indicators, and targets that represent program operations and progress in implementation. This is ideally completed by program planners who have an in-depth understanding of the program design and implementation.

program planning: The process of developing a set of activities that are designed and selected to address a particular health problem and implemented to reach a specific set of health goals.

prospective cohort study: A study design that enrolls a group of individuals when they are disease-free and follows these same individuals over time, typically long enough for some individuals to develop the disease of interest.

public health surveillance: The ongoing and systematic collection, management, analysis, and interpretation of data that is disseminated to promote public health action at a local, state, regional, or global level.

reflexivity: The process of a continual internal dialogue and critical self-evaluation of a researcher's positionality as well as active acknowledgement and explicit recognition that this position may affect the research process and outcome.

reliability: The repeatability of findings.

resilience: The capacity of a system to withstand and adapt to disturbances over time.

risk factor: A factor that raises the probability of adverse health outcomes, such as an attribute or characteristic of an individual, an exposure, causative agent, or condition that increases the likelihood of developing a disease or suffering more severely from its effects.

secondary data: Data that are already compiled, gathered, organized, and published by others, such as electronic health records, vital records, or registries.

self-efficacy: A personal and individual belief in one's own ability to be successful with the task at hand.

simple system: A system of few parts that are stable and predictable.

small for gestational age (SGA): The term for fetuses or newborns who are smaller in size than normal for their gestational age, most commonly defined as a weight below the 10th percentile for the gestational age.

SMART format: Specific, measurable, attainable, realistic, timed. Used to outline program objectives and outcomes for program planning.

social safety net programs: Programs intended to provide basic goods, services, or care to individuals in need in order to protect against poverty and hardship.

stakeholders: Individuals or groups that have an interest or concern in the program, such as members of the priority population, administrators, funders, partners, or an advisory board.

stepwise approach: A process of evaluation involving data collection, from program design to implementation, to measure utilization, coverage, impact and cost-effectiveness. Each step of data collection feeds into the next. This process is used to understand and measure program implementation details and the impact of a program.

stunting: The impaired linear growth or deficits in cognitive and socio-emotional development that children experience from chronic poor nutrition, repeated infection, and inadequate psychosocial stimulation. Defined by a height-for-age z-score less than two standard deviations below the WHO Child Growth Standards median.

summative evaluation: An evaluation used to make decisions about the program, typically by a funder, program planner, or other decision maker. Summative evaluations can inform whether to continue, change, expand, or end a project or intervention.

surveillance: The continuous and repeated collection of data with the purpose of detecting trends to initiate public health action (see nutrition surveillance).

sustainability: The capacity to meet current goals without compromising future capacity.

Sustainable Development Goals: A set of development goals from the United Nations that call on the world to approach development differently—that is, to see development across the goals as part of an *integrated whole* and that each goal, working in tandem with the other goals, is essential in order to achieve meaningful, impactful development.

system: A network of interconnected parts that operate toward a purpose.

systems science: A field developed to assess and model various contextual factors across different public health problems. The purpose of systems science is to identify critical leverage points within the system that might impact the outcome of interest.

systems thinking: A method of problem-solving that analyzes interconnected components as part of a whole system.

theory: The evidenced guidelines or principles used to develop an understanding of an unknown set of circumstances, such as health-related behaviors on individual and population levels in public and community health settings.

trans **fat:** Unsaturated fatty acids that contain at least one double bond in the *trans* configuration, which alters the physical properties of oils and biologic health effects when consumed. Created by adding hydrogen to liquid vegetable oils to create a solid or semisolid fat. (Source: https://wwwn.cdc.gov/nchs/data/nhanes/2009-2010/lab methods/TFA_F_MET.pdf)

transtheoretical model: A model of change characterized by a series of five stages: precontemplative to contemplative, then planning, action, and finally maintenance of a given behavior.

24-hour recall: A detailed report of all food and beverages consumed in the preceding 24 hours via a trained interviewer, typically using the multi-pass approach.

undernutrition: The outcome of insufficient food intake and repeated infectious diseases. Undernutrition includes being underweight for one's age, too short for one's age (stunted), dangerously thin for one's height (wasted) and deficient in vitamins and minerals (micronutrient malnutrition).

underweight: Defined by a weight-for-age z-score less than 2 standard deviations below the WHO Child Growth Standards median.

urbanization: Population migration from rural to urban areas resulting in urban growth and often characterized by changes in the built environment and food system.

validity: The credibility or believability of the research.

variables: The checks and balances or the quantifiable factors that reveal the significance of each part of the theory.

wage penalties: Lower wages due to weight stigma despite the same work when compared to a non-obese counterpart.

WASH (water, sanitation, and hygiene): An area of public health research focused on water, sanitation, and hygiene as causes of and potential solutions for communicable disease and malnutrition.

WASH infrastructure: Infrastructure to promote safe and clean water, sanitation, and hygiene.

wasting: A symptom of acute undernutrition, usually as a consequence of insufficient food intake or a high incidence of infectious diseases. Wasting impairs the functioning of the immune system and can lead to increased severity and duration of and susceptibility to infectious diseases and an increased risk for death. Defined as weight-for-height z-score less than 2 standard deviations below the WHO Child Growth Standards median.

weight stigma: The negative, prejudicial attitudes toward individuals with higher weight that leads to experiences of being devalued, derogated, and ostracized in society.

years lived with disability (YLD): A measurement of nonfatal disease states (e.g., loss of limb, moderate depression, or loss of function due to a stroke) as a component of DALY (disability-adjusted life year).

years of life lost (YLL): The number of years that a life was cut short due to a disease, which is generally straightforward to calculate for a given population.

Index

Cash Transfers for Orphans and Vulnerable Children (CT-OVC), 376
catabolism, 244
Centers for Disease Control and Prevention (CDC), 167
cerebral hypoxia, 202
cerebral palsy, 200, 364
cerebrovascular disease, 202
Chicago Public Schools (CPS), 80-81, 86
Child and Adult Care Food Program (CACFP), 332-34, *333*, 335, 338
Child Growth Standards, 237-39
Child Nutrition and WIC Reauthorization Act (2004), 337
children: dietary intake of, 43-45; diet-related behaviors, 184; diet-related health risks, 174; early learning programs, 364-65; education for, 302-3; feeding practices of, 102; food frequency questionnaires, 44; food marketing to, 182, 325, 345, 346-49; growth patterns, 103; growth problems, 136; health and morbidity of, 382; low birth weight, 199-200, 244, 255; lower respiratory infections in, 198; low-income, 365; nutrition for, 258-59; obesity in, 164-65, 167, 169, 180, 283; overweight, 164-65, 167, 295; racial and ethnic minority, 365; small for gestational age (SGA), *243*, 255; undernutrition in, 198-99; weight-status classifications, *167*. *See also* stunting
Children's Food and Beverage Advertising Initiative (CFBAI), 348
Children's Investment Fund Foundation, 103
Choices Programme, 338
cholesterol, 204, 283
chronic obstructive pulmonary disease (COPD), 197
chronosystem, 94
climate change, 223-24, 225, 296, 308
Commodity Supplemental Food Program, 334
communities: assets and needs of, 55; understanding and partnering with, 57-60
community-based interventions, 184
community-based organizations (CBOs), 81; and stunting, 258
Community Eligibility Provision (CEP), 323, 329
community gardens, 338
community health assessment (CHA): analyze and interpret data, 74-75; assessment team, 59-60; basics of, 55-57; case study, 52-54; common myths and realities about, *58*; constructing good questions, 71, 74; data collection, 63-68; direct and participant observation, 70; ethical considerations for primary data collection, 67-68; focus group constructs, *73*; goals of, 76; how to conduct, *60*; key informant interviews, 70-71; nominal group technique (NGT), 69-70; plan for

the future and disseminate findings, 75-76; planning and organizing, 60-63; poor and better assessment questions, *63*; primary data collection and analysis, 68-74; purpose of, 62; scope of, 62; secondary data collection and analysis, 63-67; secondary data gaps, *67*; secondary data sources, 65; survey constructs, *72*; surveys and focus groups, 71; terminology, 55; understanding and partnering with the community, 57-60
community health needs assessment (CHNA), 56
community kitchen, 52-53
Community Tool Box, 55, 57
comparative risk assessment (CRA), 141
congenital birth defects, 148
congestive heart failure, 175
Continuous Update Project (CUP), 139-40
coronary heart/artery disease (CHD), 20, 131, 175, 202. *See also* cardiovascular disease (CVD); heart disease
cultural diversity, 370

Danish Nutrition Council, 130
data assessment, 74-75
data collection: constructing good questions, 71, 74; direct and participant observation, 70; ethical considerations, 67-68; focus group studies, 71, *73*; information gaps, 66-67, *67*; key informant interviews, 70-71; localized data, 64; nominal group technique (NGT), 69-70; primary data collection and analysis, 68-69; reflexivity, 68; reliability, 64; secondary data collection and analysis, 63-67; secondary data sources, 65; surveys, 71, *72*; validity, 64
death: nutrition-related risk factors, 203-4; risk factors in low- and middle-income countries, 197-203
dementia, 136
Demographic and Health Survey (DHS), 8, 24, 25-26
demographic transitions, 136, 205
depression, 56, 145, 146, 180, 369
diabetes, 93, 136, 139, 140, 143, 146, 148, 203; and BPA exposure, 218; dietary factors, 155; and the food environment, 283, 284; obesity as risk factor for, 222; related to stunting, 244; and stroke, 203, 205; type 2, 177, 324
diarrheal disease, 197, 200; as cause of death, 204-5; micronutrient deficiencies as risk factor, 201-2; organisms causing, 254; reduction of deaths from, 204; and stunting, 253-54; and suboptimal breastfeeding, 200-201; undernutrition as risk factor, 201
diet: animal-based foods, 253, 260, 307; biofortification of, 260, 301; diversity in, 45, 222, 251, 253, 260, 303, 304; in Ethiopia, *257*; fruits and vegetables in,

monitoring and evaluation (M&E), 103, *104*, 105; adaptive programming, 109; adequacy assessments, 116; formative evaluations, 114; impact evaluation, 107, 118-21; implementation theory, 111-12; main purposes of, 121; plausibility assessments, 116-17; probability assessments, 117-18; process evaluation, 106, 111-12, *113-14*, 114-18; process evaluation in Cambodia, 110; program efficacy/effectiveness, 115-16; program evaluation, 105-7, 112; program logic models, 107-8; program monitoring, 108-9, 111; sample information collected, *109*; step-wise approach to, 106, *107*; summative effectiveness evaluations, *117*; summative evaluations, 114

mortality: infant, 381-82, 393; and low birth weight, 200; from lower respiratory infections, 198; neonatal, 381-82; and obesity, 177, 179; perinatal, 244, 381-82; premature, 179; undernutrition-related, 300

Multicentre Growth Reference Study, 238-39, 249, 250

National Academy of Medicine, 8

National Cancer Institute (NCI), 40, 42

National Health and Nutrition Examination Survey (NHANES), 7, 12, 15-18, 27, 40; applications to inform public health nutrition, 18-20; continuous web tutorial, *18*; examples of nutritional data collected, *19*; mobile examination center (MEC), 15, *16*; on phthalates, 218; proxy reporting for children, 44; types of nutrition data collected, 16-17, *17*

National Plans of Action for Nutrition, 259

National Programme for Prevention and Control of Cancer, Diabetes, Cardiovascular Diseases, and Stroke (India), 214-15

National School Lunch Program (NSLP), 81, 323, 328-30, 335, 338

neural tube defects, 48

neurodevelopmental disorders, 200

night blindness, 48, 119

nominal group technique (NGT), 69-70

non-emergency medical transportation (NEMT), 367

nongovernmental organizations (NGOs), 119; and stunting, 258

nutrients: assessment of, 36; deficiencies, 223; supplementation, 260

nutrition: animal source foods in Ethiopia, *257*; deficiencies in, 255, 256; diversity in, 378; in Egypt, 295-96; and the health-poverty trap, 205; maternal, 261; monitoring, 11; policies, 48; and the SDGs, 306; standards for school meals, 48; for young children, 259

nutritional supplements, 102

Nutrition Assistance for Puerto Rico, 334

nutrition-based programs: in high-income countries, 338-39, *340-43*; in the United States, 325-38

Nutrition Data System for Research (NDSR), 36

Nutrition Environment Measures Survey in Stores (NEMS-S), 280

nutrition epidemiology, 34, 38, 47, 143

nutrition expertise, 370

nutrition insecurity, 256

Nutrition Keys, 338, *339*

nutrition programs: aimed at reducing stunting, 259-60; community level, 337-38; monitoring and evaluation of, 102-3, 105-7; school-focused, 336-37; state and local, 335-36; using logic models in, 89-91. *See also* federal nutrition assistance programs

nutrition-related disease burden, 53

nutrition-sensitive approaches, 300-303; in agriculture, 301-2; challenges of, 303-6; in education and early child development, 302-3; and water, sanitation, and hygiene (WASH), 302

nutrition surveillance, 7, 26-27; as aid to impact evaluation, 118-21; in Australia, 23-24; in Bangladesh, 119-20; demographic and health survey, 25-26; in Indonesia, 119-20; in international settings (examples from high-income countries), 20-24; in international settings (examples from low- and middle-income countries), 24-25; in Korea, 23; in low- and middle-income countries, 43; oversampling of population subgroups, 15, 24; in special populations, 43-44; in the United States, 11-12, *13-14*, 15-18. *See also* dietary intake; public health surveillance

nutrition transitions, 136, 205; in Brazil, 210-13; challenges in studying, 224-25; cited in publications in PubMed, *216*; and climate change, 223-24; consequences of, 222-24; defined, 215-16; and diet, 216-17; drivers of, 220-22; and eating patterns, 218-19; and economic development, 220-21; and food packaging/processing, 217-18; and globalization, 221-22; in India, 213-15; key stages of, 215-16; and obesity, 222-23; and physical activity, 219-20; and urbanization, 221; in the United States, 215; in Western Europe, 215

obesity, 15, 18, 20, 24, 25, 27, 136, 225; and BPA exposure, 218; in Brazil, 212; causes, 20, 172-75; causes and solutions framework, *181*; in children, 164-65, 167, 169; community-based approaches, 184; consequences, 175-80, *176*; defined, 165-67; and the dual burden, 222-23; in Egypt, 295; and the food environment, 282-83, 284; global trends, 167-68; in high-income countries, 324, *325*; home-based ap-